Color Atlas of
Head and Neck Anatomy
Second Edition

Color Atlas of
Head and Neck Anatomy
Second Edition

Robert M.H. McMinn MD, PhD, FRCS (Eng.)
Emeritus Professor of Anatomy
Royal College of Surgeons of England
and University of London
London, UK

Ralph T. Hutchings
Freelance Photographer
Formerly Chief Medical Laboratory Scientific Officer
Royal College of Surgeons of England
London, UK

Bari M. Logan MA, FMA, Hon. MBIE
University Prosector
Department of Anatomy
University of Cambridge
Cambridge, UK

M Mosby-Wolfe

London Baltimore Bogotá Boston Buenos Aires Caracas Chicago Madrid Mexico City Milan Philadelphia St. Louis Sydney Tokyo Toronto Wiesbaden

Copyright © 1994 Times Mirror International Publishers Limited

Published in 1994 by Mosby–Wolfe, an imprint of Times Mirror International Publishers Limited

Reprinted in 1995

Printed in Spain by Grafos S.A. Arte sobre papel, Barcelona, Spain

ISBN 0 7234 1994 9

For full details of all Times Mirror International Publishers Limited titles please write to Times Mirror International Publishers Limited, Lynton House, 7–12 Tavistock Square, London WC1H 9LB, England.

A CIP catalogue record for this book is available from the British Library.

Library of Congress Cataloging-in-Publication Data has been applied for.

Contents

Preface

For this new edition, explanatory commentaries and orientation diagrams have been provided to help readers to understand exactly what they are looking at, and to offer guidance on what is most important. There are over 50 new illustrations, including examples of the new imaging techniques which are now routinely used in clinical investigations and which provide such an important link between the academic and applied aspects of anatomy. In view of the popularity of the atlas with students of dentistry, we have included an appendix on the anatomical background to dental anaesthesia.

Despite the additions and changes, the atlas remains entirely compatible for use with Berkovitz and Moxham's *A Textbook of Head and Neck Anatomy*, since all existing key numbers have been retained and any new ones are additional.

We hope the atlas will continue to meet the needs of all those students in medical and paramedical disciplines who need a visual presentation of the anatomy of the head and neck—an intricate and fascinating part of the human body.

Acknowledgements

For new radiographs and imaging material we are indebted to the following:

- Professor R. Ger and Dr P.H. Abrahams for Figs 156F, 204A and 205B (Churchill Livingstone).
- Professor J. Weir and Dr P.H. Abrahams for Figs 210A, 211B, 212A and 213B (Churchill Livingstone).
- Dr N.R. Moore for Figs 180B, 193C, 194A and 194B.
- Dr M.D. Hourihan for Figs 214A and 215B.

For advice on dental matters we are grateful to Dr Brian Berkovitz and Professor David Langdon. We also thank Dave Burin of Mosby–Wolfe for all editorial duties and Dr David Johnson for proofreading.

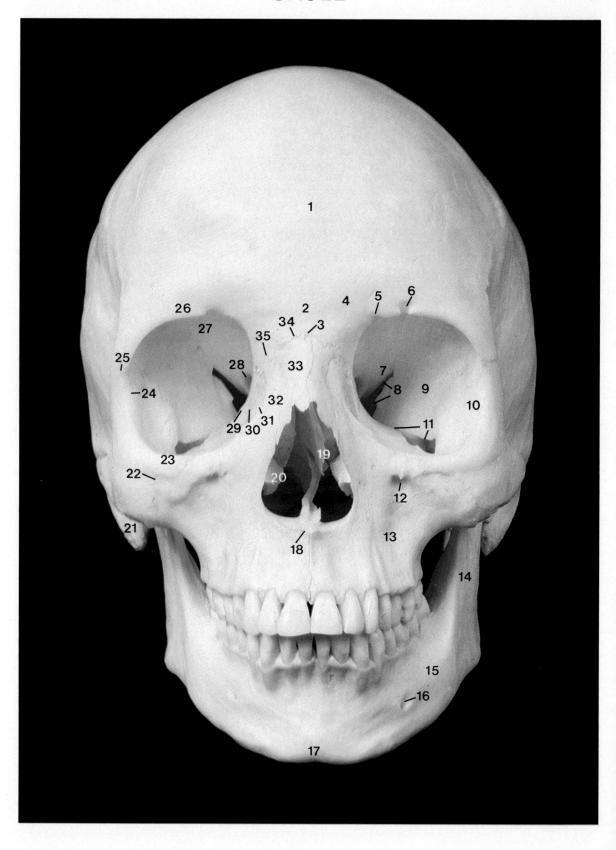

SKULL
From the front
This is the standard view from the front. The most obvious features are the two orbits and the central opening of the nasal cavity.

1	Frontal bone
2	Glabella
3	Nasion
4	Superciliary arch
5	Frontal notch
6	Supra-orbital foramen
7	Lesser wing of sphenoid bone
8	Superior orbital fissure
9	Greater wing of sphenoid bone
10	Zygomatic bone
11	Inferior orbital fissure
12	Infra-orbital foramen
13	Maxilla
14	Ramus
15	Body
16	Mental foramen
17	Mental protuberance
18	Anterior nasal spine
19	Nasal septum
20	Inferior nasal concha
21	Mastoid process
22	Zygomaticomaxillary suture
23	Infra-orbital margin
24	Marginal tubercle
25	Frontozygomatic suture
26	Supra-orbital margin
27	Orbital part of frontal bone
28	Optic canal
29	Posterior lacrimal crest
30	Fossa for lacrimal sac
31	Anterior lacrimal crest
32	Frontal process of maxilla
33	Nasal bone
34	Frontonasal suture
35	Frontomaxillary suture

14, 15, 16, 17 of mandible

• The term skull includes the mandible, while the cranium is the skull without the mandible; these definitions, however, are not always strictly observed.

• The calvaria (a term not often used) is the upper part of the skull that encloses the brain (i.e. the cranial cavity) and has a roof or skull cap (cranial vault), and a floor—the base of the skull.

• The anterior part of the skull forms the facial skeleton.

• *The cavities of the skull:*
Cranial cavity, containing the brain and its membranes.
Nasal cavity, divided into right and left halves by the nasal septum (19, seen here through the pear-shaped opening, the anterior nasal or piriform aperture).
Orbital cavities or orbits, right and left, which contain the eyes.

• *The bones of the skull:*

Unpaired	*Paired*
Frontal bone	Maxilla
Ethmoid bone	Nasal bone
Sphenoid bone	Lacrimal bone
Vomer	Inferior nasal concha
Occipital bone	Palatine bone Temporal bone
Mandible	Zygomatic bone Parietal bone

For details of individual bones, see pages 34–53.

• The supra-orbital, infra-orbital and mental foramina (6, 12 and 16) lie in approximately the same vertical plane.

• The supra-orbital foramen (or notch, 6) in the frontal bone lies just above (or at) the supra-orbital margin (26) about 2.5 cm from the midline.

• The infra-orbital foramen (12) in the maxilla is 0.5 cm below the infra-orbital margin (23), directly in line below the pupil (with the eye looking straight ahead) and in the long axis of the upper second premolar tooth.

• The mental foramen (16) in the mandible lies either below the apex of the lower second premolar tooth or in the interval between the apices of the first and second premolars (as on page 34, B10).

• *Ossification of the skull:*
Bones developed by endochondral ossification:
Ethmoid bone
Inferior nasal concha
Sphenoid bone (except for lateral part of greater wing)
Petromastoid and styloid parts of temporal bone
Occipital bone (below superior nuchal line)
The rest of the skull bones develop by intramembranous ossification.

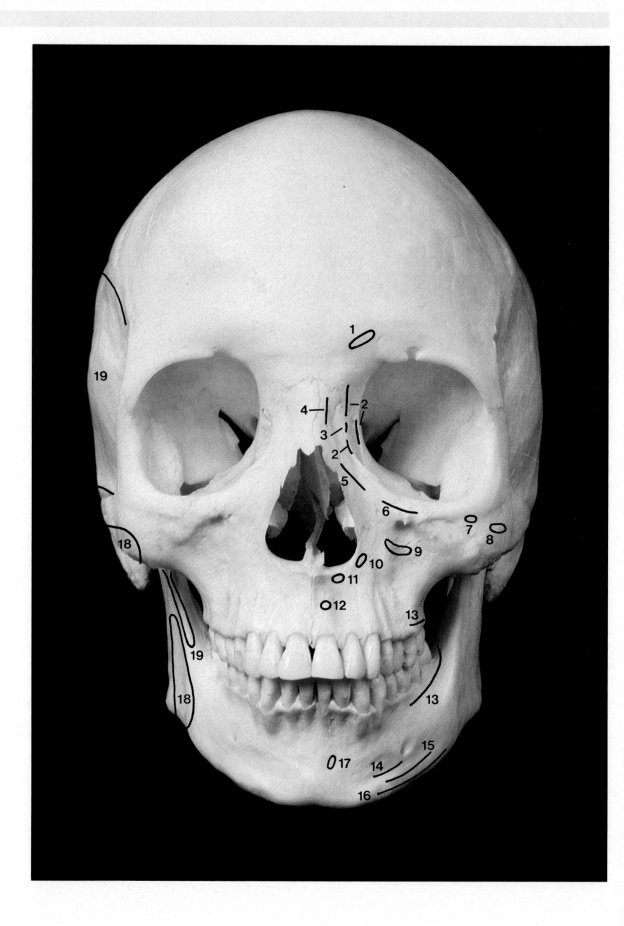

SKULL
From the front
Muscle attachments

The attachments of the muscles belonging to the group commonly called the muscles of the face or muscles of facial expression are shown on the left side of the skull. On the right side are shown parts of the attachments of temporalis and masseter, which belong to the muscles of mastication and are seen more extensively in the lateral view (page 16).

1	Corrugator supercilii
2	Orbicularis oculi
3	Medial palpebral ligament
4	Procerus
5	Levator labii superioris alaeque nasi
6	Levator labii superioris
7	Zygomaticus minor
8	Zygomaticus major
9	Levator anguli oris
10	Nasalis (transverse part)
11	Nasalis (alar part)
12	Depressor septi
13	Buccinator
14	Depressor labii inferioris
15	Depressor anguli oris
16	Platysma
17	Mentalis
18	Masseter
19	Temporalis

• Orbicularis oculi (2) is attached partly in front of and partly behind the fossa for the lacrimal sac (page 14, 39).

• The attachment of levator labii superioris (6) is above the infra-orbital foramen (page 10, 12), and that of levator anguli oris (9) below the foramen.

• The attachment of depressor labii inferioris (14) is in front of the mental foramen (page 10, 16), and that of depressor anguli oris (15) below the foramen.

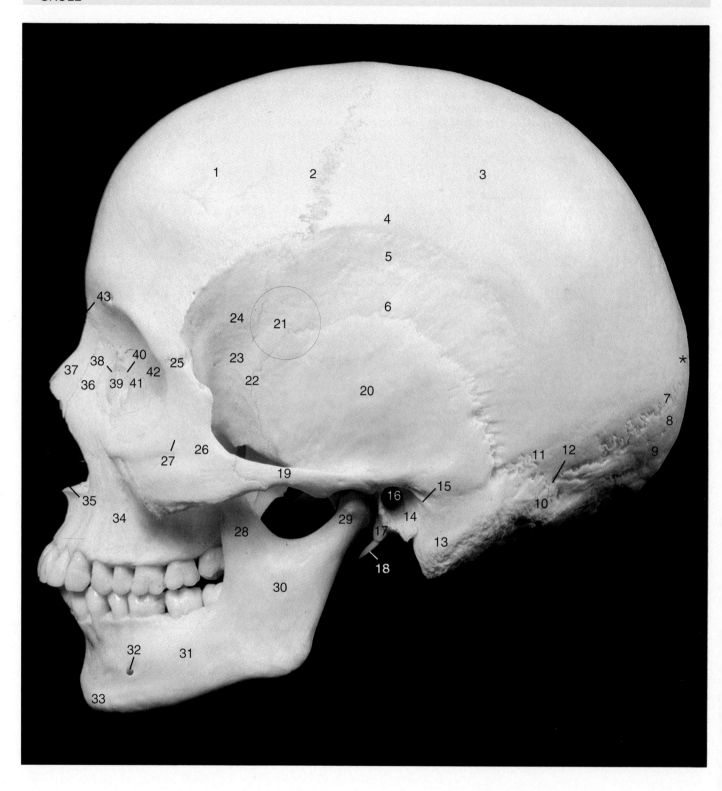

SKULL
From the left

This is the standard view from the side. Prominent features include the zygomatic bone (cheek bone, 26) and zygomatic arch (19), the ramus of the mandible (30) with the coronoid and condylar processes (28 and 29), the external acoustic meatus (16) and the mastoid process (13). An asterisk (★) marks the most posterior part of the skull (the occiput), which is above and behind the external occipital protuberance (9)

1	Frontal bone
2	Coronal suture
3	Parietal bone
4	Superior ⎫ temporal line
5	Inferior ⎭
6	Squamosal suture
7	Lambdoid suture
8	Occipital bone
9	External occipital protuberance
10	Occipitomastoid suture
11	Parietomastoid suture
12	Asterion
13	Mastoid process
14	Tympanic part of temporal bone
15	Suprameatal triangle
16	External acoustic meatus
17	Sheath of styloid process
18	Styloid process
19	Zygomatic arch
20	Squamous part of temporal bone
21	Pterion
22	Sphenosquamosal suture
23	Greater wing of sphenoid bone
24	Sphenofrontal suture
25	Frontozygomatic suture
26	Zygomatic bone
27	Zygomaticofacial foramen
28	Coronoid process ⎫
29	Condylar process ⎪
30	Ramus ⎬ of mandible
31	Body ⎪
32	Mental foramen ⎪
33	Mental protuberance ⎭
34	Maxilla
35	Anterior nasal spine
36	Frontal process of maxilla
37	Nasal bone
38	Anterior lacrimal crest
39	Fossa for lacrimal sac
40	Posterior lacrimal crest
41	Lacrimal bone
42	Orbital part of ethmoid bone
43	Nasion

• Some anatomical points of the skull:

Nasion (43): the point of articulation between the two nasal bones and the frontal bone.

Inion (9): the central point of the external occipital protuberance.

Bregma (page 20, 10): the junction of the sagittal and coronal sutures (i.e. between the frontal and the two parietal bones). In the newborn skull the anterior fontanelle is in this region (page 74, A1 and D1).

Lambda (page 18, 3): the junction of the sagittal and lambdoid sutures (i.e. between the occipital and the two parietal bones). In the newborn skull the posterior fontanelle is in this region (page 74, C30 and D30).

Pterion (21): an H-shaped area (not a single point) where the frontal, parietal, squamous part of the temporal and greater wing of the sphenoid bones articulate. It is an important landmark since it overlies the anterior branch of the middle meningeal artery (page 30, 2), which may be ruptured by blows on the side of the head, giving rise to extradural haemorrhage (page 161). In the newborn skull the sphenoidal fontanelle is in this region (page 74, B27).

Asterion (12): the junction of the lambdoid, parietomastoid and occipitomastoid sutures (i.e. between the occipital, parietal and temporal bones). In the newborn skull the mastoid fontanelle is in this region (page 74, B20).

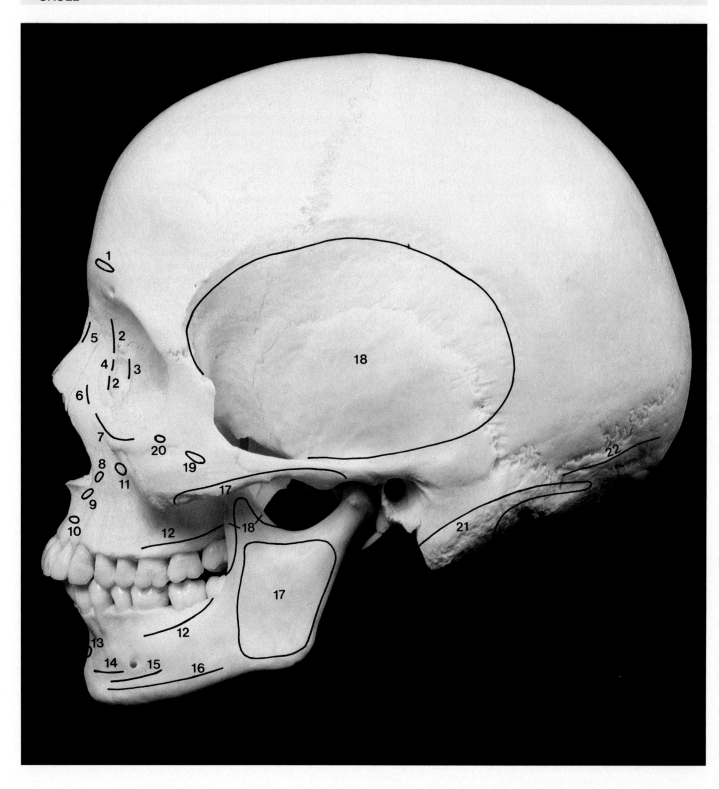

SKULL
From the left
Muscle attachments

1 Corrugator supercilii
2 Orbicularis oculi (orbital and palpebral parts)
3 Orbicularis oculi (lacrimal part)
4 Medial palpebral ligament
5 Procerus
6 Levator labii superioris alaeque nasi
7 Levator labii superioris
8 Nasalis (transverse part)
9 Nasalis (alar part)
10 Depressor septi
11 Levator anguli oris
12 Buccinator
13 Mentalis
14 Depressor labii inferioris
15 Depressor anguli oris
16 Platysma
17 Masseter
18 Temporalis
19 Zygomaticus major
20 Zygomaticus minor
21 Sternocleidomastoid
22 Occipital belly of occipitofrontalis

• The buccinator (12) has bony attachments to the upper and lower jaws opposite the three molar teeth.

• The medial palpebral ligament (4) and the orbital and palpebral parts of orbicularis oculi (2) are attached to the anterior lacrimal crest; the lacrimal part of orbicularis oculi (3) is attached to the posterior lacrimal crest.

• The area occupied by the upper attachment of temporalis (18) is the temporal fossa. The lowest fibres of the muscle run horizontally (page 114, A2) and turn down over the front of the root of the zygomatic process of the temporal bone to reach the mandibular attachment (see the second note on page 115).

• The attachment of sternocleidomastoid (21) to the mastoid process extends well back on to the occipital bone, a feature not expected from the name of the muscle—which suggests it is limited above to the mastoid process alone.

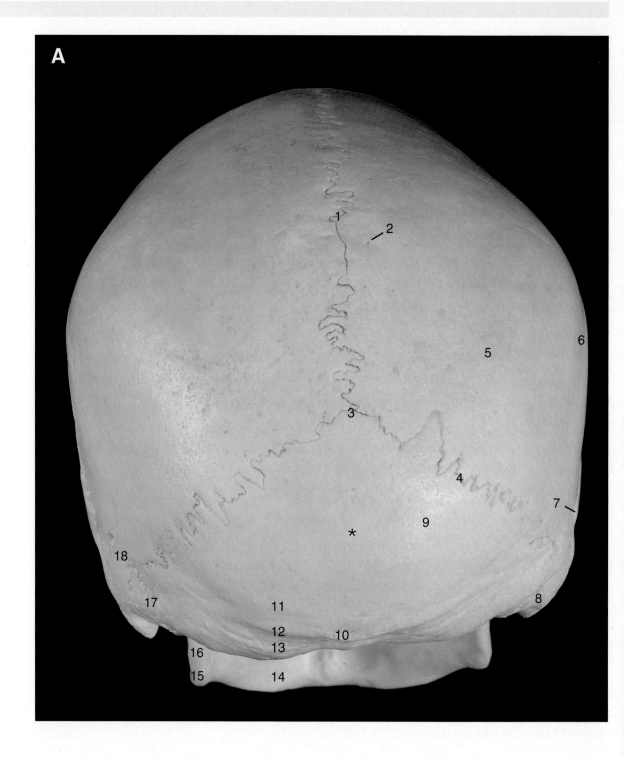

SKULL

From behind

A With the mandible in place

B A different specimen without the mandible

This is the standard view from behind, showing the sagittal and lambdoid sutures (1 and 4) and the external occipital protuberamce (10). An asterisk (★) marks the occiput (as on page 14). In the skull in B there are some sutural bones (19) and there has been bony fusion in some sutural areas.

• Sutural bones (B19) arise from separate centres of ossification that may occur within cranial sutures. They are commonest in the lambdoid suture (4) and have no clinical significance.

• The occiput (★) is the most posterior part of the skull; it is situated in the midline of the occipital bone a few centimeters above the external occipital protuberance (10 and page 14, 8), and is the part struck when falling on the back of the head.

1	Sagittal suture	11	Supreme ⎫
2	Parietal foramen	12	Superior ⎬ nuchal line
3	Lambda	13	Inferior ⎭
4	Lambdoid suture	14	Body ⎫
5	Parietal bone	15	Angle ⎬ of mandible
6	Parietal tuberosity	16	Ramus ⎭
7	Temporal bone	17	Occipitomastoid suture
8	Mastoid process	18	Parietomastoid suture
9	Squamous part of occipital bone	19	Sutural bones
10	External occipital protuberance (inion)		

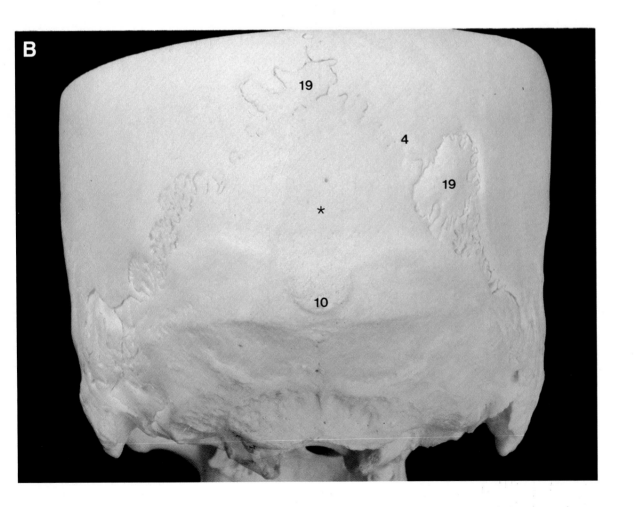

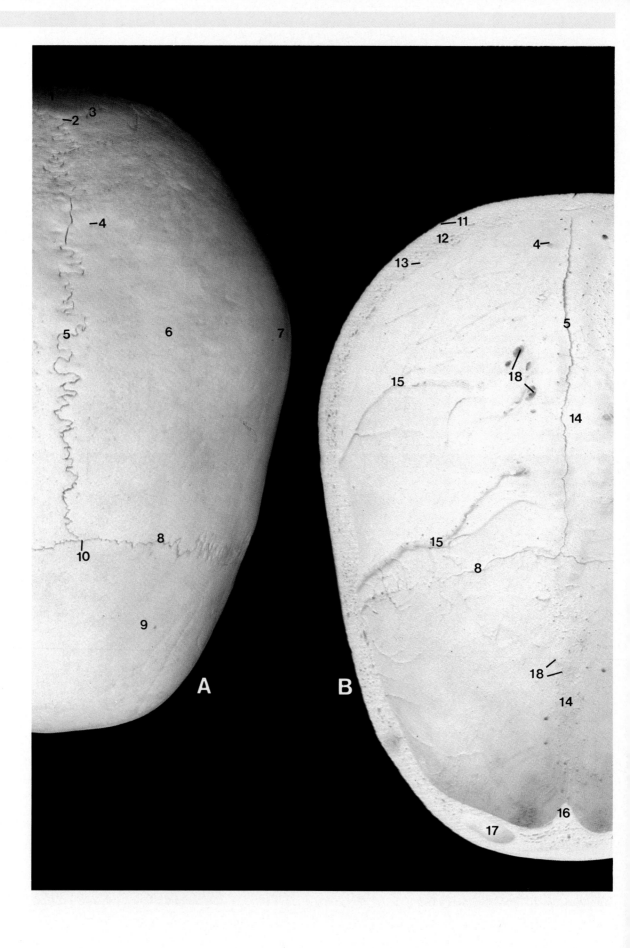

1	Occipital bone
2	Lambda
3	Lambdoid suture
4	Parietal foramen
5	Sagittal suture
6	Parietal bone
7	Parietal tuberosity
8	Coronal suture
9	Frontal bone
10	Bregma
11	Outer table
12	Diploë of parietal bone
13	Inner table
14	Groove for superior sagittal sinus
15	Grooves for middle meningeal vessels
16	Frontal crest
17	Frontal sinus
18	Depressions for arachnoid granulations

VAULT OF SKULL
A External surface (left half)
B Internal surface (left half)
C Diploë of the right parietal bone

The standard view from above is shown in A, with the sagittal suture (5) in the midline and the coronal suture at the front (8). Internally in B there are grooves and impressions for the superior sagittal sinus (14; page 158, 2), the middle meningeal vessels (15; page 161, B16 and 17) and arachnoid granulations (page 170, 6).

In C the outer layer (outer table) of compact bone has been dissected away to show the 'honeycomb' of cancellous (spongy) bone, known in the skull as the diploë.

• The vertex of the skull is the central uppermost part, approximately where the sagittal suture is labelled (5).

• The parietal tuberosity (7) is the most lateral part of the cranial vault; it is particularly prominent in this specimen.

• Suture lines on the inside of the skull (as in B5 and 8) are less convoluted than on the outside (as in A5 and 8).

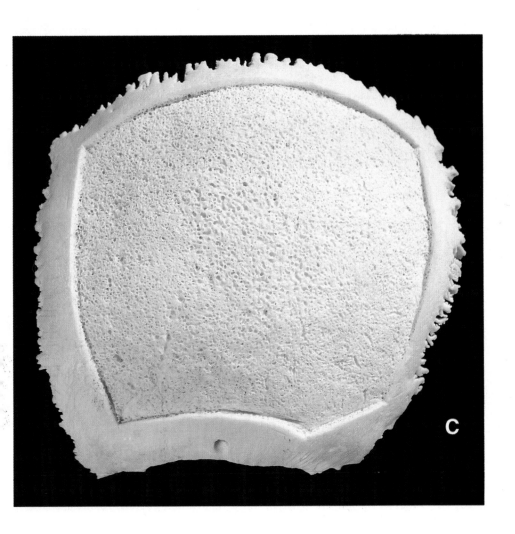

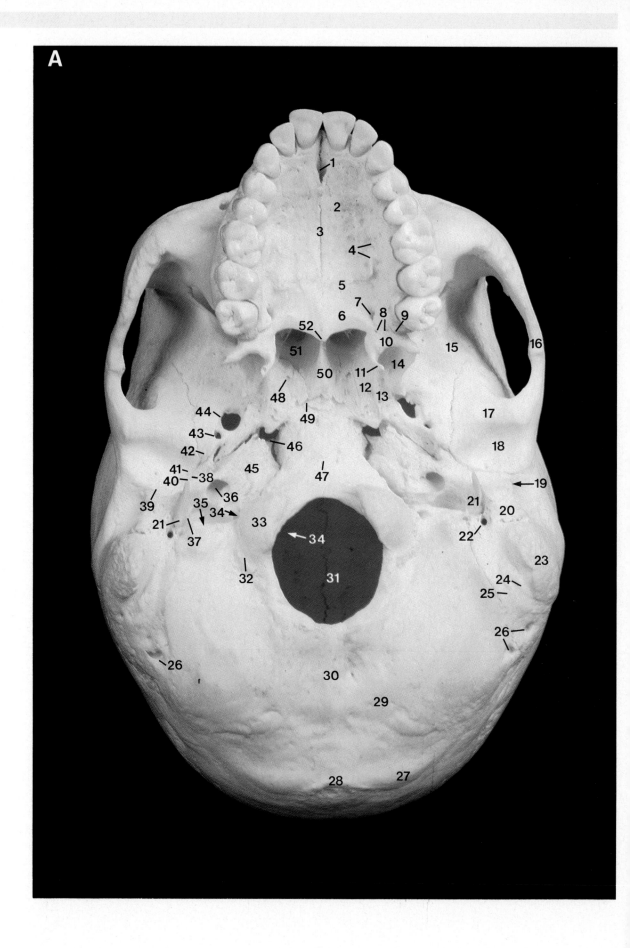

BASE OF SKULL
External surface
A From below
B From below and behind

In A, the standard view of the external surface of the base, the most important foramina (apart from the very large foramen magnum, 31) are the foramen lacerum (46), foramen ovale (44, unusually round where labelled but of more typical oval shape on the unlabelled opposite side), foramen spinosum (43), the stylomastoid foramen (22), the jugular foramen (35) and the carotid canal (36).

The angled view in B shows parts of the nasal conchae (58–60), visible through the posterior nasal apertures (choanae, A51).

• The palatine processes of the maxillae (2) and the horizontal plates of the palatine bones (6) form the hard palate.

1	Incisive fossa	31	Foramen magnum
2	Palatine process of maxilla	32	Condylar canal
3	Median palatine suture	33	Occipital condyle
4	Palatine grooves and spines	34	Hypoglossal canal
5	Transverse palatine suture	35	Jugular foramen
6	Horizontal plate of palatine bone	36	Carotid canal
7	Greater palatine foramen	37	Sheath of styloid process
8	Lesser palatine foramina	38	Petrotympanic fissure
9	Tuberosity of maxilla	39	Squamotympanic fissure
10	Pyramidal process of palatine bone	40	Tegmen tympani
11	Pterygoid hamulus	41	Petrosquamous fissure
12	Medial pterygoid plate	42	Spine of sphenoid bone
13	Scaphoid fossa	43	Foramen spinosum
14	Lateral pterygoid plate	44	Foramen ovale
15	Infratemporal crest	45	Apex of petrous part of temporal bone
16	Zygomatic arch	46	Foramen lacerum
17	Articular tubercle	47	Pharyngeal tubercle
18	Mandibular fossa	48	Palatovaginal canal
19	External acoustic meatus	49	Vomerovaginal canal
20	Tympanic part of temporal bone	50	Vomer
21	Styloid process	51	Posterior nasal aperture (choana)
22	Stylomastoid foramen	52	Posterior nasal spine
23	Mastoid process	53	Infratemporal surface ⎤ of maxilla
24	Mastoid notch	54	Zygomatic process ⎦
25	Occipital groove	55	Zygomaticomaxillary suture
26	Mastoid foramen (double on left)	56	Zygomaticotemporal foramen
27	Superior nuchal line	57	Inferior orbital fissure
28	External occipital protuberance	58	Inferior ⎤
29	Inferior nuchal line	59	Middle ⎬ nasal concha
30	External occipital crest	60	Superior ⎦

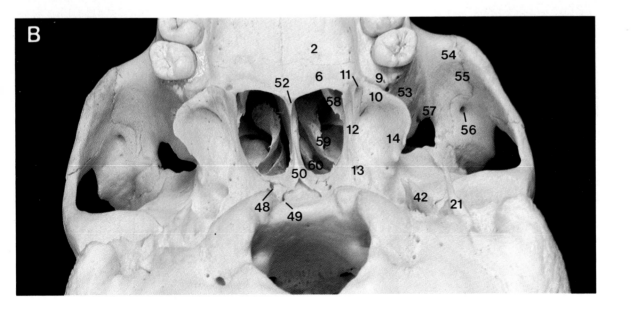

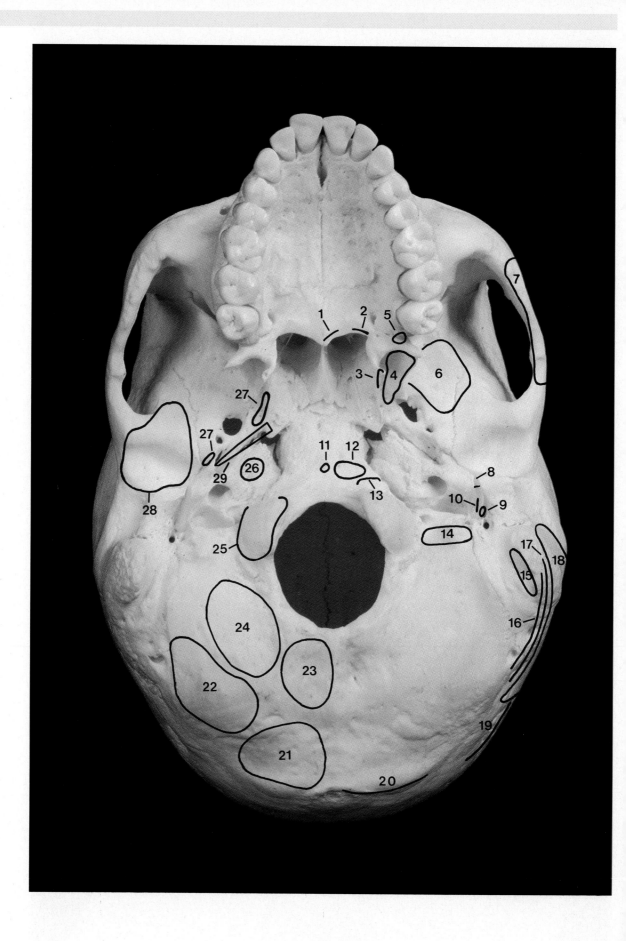

BASE OF SKULL
External surface
Muscle attachments

The main origins of the medial and lateral pterygoid muscles (4 and 6) are from the respective sides of the lateral pterygoid plate, with the lateral pterygoid also arising from the infratemporal surface of the greater wing of the sphenoid (6). The uppermost part of the superior constrictor of the pharynx (3) is attached to the lower part of the posterior border of the medial pterygoid plate. Sternocleidomastoid (18) is on the outer side of the mastoid process, with the posterior belly of digastric (15) on the inner side. Trapezius (20) reaches the back of the skull behind semispinalis (21) and the suboccipital muscles (22–24).

1	Musculus uvulae
2	Palatopharyngeus
3	Superior constrictor of pharynx
4	Medial pterygoid (deep head)
5	Medial pterygoid (superficial head)
6	Lateral pterygoid (upper head)
7	Masseter
8	Styloglossus
9	Stylohyoid
10	Stylopharyngeus
11	Pharyngeal raphe
12	Longus capitus
13	Rectus capitis anterior
14	Rectus capitis lateralis
15	Posterior belly of digastric
16	Longissimus capitis
17	Splenius capitis
18	Sternocleidomastoid
19	Occipital belly of occipitofrontalis
20	Trapezius
21	Semispinalis capitis
22	Superior oblique
23	Rectus capitis posterior minor
24	Rectus capitis posterior major
25	Capsule of atlanto-occipital joint
26	Levator veli palatini
27	Tensor veli palatini
28	Capsule of temporomandibular joint
29	Cartilaginous part of auditory tube

•Principal skull foramina and their contents:
(for more precise details see pages 231–232)

Supra-orbital foramen
  Supra-orbital nerve and vessels
Infra-orbital foramen
  Infra-orbital nerve and vessels
Mental foramen
  Mental nerve and vessels
Mandibular foramen
  Inferior alveolar nerve and vessels
Optic canal
  Optic nerve
  Ophthalmic artery
Superior orbital fissure
  Ophthalmic nerve and veins
  Oculomotor, trochlear and abducent nerves
Inferior orbital fissure
  Maxillary nerve
Sphenopalatine foramen
  Sphenopalatine artery
  Nasal branches of pterygopalatine ganglion
Foramen rotundum
  Maxillary nerve
Foramen ovale
  Mandibular and lesser petrosal nerves
Foramen spinosum
  Middle meningeal vessels
Foramen lacerum
  Internal carotid artery (entering from behind and emerging above)
  Greater petrosal nerve (entering from behind and leaving anteriorly as the nerve of the pterygoid canal)
Carotid canal
  Internal carotid artery and nerve
Jugular foramen
  Inferior petrosal sinus
  Glossopharyngeal, vagus and accessory nerves
  Internal jugular vein (emerging below)
Internal acoustic meatus
  Facial and vestibulocochlear nerves
  Labyrinthine artery
Hypoglossal canal
  Hypoglossal nerve
Stylomastoid foramen
  Facial nerve
Foramen magnum
  Medulla oblongata and meninges
  Vertebral and anterior and posterior spinal arteries
  Accessory nerves (spinal parts)

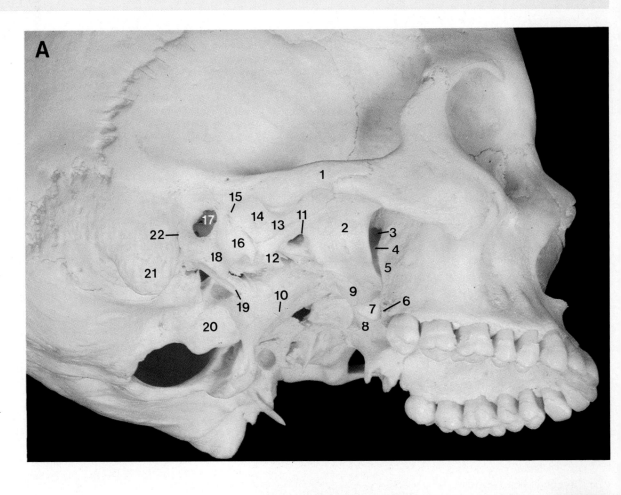

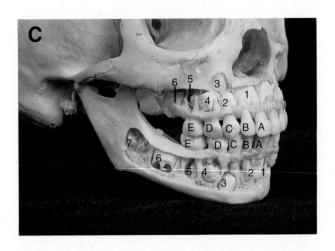

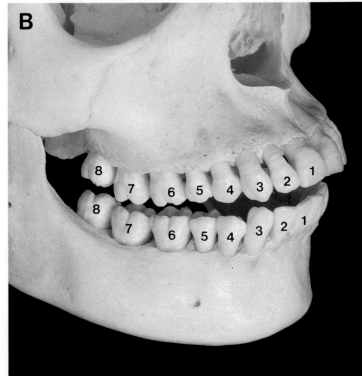

BASE OF SKULL
Infratemporal region and teeth
A The right infratemporal region, obliquely from below

1 Zygomatic arch
2 Lateral pterygoid plate
3 Sphenopalatine foramen
4 Pterygomaxillary fissure
5 Infratemporal surface of maxilla
6 Tuberosity of maxilla
7 Pyramidal process of palatine bone
8 Pterygoid hamulus
9 Medial pterygoid plate
10 Pharyngeal tubercle
11 Foramen ovale
12 Spine of sphenoid bone
13 Articular tubercle
14 Mandibular fossa
15 Squamotympanic fissure
16 Tympanic part of temporal bone
17 External acoustic meatus
18 Sheath of styloid process
19 Styloid process
20 Occipital condyle
21 Mastoid process
22 Tympanomastoid fissure

The main reason for examining the tilted view in A is to note the pterygomaxillary fissure (4), behind the maxilla (5) and in front of the pterygoid process whose lateral pterygoid plate (2) is shown throughout its length. In the depth of the fissure, i.e. in the medial wall of the pterygopalatine fossa (pages 70 and 71), the sphenopalatine foramen (3) is seen. (In the normal lateral view, as in page 14, the fissure and plate are largely obscured by the zygomatic arch and the coronoid process of the mandible—see page 14, 19 and 28).

In B–D, the teeth are labelled by numbers or letters according to dental convention (see notes). B shows adult teeth (numbered), while in C, from the skull of a 4-year-old child, the unerupted teeth of the permanent dentition have been displayed by dissecting away bone from the jaws which still contain the erupted deciduous teeth (lettered). In D individual upper and lower adult teeth are shown from their outer (labial or buccal) sides, to illustrate their roots.

• The corresponding teeth of the upper and lower jaws have corresponding names. In dentistry the teeth are often referred to by the numbers 1–8 as listed, rather than by name. Thus 'right upper six' refers to the right upper first molar.

• In the deciduous dentition of the child ('milk teeth'), there are central and lateral incisors and canines in corresponding positions to the permanent teeth of the same name, but the first and second deciduous molars are in the positions of the first and second permanent premolars. To distinguish them from the permanent teeth, the deciduous teeth are given letters instead of numbers (as in C).

B Permanent dentition, right side

1 Central ⎫
2 Lateral ⎭ incisor
3 Canine
4 First ⎫
5 Second ⎭ premolar
6 First ⎫
7 Second ⎬ molar
8 Third ⎭

C Erupted and unerupted teeth, right side, in the skull of a child aged 4. Deciduous teeth lettered; permanent teeth numbered, as in B

A Central ⎫
B Lateral ⎭ incisor
C Canine
D First ⎫
E Second ⎭ molar

D Adult right upper and lower teeth, from the right

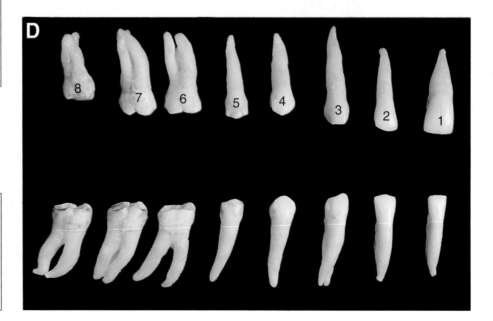

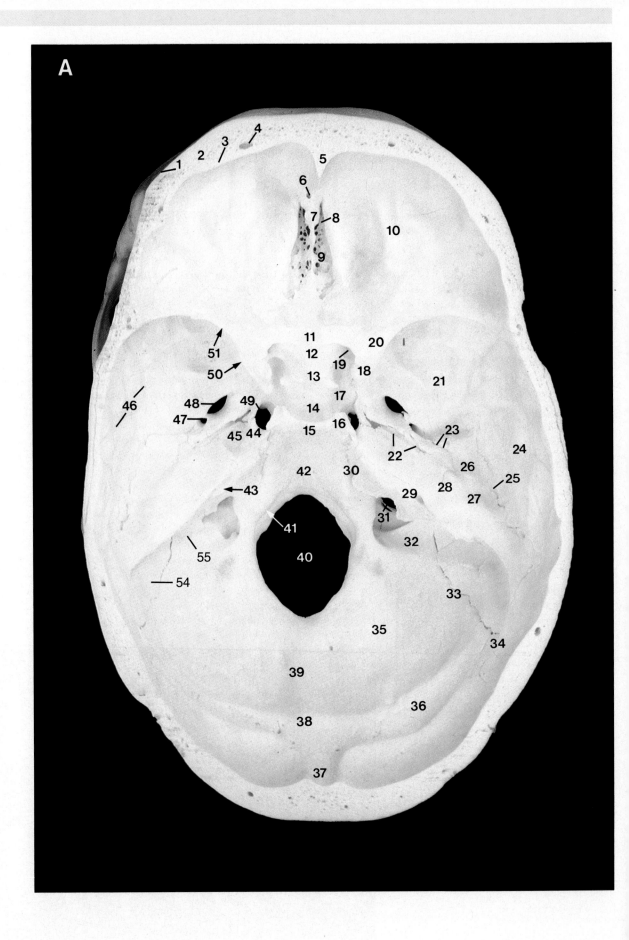

BASE OF SKULL
Internal surface—Anterior, middle and posterior cranial fossae
A From above
B The right half of the middle cranial fossa, from above, right and behind
C The left half of the middle cranial fossa, from above

The standard view directly from above is shown in A. In B the skull has been tilted downwards and forwards to bring into view the right superior orbital fissure (51) and foramen rotundum (50) which are not seen when looking straight down from above. The specimen in C shows the left venous and petrosal foramina (52 and 53) which are not often present.

• For details of the bones of the cranial fossae see pages 64-67.

• The foramina rotundum, ovale and spinosum (50, 48 and 47) are always present within the greater wing of the sphenoid bone; the venous (emissary sphenoidal) foramen (of Vesalius, C52) and the petrosal (innominate) foramen (C53) are occasional additions.

• The openings in the *anterior cranial fossa* are:
  the foramen caecum (6)
  the foramina of the cribriform plate of the ethmoid bone (9)

• The openings in the *middle cranial fossa* are:
  the optic canal (19)
  the superior orbital fissure (51)
  the foramen rotundum (50)
  the foramen ovale (48)
  the foramen spinosum (47)
  the venous (emissary sphenoidal) foramen (of Vesalius) (52) (occasional)
  the petrosal (innominate) foramen (53) (occasional)
  the foramen lacerum (49)
  the hiatus for the greater and lesser petrosal nerves (22 and 23)

• The openings in the *posterior cranial fossa* are:
  the foramen magnum (40)   the jugular foramen (31)
  the internal acoustic meatus (43)   the hypoglossal canal (41)
  the aqueduct of the vestibule (55) the mastoid foramen (54)

• For the contents of skull foramina see pages 25 and 231–232.

1 Outer table	21 Greater wing of sphenoid bone	38 Internal occipital protuberance
2 Diploë	22 Hiatus and groove for greater petrosal nerve	39 Internal occipital crest
3 Inner table	23 Hiatus and groove for lesser petrosal nerve	40 Foramen magnum
4 Frontal sinus (upper extremity)	24 Squamous part of temporal bone	41 Hypoglossal canal
5 Frontal crest	25 Petrosquamous fissure	42 Clivus
6 Foramen caecum	26 Tegmen tympani	43 Internal acoustic meatus
7 Crista galli	27 Arcuate eminence	44 Apex of petrous part of temporal bone
8 Groove for anterior ethmoidal nerve and vessels	28 Petrous part of temporal bone	45 Trigeminal impression
9 Cribriform plate of ethmoid bone	29 Groove for superior petrosal sinus	46 Grooves for middle meningeal vessels
10 Orbital part of frontal bone	30 Groove for inferior petrosal sinus and petro-occipital suture	47 Foramen spinosum
11 Jugum of sphenoid bone	31 Jugular foramen	48 Foramen ovale
12 Prechiasmatic groove	32 Groove for sigmoid sinus	49 Foramen lacerum
13 Tuberculum sellae	33 Occipitomastoid suture	50 Foramen rotundum
14 Pituitary fossa (sella turcica)	34 Mastoid (postero-inferior) angle of parietal bone	51 Superior orbital fissure
15 Dorsum sellae	35 Occipital bone	52 Venous (emissary sphenoidal) foramen (of Vesalius)
16 Posterior clinoid process	36 Groove for transverse sinus	53 Petrosal (innominate) foramen
17 Carotid groove	37 Groove for superior sagittal sinus	54 Mastoid emissary foramen
18 Anterior clinoid process		55 Aqueduct of vestibule
19 Optic canal		
20 Lesser wing of sphenoid bone		

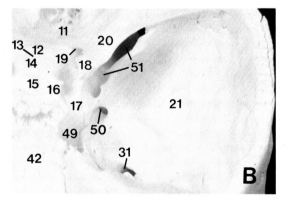

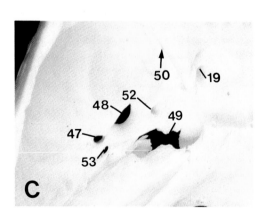

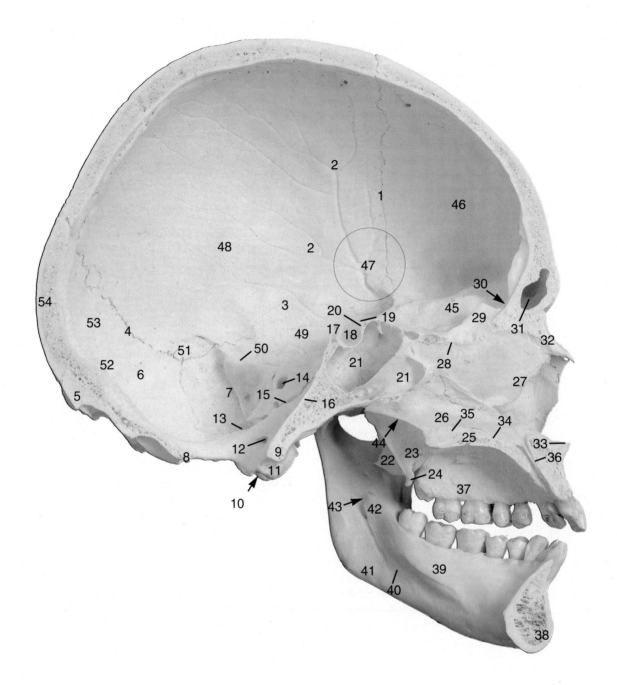

INTERIOR OF SKULL
Left half, in a median sagittal section
The inside of the left half of the skull is seen from the right, with the bony part of the nasal septum intact (the vomer, 26, and the perpendicular plate of the ethmoid bone, 27). The encircled area (47) indicates the position of pterion (see the notes on pages 15 and 161).

• The grooves for the middle meningeal vessels (2) on the inside of the cranial vault pass upwards and backwards.

• The groove for the transverse sinus (6) runs forwards on the occipital bone, crosses the mastoid angle of the parietal bone (51) and then turns downwards on the temporal bone to become the groove for the sigmoid sinus (7) which leads into the jugular foramen (13; compare with the views in page 28, A36, 34, 32 and 31).

• The pituitary fossa (18) lies above the sphenoidal sinus (21).

• The hypoglossal canal (12) in the occipital bone is above the occipital condyle (11), with the internal acoustic meatus (14) at a higher level in the temporal bone. In this view the occipital condyle obscures the mastoid process (10).

1 Coronal suture
2 Grooves for middle meningeal vessels
3 Squamosal suture
4 Lambdoid suture
5 External occipital protuberance
6 Groove for transverse sinus
7 Groove for sigmoid sinus
8 Posterior | margin of foramen magnum
9 Anterior |
10 Mastoid process
11 Occipital condyle
12 Hypoglossal canal
13 Jugular foramen
14 Internal acoustic meatus
15 Groove for inferior petrosal sinus
16 Clivus
17 Dorsum sellae
18 Pituitary fossa
19 Anterior clinoid process
20 Optic canal
21 Sphenoidal sinus
22 Lateral | pterygoid plate
23 Medial |
24 Pterygoid hamulus
25 Hard palate
26 Vomer
27 Perpendicular plate | of ethmoid bone
28 Cribriform plate |

29 Crista galli
30 Foramen caecum
31 Frontal sinus
32 Nasal bone
33 Anterior nasal spine
34 Nasal crest of maxilla
35 Nasal crest of palatine bone
36 Incisive canal
37 Alveolar process of maxilla
38 Mental protuberance
39 Mylohyoid line of mandible
40 Groove for mylohyoid nerve
41 Angle of mandible
42 Lingula
43 Mandibular foramen
44 Posterior nasal aperture (choana)
45 Orbital part | of frontal bone
46 Squamous part |
47 Pterion (encircled)
48 Parietal bone
49 Squamous part of temporal bone
50 Groove for superior petrosal sinus
51 Mastoid (posterior inferior) angle of parietal bone
52 Internal occipital protuberance
53 Occipital bone
54 Occiput

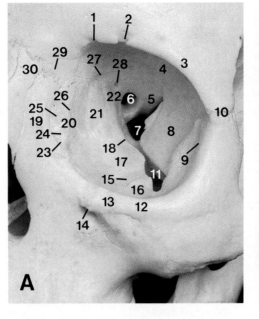

A

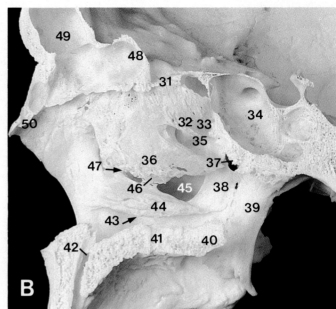

B

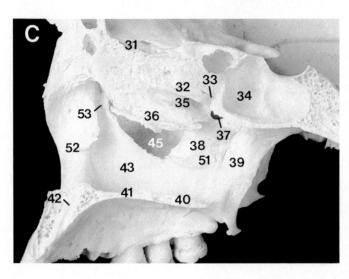

C

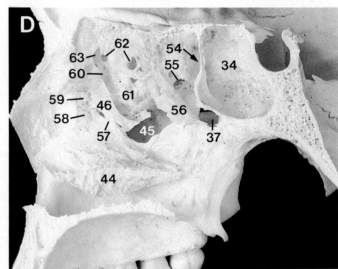

D

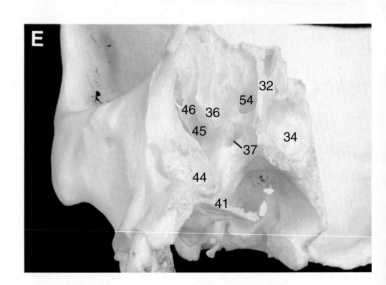

E

CAVITIES OF SKULL
Orbit and nasal cavity
A Left orbit
B Right half of the nasal cavity, with the lateral wall intact
C Lateral wall, with the inferior nasal concha removed
D Lateral wall, with the middle nasal concha removed
E Oblique view, from the front and the left, with the nasal septum removed.

In A, looking into the left orbit slightly from the left and above, the roof, lateral wall, floor and medial wall can all be seen. The bones taking part in these boundaries are bracketed together in the key, and are described further on pages 54–59.

B–E all show the lateral wall of the right half of the nasal cavity. In B the wall is complete. Removal of the inferior nasal concha (B44) in C enables more of the medial wall of the maxilla to be seen (43). Removal of the middle nasal concha (B36) in D displays the ethmoidal bulla (61) and semilunar hiatus (60). The oblique view in E shows the opening in the anterior wall of the sphenoidal sinus (54).

• For further details of the bones of the orbit see pages 54–59, and of the nose pages 54 and 60–63.

• In B the crista galli (48) is large and the frontal sinus (49) has extended into it.

1 Frontal notch	33 Spheno-ethmoidal recess
2 Supra-orbital foramen	34 Sphenoidal sinus
3 Supra-orbital margin	35 Superior meatus
4 Orbital part of frontal bone ⎫ forming roof	36 Middle nasal concha
5 Lesser wing of sphenoid bone ⎭	37 Sphenopalatine foramen
6 Optic canal	38 Perpendicular plate of palatine bone
7 Superior orbital fissure	39 Medial pterygoid plate
8 Greater wing of sphenoid bone ⎫	40 Horizontal plate of palatine bone
9 Zygomatic bone (with leader to ⎬ forming lateral wall	41 Palatine process of maxilla
marginal tubercle) ⎭	42 Incisive canal
10 Frontozygomatic suture	43 Inferior meatus and medial wall of maxilla
11 Inferior orbital fissure	44 Inferior nasal concha
12 Infra-orbital margin	45 Maxillary hiatus
13 Zygomaticomaxillary suture	46 Uncinate process of ethmoid bone
14 Infra-orbital foramen	47 Middle meatus
15 Infra-orbital groove	48 Crista galli
16 Zygomatic bone ⎫	49 Frontal sinus
17 Maxilla ⎬ forming floor	50 Nasal bone
18 Orbital process of palatine bone ⎭	51 Conchal crest of perpendicular plate of palatine bone
19 Frontal process of maxilla ⎫	52 Conchal crest of maxilla
20 Lacrimal bone ⎬ forming medial wall	53 Nasolacrimal canal
21 Orbital plate of ethmoid bone ⎬	54 Aperture of sphenoidal sinus into spheno-ethmoidal recess
22 Body of sphenoid bone ⎭	55 Aperture of posterior ethmoidal air cell into superior meatus
23 Anterior lacrimal crest	56 Base of middle nasal concha
24 Lacrimal groove	57 Ethmoidal process ⎫ of inferior nasal concha
25 Fossa for lacrimal sac	58 Lacrimal process ⎭
26 Posterior lacrimal crest	59 Descending process of lacrimal bone
27 Anterior ⎫ ethmoidal foramen	60 Semilunar hiatus
28 Posterior ⎭	61 Ethmoidal bulla
29 Frontomaxillary suture	62 Apertures of middle ethmoidal air cells
30 Nasal bone	63 Frontonasal duct
31 Cribriform plate of ethmoid bone	
32 Superior nasal concha	

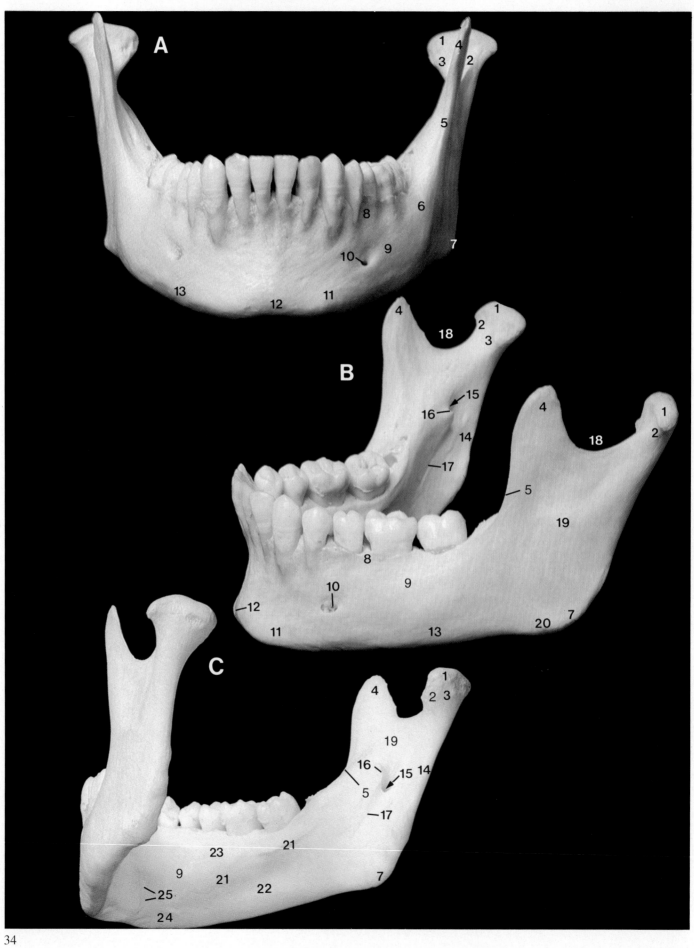

MANDIBLE

A From the front
B From the left and above
C From the left and below
D From above

The mandible is the bone of the lower jaw, bearing the lower teeth and forming the temporomandibular joints with the temporal bones. In this mandible the third molar teeth are unerupted (B and D, 26)

• The main features of the **mandible** are:
  the body (9) with the lower teeth
  the ramus (19) passing upwards, with the mandibular foramen (C15)
    on its medial side
  the coronoid process (4) at the upper anterior end of the ramus (19)
  the condylar process (condyle) comprising the head (1) and neck (2)
    at the upper posterior end of the ramus (19)
  the angle (7) at the lower posterior end of the ramus (19)

1	Head	**14**	Posterior border of ramus
2	Neck	**15**	Mandibular foramen
3	Pterygoid fovea	**16**	Lingula
4	Coronoid process	**17**	Mylohyoid groove
5	Anterior border of ramus and coronoid notch	**18**	Mandibular notch
6	Oblique line	**19**	Ramus
7	Angle	**20**	Inferior border of ramus
8	Alveolar part	**21**	Mylohyoid line
9	Body	**22**	Submandibular fossa
10	Mental foramen	**23**	Sublingual fossa
11	Mental tubercle	**24**	Digastric fossa
12	Mental protuberance	**25**	Superior and inferior mental spines
13	Base	**26**	Unerupted third molar tooth

1, 2, 3 forming condylar process

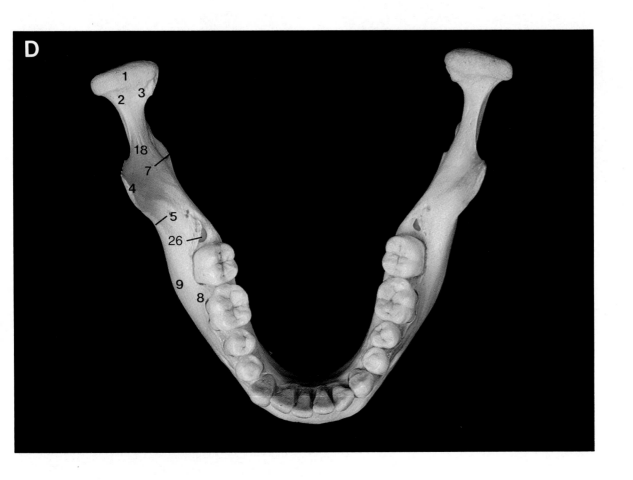

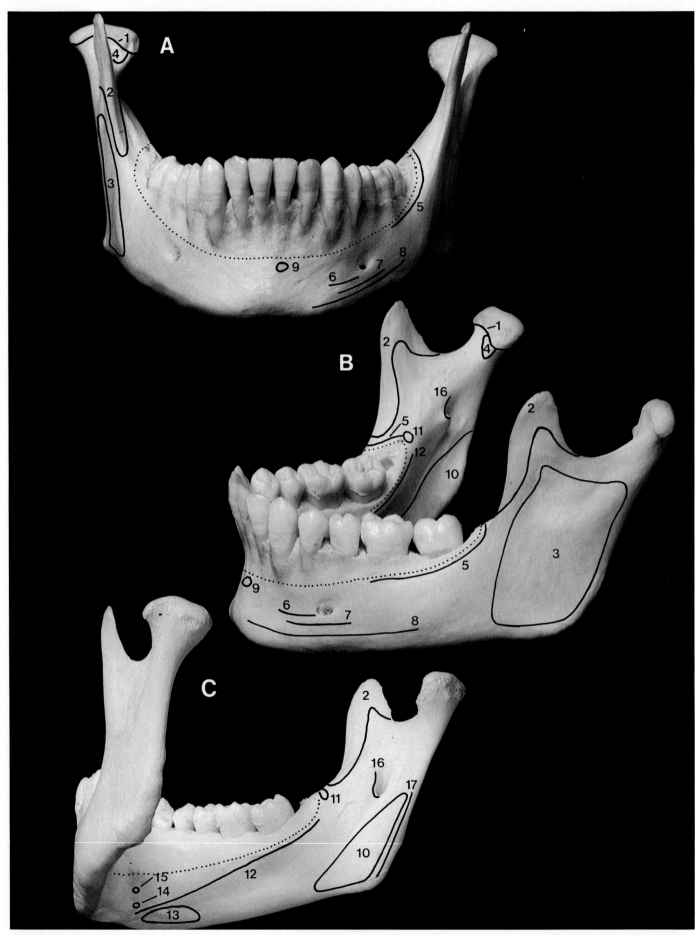

MANDIBLE
Muscle attachments and age changes
A From the front
B From the left and above
C From the left and below
D Mandible in old age, from the right

In C the yellow marker indicates where the lingual nerve lies in contact with the periosteum—below and behind the third molar tooth (here unerupted). The side view of the edentulous (toothless) mandible in old age (D) should be compared with B and C. Note that the angle between the ramus and the body has become more obtuse, and that alveolar bone has become resorbed so that the mental foramen comes to lie nearer the upper surface of the edentulous body.

• The attachment of the buccinator muscle (5, to the alveolar bone opposite the molar teeth—the third molar is here unerupted) extends back to the pterygomandibular raphe (11).

• The attachment of the temporalis tendon (2) extends from the lowest part of the mandibular notch, over the coronoid process, and down the front of the ramus almost as far as the third molar tooth (here unerupted).

1	Capsule of temporomandibular joint
2	Temporalis
3	Masseter
4	Lateral pterygoid
5	Buccinator
6	Depressor labii inferioris
7	Depressor anguli oris
8	Platysma
9	Mentalis
10	Medial pterygoid
11	Pterygomandibular raphe and superior constrictor of pharynx
12	Mylohyoid
13	Anterior belly of digastric
14	Geniohyoid
15	Genioglossus
16	Sphenomandibular ligament
17	Stylomandibular ligament

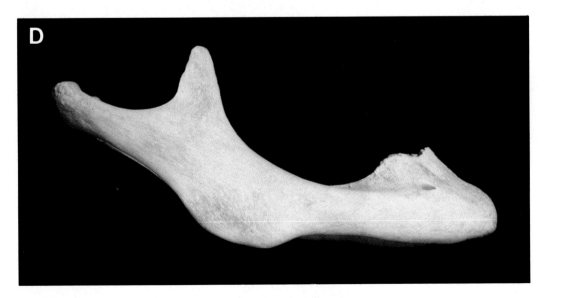

D

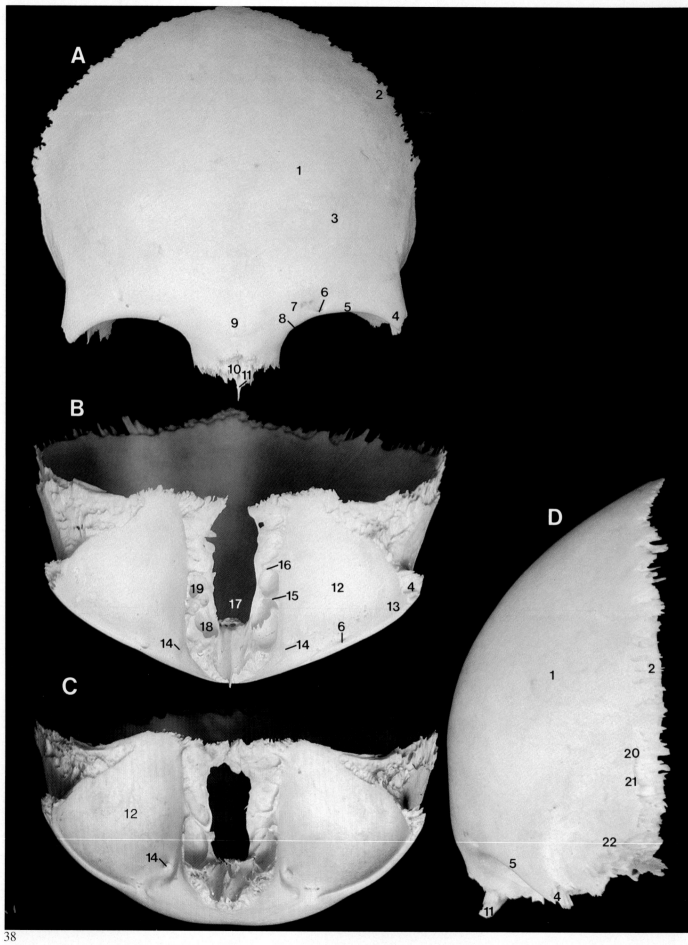

FRONTAL BONE
A External surface, from the front
B From below
C From below
D From the left
E Internal surface, from above and behind
F External surface, from the front

The frontal bone is at the top and front of the skull, forming the forehead and containing the frontal sinuses. In the specimen shown in C, the orbital parts (12) have become joined together at the back of the ethmoidal notch (B17). In F the midline frontal (metopic) suture (25) has persisted.

• The main features of the *frontal bone* are:

the squamous part (1) curving upwards and backwards above the nose and orbits
the orbital parts (12) passing backwards as the roofs of the orbits
the nasal part (10) with the nasal spine (11) passing downwards.

• In the intact skull, the ethmoidal notch (B17) is filled by the cribriform plate of the ethmoid bone and crista galli (page 28, A7 and 9; page 40, A2 and 3).

1 Squamous part		**14** Trochlear fovea (tubercle in C)
2 Parietal margin		**15** Anterior ethmoidal foramen
3 Frontal tuberosity		**16** Posterior ethmoidal foramen
4 Zygomatic process		**17** Ethmoidal notch
5 Supra-orbital margin		**18** Frontal sinus
6 Supra-orbital foramen		**19** Roof of ethmoidal air cells
7 Superciliary arch		**20** Superior temporal line
8 Position of frontal notch or foramen		**21** Inferior temporal line
9 Glabella		**22** Temporal surface
10 Nasal part		**23** Frontal crest
11 Nasal spine		**24** Foramen caecum
12 Orbital part		**25** Frontal (metopic) suture
13 Fossa for lacrimal gland		

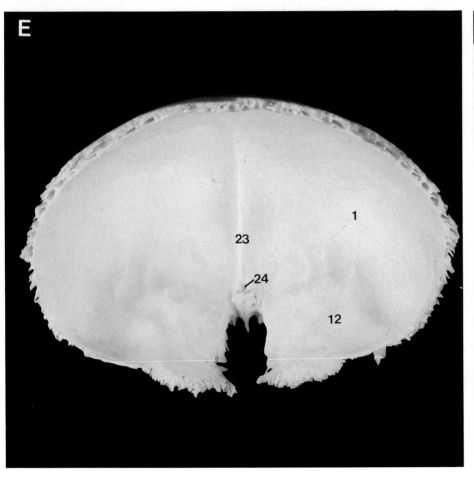

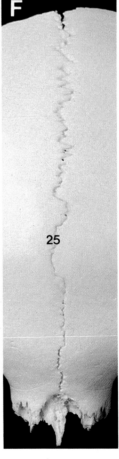

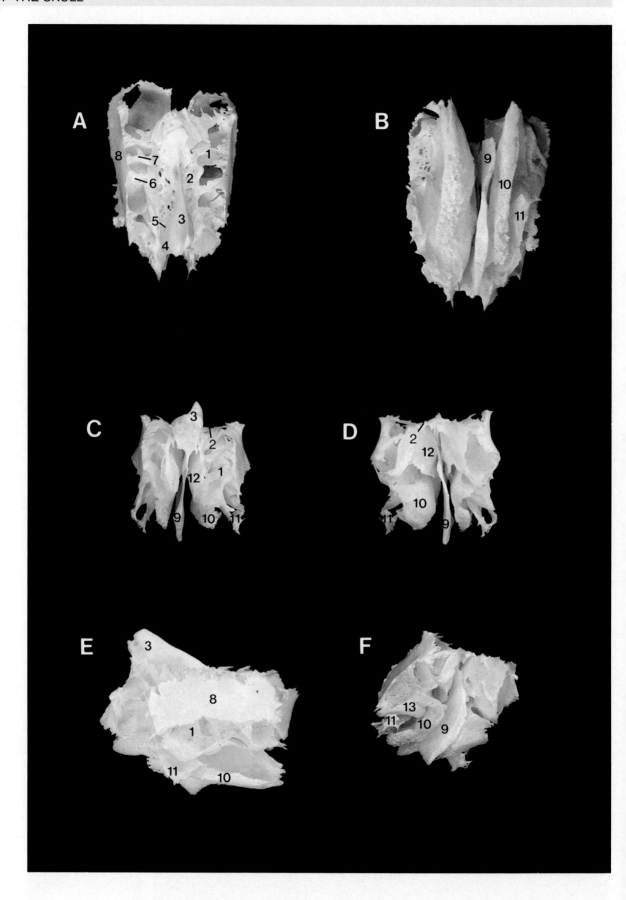

ETHMOID BONE

A From above
B From below
C From the front
D From behind
E From the left
F From the left, below and behind

The ethmoid bone is in the centre of the skull between the orbits, containing the ethmoidal sinuses and forming parts of the nasal and orbital cavities. The specimen in F has been tilted obliquely upwards to show how the (left) ethmoidal bulla (F13) is overlapped by the middle nasal concha (F10).

1	Ethmoidal labyrinth and air cells
2	Cribriform plate
3	Crista galli
4	Ala of crista galli
5	Slit for anterior ethmoidal nerve and vessels
6	Groove for anterior ethmoidal nerve and vessels
7	Groove for posterior ethmoidal nerve and vessels
8	Orbital plate
9	Perpendicular plate
10	Middle nasal concha
11	Uncinate process
12	Superior nasal concha
13	Ethmoidal bulla

• The main features of the *ethmoid bone* are:
the perpendicular plate (B, C, D and F, 9) with the crista galli (A and C, 3) at the upper end
the cribriform plate (A, C and D, 2) on each side at right angles to the perpendicular plate
the ethmoidal labyrinth (sinus, A and C, 1) on each side hanging down from the outer edge of the cribriform plate
superior and middle nasal conchae (C and D, 12 and 10) on the medial side of each labyrinth

• The crista galli and cribriform plates (A3 and 2) form the central part of the floor of the anterior cranial fossa (page 28, A7 and 9).

• The perpendicular plate forms part of the bony nasal septum (page 31, 27).

• The superior and middle nasal conchae (C and D, 12 and 10) project from the medial wall of the ethmoidal labyrinth as part of the lateral wall of the nasal cavity (page 32, B32 and 36). (The inferior nasal concha is a separate bone, not part of the ethmoid: page 32, B44 and page 48, G and H.)

• The lateral wall of the ethmoidal labyrinth is the orbital plate (A and E, 8), forming part of the medial wall of the orbit (page 32, A21 and page 59, D and E, 20). This orbital plate is paper-thin and hence often called the lamina papyracea; the outlines of ethmoidal air cells are usually visible through it (as in E8).

• The ethmoidal bulla (F13, a bulging air cell) is under cover of the middle nasal concha (F10). When this concha is removed (as in page 32, D) a groove is seen between the bulla and the uncinate process of the ethmoid (F10 and 11). This groove, lined by mucous membrane in the intact nasal cavity, is the semilunar hiatus (page 32, D60, between 61 and 46, and page 128, B12, between 11 and 14).

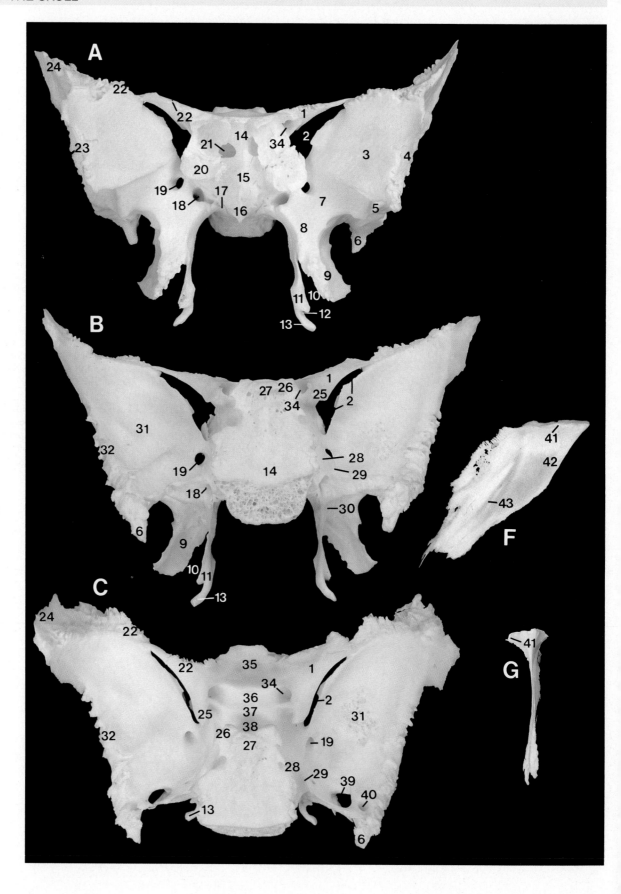

SPHENOID BONE

A From the front
B From behind
C From above and behind
D From below
E From the right

The sphenoid bone is in the middle of the base of the skull, extending to each side and containing the pituitary fossa and the sphenoidal sinuses.

VOMER

F From the left
G From behind

The vomer is in the midline of the base of the skull, forming the posterior part of the nasal septum.

• The main features of the *sphenoid bone* are:

the body (A14) containing the two sphenoidal air sinuses with their apertures anteriorly (A21)
the pituitary fossa (C and E, 38) indenting the upper surface of the body
the lesser wing (1) on each side passing laterally with the optic canal between its roots (C34)
the greater wing (A3; B31) on each side passing laterally below the lesser wing, with the superior orbital fissure (A and B, 2) between the lesser and greater wings, and the foramina rotundum, ovale and spinosum within the greater wing
the pterygoid process (A8) on each side passing downwards to divide into the medial and lateral pterygoid plates (A and B, 9 and 11)

• The posterior part of the body which joins the occipital bone at the spheno-occipital synchondrosis (page 67) is commonly known as the basisphenoid (B14 and the lower 14 in D).

• The main features of the *vomer* are the alae (41) which project laterally at the upper margin.

1	Lesser wing	15	Crest	30	Scaphoid fossa
2	Superior orbital fissure	16	Rostrum	31	Cerebral surface of greater wing
3	Orbital surface	17	Vaginal process	32	Squamous margin
4	Temporal surface	18	Pterygoid canal	33	Groove for auditory tube
5	Infratemporal crest	19	Foramen rotundum	34	Optic canal
6	Spine	20	Concha	35	Jugum
7	Maxillary surface	21	Aperture of sphenoidal sinus	36	Prechiasmatic groove
8	Pterygoid process	22	Frontal margin	37	Tuberculum sellae
9	Lateral pterygoid plate	23	Zygomatic margin	38	Pituitary fossa (sella turcica)
10	Pterygoid notch	24	Parietal margin	39	Foramen ovale
11	Medial pterygoid plate	25	Anterior clinoid process	40	Foramen spinosum
12	Groove of pterygoid hamulus	26	Posterior clinoid process	41	Ala
13	Pterygoid hamulus	27	Dorsum sellae	42	Posterior border
14	Body	28	Carotid groove	43	Groove for nasopalatine nerve and vessels
		29	Lingula		

(3, 4, 5, 6, 7) of greater wing

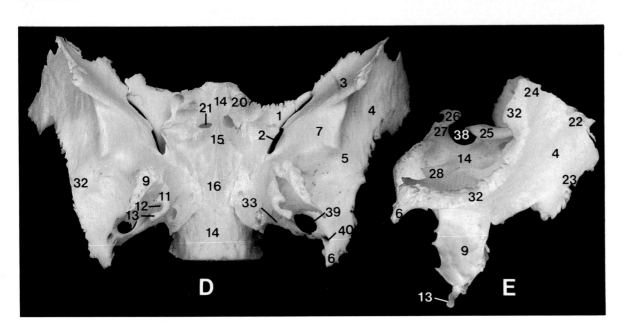

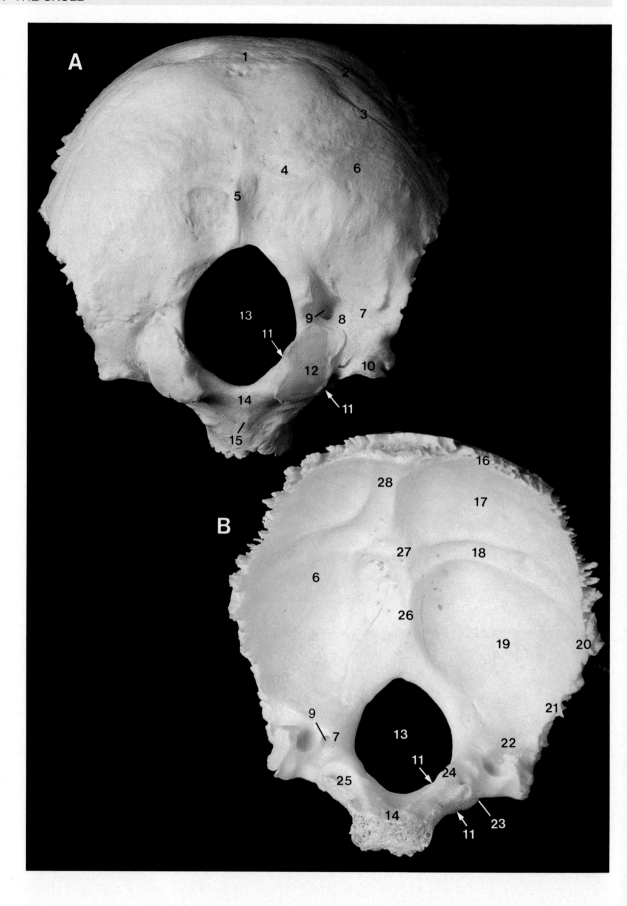

OCCIPITAL BONE
A External surface, from below
B Internal surface
C External surface, from the right and below
The occipital bone is at the back of the base of the skull, containing the foramen magnum and bearing the condyles for the atlanto-occipital joints by which the skull is attached to the vertebral column.

• The main features of the *occipital bone* are:
    the foramen magnum (13) in the lower part
    the squamous part (6) curving upwards and backwards behind the foramen magnum
    the lateral parts (7), with condyles on the lower surfaces (A and C, 12)
    the basilar part (A and B, 14) in front of the foramen magnum

1	External occipital protuberance	15	Pharyngeal tubercle
2	Supreme nuchal line	16	Lambdoid margin
3	Superior nuchal line	17	Cerebral fossa
4	Inferior nuchal line	18	Groove for transverse sinus
5	External occipital crest	19	Cerebellar fossa
6	Squamous part	20	Lateral angle
7	Lateral part	21	Mastoid margin
8	Condylar fossa	22	Groove for sigmoid sinus
9	Condylar canal	23	Jugular notch
10	Jugular process	24	Jugular tubercle
11	Hypoglossal canal	25	Groove for inferior petrosal sinus
12	Condyle	26	Internal occipital crest
13	Foramen magnum	27	Internal occipital protuberance
14	Basilar part	28	Groove for superior sagittal sinus

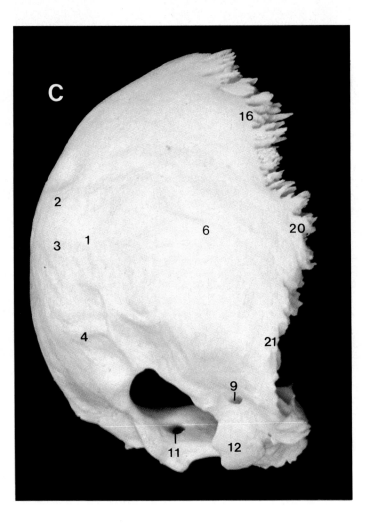

• The anterior end of the basilar part (B14) which joins the sphenoid bone at the spheno-occipital synchondrosis (page 67) is commonly known as the basi-occiput (compare with the basisphenoid—see the note on page 43).

• The hypoglossal canal (A and C, 11) passes approximately above the middle of the occipital condyle (A12), but is only seen when viewed from the side (as in C, 11). The hypoglossal nerve runs through it.

• The condylar canal (A9), which is not always present, opens behind the occipital condyle. An emissary vein passes through it connecting the sigmoid sinus (inside the skull) to veins in the suboccipital region (outside the skull).

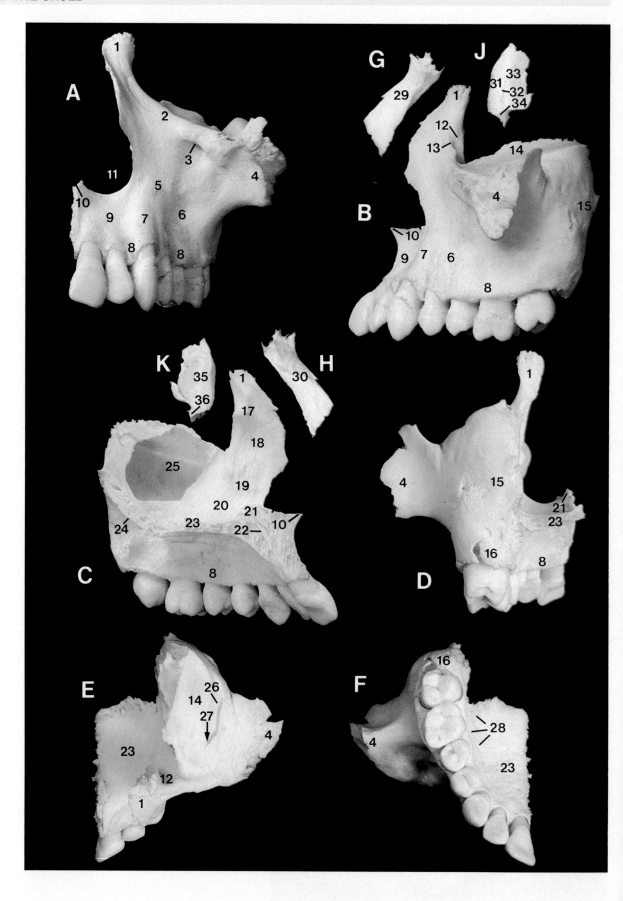

MAXILLA, left
A From the front
B From the lateral side
C From the medial side
D From behind
E From above
F From below
The maxilla forms half of the upper jaw, bearing the upper teeth of one side and containing the maxillary sinus. In this specimen the third molar tooth is unerupted (D and F, 16).

NASAL BONE, left
G From the lateral side
H From the medial side
The nasal bone forms with its fellow the bridge of the nose

LACRIMAL BONE, left
J From the lateral side
K From the medial side
The lacrimal bone is at the front of the medial wall of the orbit

1 Frontal process
2 Infra-orbital margin
3 Infra-orbital foramen
4 Zygomatic process
5 Anterior surface
6 Canine fossa
7 Canine eminence
8 Alveolar process
9 Incisive fossa
10 Anterior nasal spine
11 Nasal notch
12 Lacrimal groove
13 Anterior lacrimal crest
14 Orbital surface
15 Infratemporal surface
16 Tuberosity (over unerupted third molar tooth)
17 Ethmoidal crest
18 Middle meatus
19 Conchal crest
20 Inferior meatus
21 Nasal crest
22 Incisive canal
23 Palatine process
24 Greater palatine groove
25 Maxillary hiatus and sinus
26 Infra-orbital groove
27 Infra-orbital canal
28 Palatine grooves and spines
29 Lateral surface and vascular foramen
30 Internal surface and ethmoidal groove
31 Lacrimal groove
32 Posterior lacrimal crest
33 Orbital surface
34 Lacrimal hamulus
35 Nasal surface
36 Descending process

• The main features of the *maxilla* are:

the maxillary sinus with the hiatus in the medial wall (C25)
the alveolar process (A–D, 8) at the lower margin with the upper teeth
the frontal process (A–D, 1) passing upwards
the palatine process (C–F, 23) passing medially
the zygomatic process (A, B, D and F, 4) passing laterally

• In the intact skull, the two maxillae unite with one another below the nasal notch (A11), but the frontal processes (A1) are separated from one another by the two nasal bones (page 10, 33)

• The palatine process (F23) articulates at the back with the horizontal plate of the palatine bone (page 48, F15). They both articulate with their fellows of the opposite side to form the hard palate (page 23, A2 and 6).

• For articulations forming the lateral wall of the nasal cavity, see pages 60–61.

• The main features of the *nasal bone* are:

the smooth lateral surface (G29)
the ethmoidal groove (H30) on the internal surface

• The main features of the *lacrimal bone* are:

the orbital (lateral) surface with the lacrimal groove (J31) at the front
the descending process (K36) pointing downwards

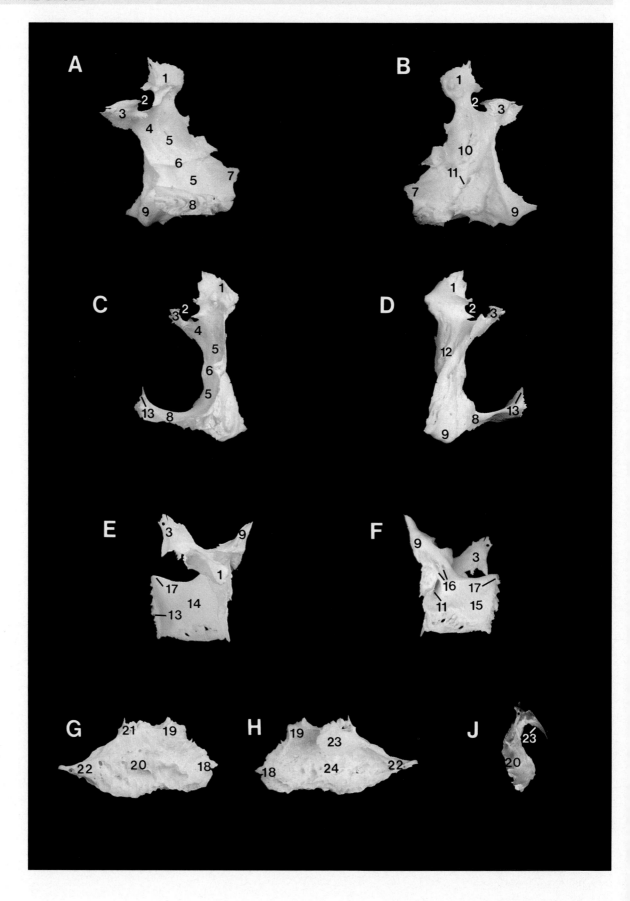

PALATINE BONE, left
A From the medial side
B From the lateral side
C From the front
D From behind
E From above
F From below
The palatine bone is at the back of the lateral wall of the nasal cavity and forms part of the roof of the mouth (hard palate).

INFERIOR NASAL CONCHA, left
G From the medial side
H From the lateral side
J From the front
The inferior nasal concha is in the lower part of the lateral wall of the nasal cavity

1	Orbital process
2	Sphenopalatine notch
3	Sphenoidal process
4	Ethmoidal crest
5	Perpendicular plate, nasal surface
6	Conchal crest
7	Maxillary process
8	Horizontal plate
9	Pyramidal process
10	Perpendicular plate, maxillary surface
11	Greater palatine groove
12	Perpendicular plate
13	Nasal crest
14	Horizontal plate, nasal surface
15	Horizontal plate, palatal surface
16	Lesser palatine canals
17	Posterior nasal canals
18	Anterior end
19	Lacrimal process
20	Medial surface
21	Ethmoidal process
22	Posterior end
23	Maxillary process
24	Lateral surface

• The main features of the ***palatine bone*** are:

the perpendicular plate (A and C, 5; B10), the largest part of the bone
the orbital and sphenoidal processes (A–D, 1 and 3) at the upper end of the perpendicular plate, with the sphenopalatine notch in between (A–D, 2)
the horizontal plate (C and D, 8) passing medially at the lower end of the perpendicular plate
the maxillary process (A and B, 7) passing forwards at the lower end of the perpendicular plate
the pyramidal process (A, B and D–F, 9) passing backwards at the lower end of the perpendicular plate

• The upper surface of the orbital process of the palatine bone (E1) forms the most posterior part of the floor of the orbit (page 32, A18).

• The sphenopalatine notch (A2), at the upper end of the perpendicular plate (A5) between the orbital and sphenoidal processes (A1 and 3), is converted into the sphenopalatine foramen (in the lateral wall of the nasal cavity) by articulation with the body of the sphenoid bone (page 70, B6).

• For articulations forming the lateral wall of the nose see pages 60–61, and the floor of the orbit, pages 58–59.

• The main features of the ***inferior nasal concha*** are:

the convex medial surface (G20) with a sharp posterior end (G22)
the lacrimal and ethmoidal processes (G19 and 21), passing upwards
the maxillary process (H and J, 23) passing downwards on the lateral side

• The anterior and posterior ends of the lateral surface (H18 and 22) articulate with the conchal crests of the maxilla and palatine bone, respectively (page 46, C17 and page 48, A6).

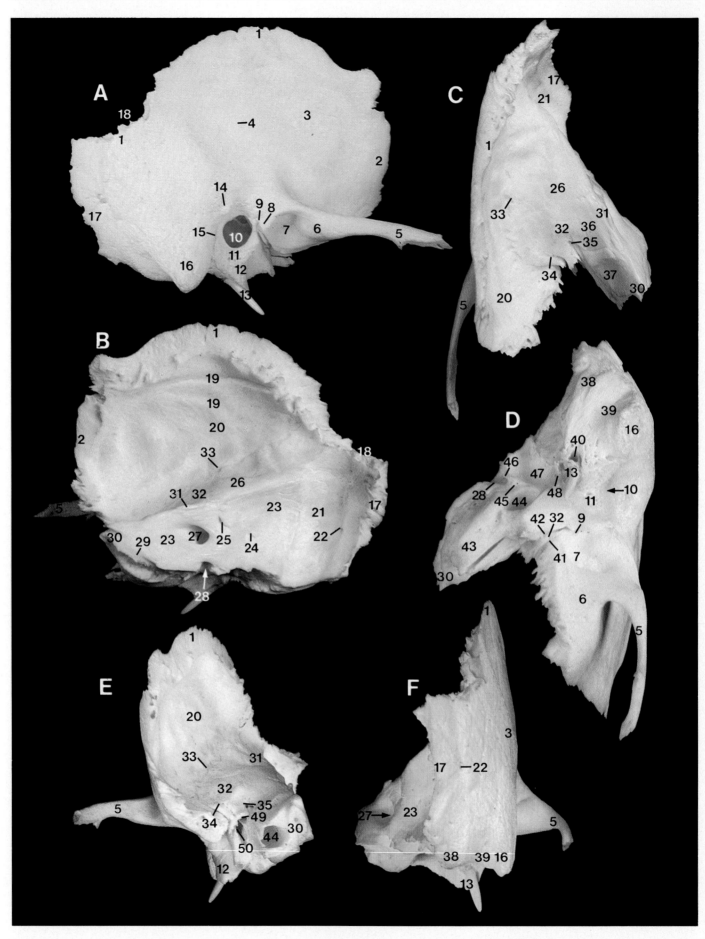

TEMPORAL BONE, right
A **From the lateral side**
B **From the medial side**
C **From above**
D **From below**
E **From the front**
F **From behind**
G **From the medial side and above**
The temporal bone is at the side and base of the skull, containing the ear and making the temporomandibular joint with the mandible.

• The main features of the *temporal bone* are:
  the petrous part (C31; D43) including the mastoid process (A and F, 16)
  the squamous part (A and F, 3) passing upwards but including the mandibular fossa (A and D, 7) facing downwards and the zygomatic process (A and D, 5) passing forwards
  the styloid process (A and F, 13) passing downwards and forwards
  the tympanic part (A11) surrounding the external acoustic meatus (A10) opening laterally
  the internal acoustic meatus (B27) in the petrous part opening medially

1	Parietal margin	27	Internal acoustic meatus
2	Sphenoidal margin	28	External opening of cochlear canaliculus in jugular notch
3	Temporal surface of squamous part	29	Groove for inferior petrosal sinus
4	Groove for middle temporal artery	30	Apex of petrous sinus
5	Zygomatic process	31	Superior margin of petrous part and groove for superior petrosal sinus
6	Articular tubercle		
7	Mandibular fossa	32	Tegmen tympani
8	Postglenoid tubercle	33	Petrosquamous fissure (upper part)
9	Squamotympanic fissure	34	Hiatus and groove for lesser petrosal nerve
10	External acoustic meatus	35	Hiatus and groove for greater petrosal nerve
11	Tympanic part	36	Anterior surface of petrous part
12	Sheath of styloid process	37	Trigeminal impression
13	Styloid process	38	Occipital groove
14	Suprameatal pit and spine (suprameatal triangle)	39	Mastoid notch
15	Tympanomastoid fissure	40	Stylomastoid foramen
16	Mastoid process	41	Petrosquamous fissure (lower part)
17	Occipital margin	42	Petrotympanic fissure
18	Parietal notch	43	Inferior surface of petrous part
19	Groove for parietal branches of middle meningeal vessels	44	Carotid canal
20	Cerebral surface of squamous part	45	Tympanic canaliculus
21	Groove for sigmoid sinus	46	Intrajugular process
22	Mastoid foramen	47	Jugular fossa
23	Posterior surface of petrous part	48	Mastoid canaliculus
24	External opening of aqueduct of vestibule	49	Semicanal for tensor tympani
25	Subarcuate fossa	50	Semicanal for auditory tube
26	Arcuate eminence	51	Groove for petrosquamous sinus

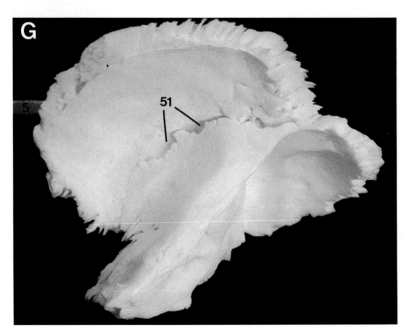

G

• The suprameatal triangle (A14) overlies the mastoid antrum (page 148, F50) which lies medially about 1.25 cm from the surface.
• The mastoid foramen (F22, above and behind the mastoid process, F16) transmits an emissary vein from the sigmoid sinus to the posterior auricular or occipital vein.
• The mastoid canaliculus (D48, in the lateral part of the jugular fossa, D47) transmits the auricular branch of the vagus nerve.
• The arcuate eminence (B26) in the petrous part overlies the anterior semicircular canal.
• In G the petrosquamous fissure (51) has remained open, so forming a groove for the petrosquamous sinus. The fissure is normally almost closed, as in B33. The sinus is present in fetal life but usually disappears in the adult; if it persists it may receive small veins from the tympanic cavity and form a venous communication between the inside and the outside of the skull.
• For further details of the temporal bone and ear see pages 148–151.

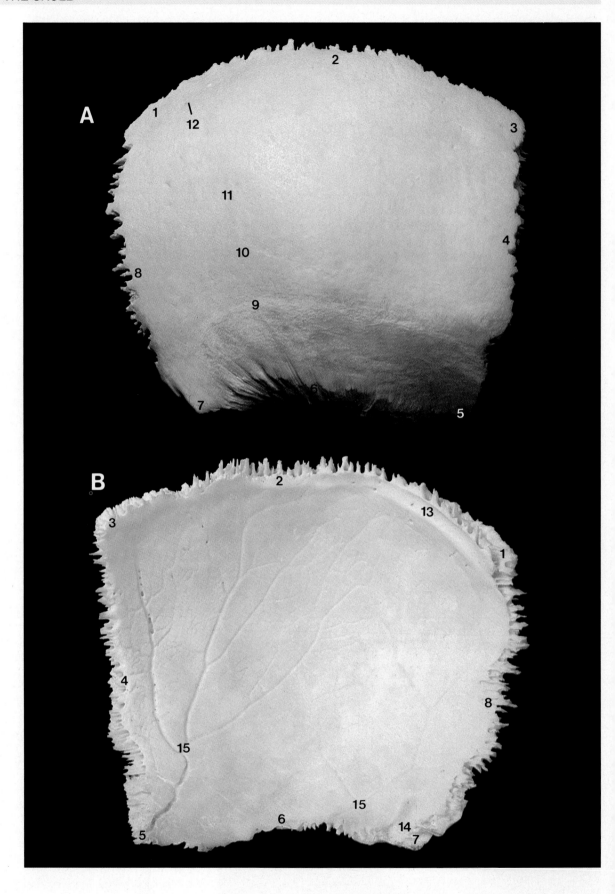

1 Occipital (posterosuperior) angle
2 Sagittal (superior) margin
3 Frontal (anterosuperior) angle
4 Frontal (anterior) margin
5 Sphenoidal (antero-inferior) angle
6 Squamous (inferior) margin
7 Mastoid (postero-inferior) angle
8 Occipital (posterior) margin
9 Inferior temporal line
10 Superior temporal line
11 Parietal tuberosity
12 Parietal foramen
13 Groove for part of superior sagittal sinus
14 Groove for sigmoid sinus at mastoid angle
15 Grooves for middle meningeal vessels
16 Frontal process
17 Temporal margin
18 Temporal process
19 Lateral surface
20 Maxillary margin
21 Zygomaticofacial foramen
22 Orbital margin
23 Orbital surface
24 Zygomaticofacial foramen
25 Temporal surface
26 Zygomaticotemporal foramen
27 Sphenoidal margin
28 Marginal tubercle

PARIETAL BONE, right
A External surface
B Internal surface
The parietal bone at the side and top of the skull

ZYGOMATIC BONE, left
C Lateral surface
D From the medial side
E From the front
F From behind
The zygomatic bone is at the front and side of the skull, forming the prominence of the cheek

• The main features of the ***parietal bone*** are:

the convex external surface (A)
the concave internal surface with grooves for the middle meningeal vessels (B15) passing upwards and backwards, and the groove for the sigmoid sinus (B14) at the mastoid (postero-inferior) angle

• To assist in orientation of the parietal bone, note that grooves for the middle meningeal vessels run upwards and backwards (B15), and that the groove for a small part of the sigmoid sinus is at the mastoid (postero-inferior) angle (B14).

• The main features of the ***zygomatic bone*** are:

the slightly convex lateral surface (C19)
the smoothly curved orbital margin (C22) and orbital surface (D23)
the frontal process (C and D, 16) passing upwards
the temporal process (C and D, 18) passing backwards

• Official nomenclature does not recognise the margins of the zygomatic bone (C17 and 22) but they are helpful terms for orientation.

• The marginal tubercle (Whitnall's tubercle, D28) lies just inside the orbital margin below the frontozygomatic suture (in the intact skull), and it can often be felt with the fingertip even if not readily visible. It receives the attachment of the lateral palpebral raphe (from orbicularis oculi) and the lateral palpebral ligament.

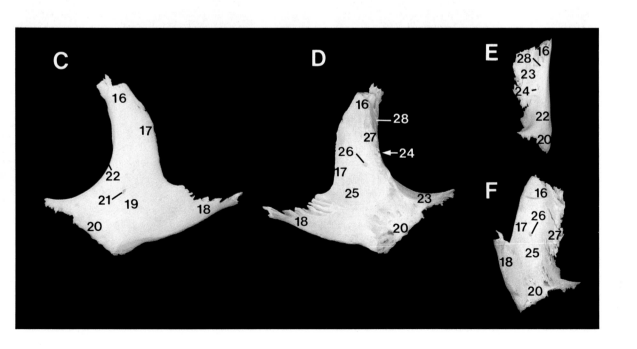

SKULL BONE ARTICULATIONS

Because of the irregular nature of the bone margins that take part in skull sutures, close and precise re-articulation of bones is not usually possible, but the illustrations on pages 54–73 indicate the way that individual skull bones become assembled together to form the complete skull.

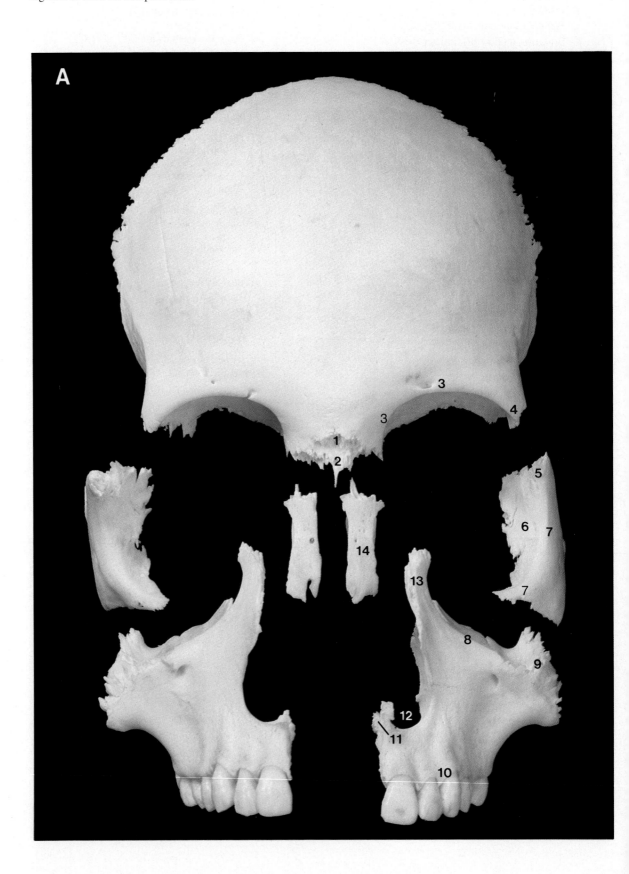

FACIAL SKELETON
Orbital and anterior nasal appertures
A and B The frontal, nasal and zygomatic bones and the maxillae,
from the front, separated and articulated

1 Nasal part	
2 Nasal spine	of frontal bone
3 Supra-orbital margin	
4 Zygomatic process	
5 Frontal process	
6 Orbital surface	of zygomatic bone
7 Orbital margin	
8 Infra-orbital margin	
9 Zygomatic process	
10 Alveolar process	of maxilla
11 Anterior nasal spine	
12 Nasal notch	
13 Frontal process	
14 Nasal bone	

• The orbital aperture (aditus of the orbit) is bounded above by the supra-orbital margin of the frontal bone (3), laterally by the zygomatic bone (7) and the zygomatic process of the frontal bone (4), below by the zygomatic bone (7) and the infra-orbital margin of the maxilla (8), and medially by the frontal bone (3) and the anterior lacrimal crest of the orbital process of the maxilla (13).

• The anterior nasal (piriform) aperture is bounded largely by the nasal notches of the maxillae (12), with the lower margins of the nasal bones above (14).

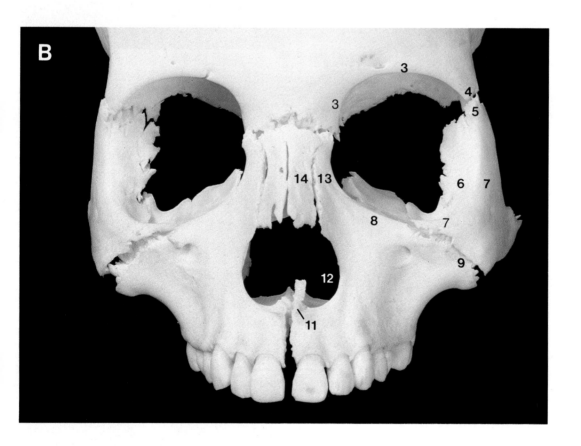

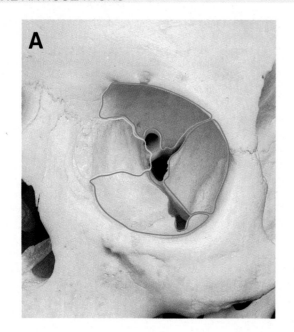

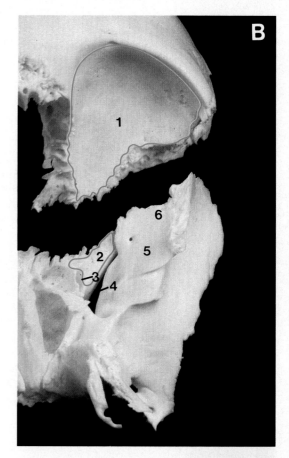

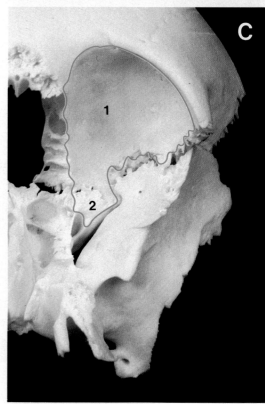

1 Orbital part of frontal bone		
2 Lesser wing		
3 Optic canal		
4 Superior orbital fissure		
5 Greater wing		
6 Frontal margin of greater wing		
7 Lesser wing		of sphenoid bone
8 Lateral wall of body		
9 Pterygoid process		
10 Foramen rotundum		
11 Superior orbital fissure		
12 Orbital surface of greater wing		
13 Zygomatic margin		
14 Orbital surface		
15 Frontal process		of zygomatic bone
16 Marginal tubercle		
17 Orbital margin		
18 Infra-orbital margin		of maxilla
19 Orbital surface		
20 Inferior orbital fissure		

ORBIT
Roof and lateral wall of the left orbit
A   The left orbit, from the front, left and above (as in page 32, A)
**B and C   Parts of the frontal and sphenoid bones, from below,
          separated and articulated, forming the roof of the orbit**
**D and E   Part of the sphenoid bone and the zygomatic bone, from
          the front (with the maxilla in E), separated and
          articulated, forming the lateral wall of the orbit**

Walls of the orbit:
Red—roof	**Green—floor**
Blue—lateral wall	**Yellow—medial wall**

• The roof of the orbit is formed mainly by the orbital part of the frontal bone (B and C, 1), with the lesser wing of the sphenoid bone (2) in the most posterior part. (The greater wing, B5, forms part of the lateral wall of the orbit.)

• The lateral wall of the orbit is formed by the orbital surfaces of the greater wing of the sphenoid (12) and the zygomatic bone (14). (The zygomatic bone also forms part of the floor of the orbit, with the maxilla—see next page.)

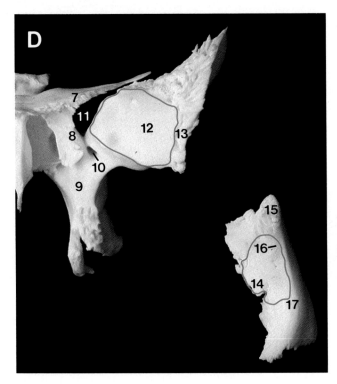

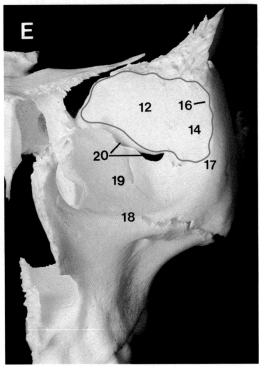

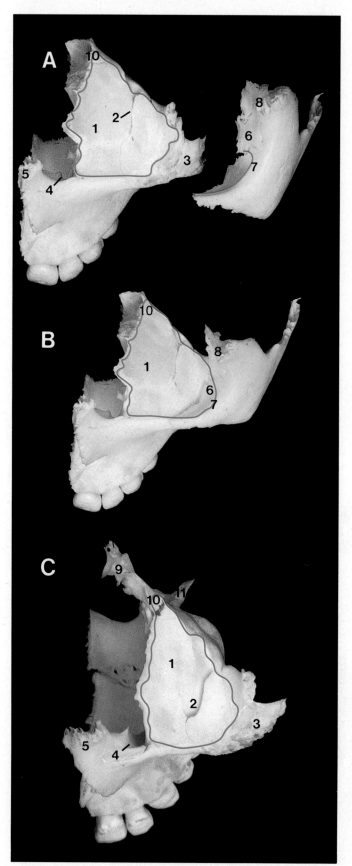

ORBIT
Floor and medial wall of the left orbit
A, B and C The left maxilla and the zygomatic and palatine bones, from above and in front, separated and articulated, forming the floor of the orbit

Wall of the orbit: **Green—floor**

In A and B the orbital process of the palatine bone (10) remains adherent to the maxilla; the whole palatine bone is shown in C. The sphenoid bone, part of whose body forms the most posterior part of the medial wall, is not shown here (see page 32, A22).

1 Orbital surface	
2 Infra-orbital groove	
3 Zygomatic process	of maxilla
4 Lacrimal groove	
5 Frontal process	
6 Orbital surface	
7 Orbital margin	of zygomatic bone
8 Frontal process	
9 Sphenoidal process	
10 Orbital process	of palatine bone
11 Pyramidal process	

D and E The left maxilla and the lacrimal bone and the ethmoid bone, from the left, separated and articulated, forming the medial wall of the orbit

Wall of the orbit: Yellow—medial wall

• The floor of the orbit is formed by the orbital surface of the maxilla (1) and zygomatic bone (6), with the orbital process of the palatine bone (10) in the most posterior part.

• The upper opening of the nasolacrimal canal (E21), formed by the maxilla and lacrimal bones, is at the front of the junction between the floor and lateral wall of the orbit (see also pages 62 and 63).

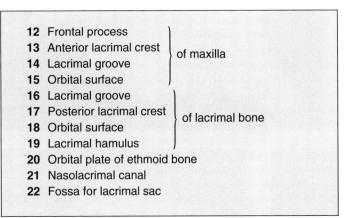

12	Frontal process	
13	Anterior lacrimal crest	of maxilla
14	Lacrimal groove	
15	Orbital surface	
16	Lacrimal groove	
17	Posterior lacrimal crest	of lacrimal bone
18	Orbital surface	
19	Lacrimal hamulus	
20	Orbital plate of ethmoid bone	
21	Nasolacrimal canal	
22	Fossa for lacrimal sac	

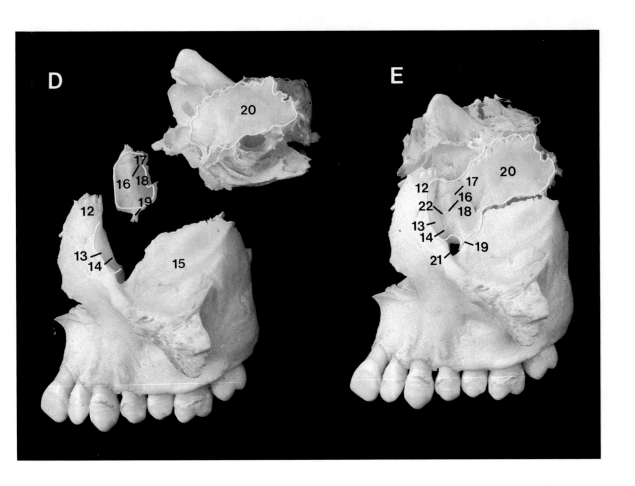

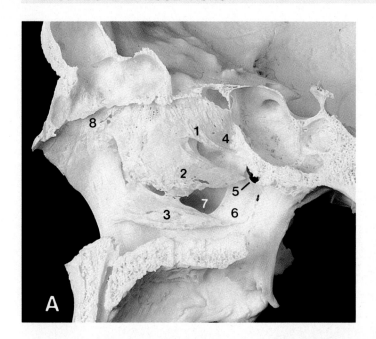

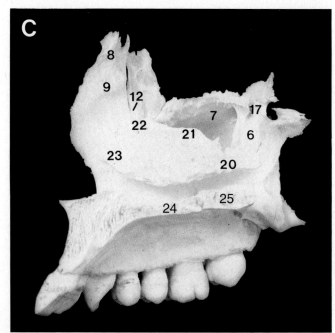

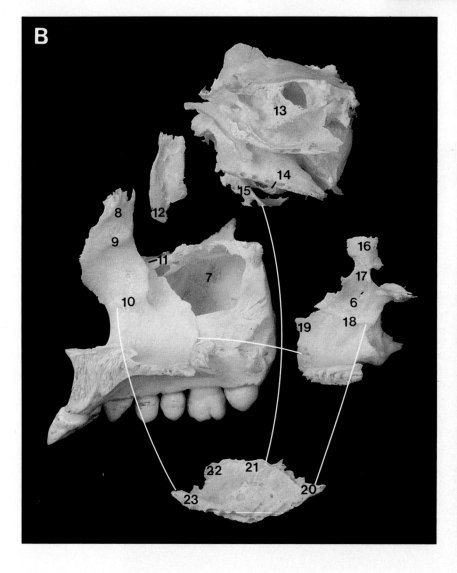

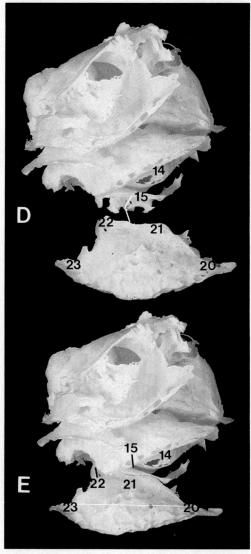

NASAL CAVITY
Right roof, floor and lateral wall

A The right half of the nasal cavity, in the intact skull (as in page 32, B)

B The right maxilla, the lacrimal, ethmoid and palatine bones and the inferior nasal concha, from the left

C The right maxilla with the lacrimal and palatine bones and the inferior nasal concha articulated

D and E The ethmoid bone and the right inferior nasal concha, separated and articulated

The white lines in B indicate which parts of the palatine bone and inferior nasal concha overlap and articulate with one another and with the maxilla, as shown in C. In E the uncinate process of the ethmoid bone (15) articulates with the ethmoidal process of the inferior concha (21).

1	Superior ⎫
2	Middle ⎬ nasal concha
3	Inferior ⎭
4	Spheno-ethmoidal recess
5	Sphenopalatine foramen
6	Perpendicular plate of palatine bone
7	Maxillary hiatus
8	Frontal process ⎫
9	Ethmoidal crest ⎬ of maxilla
10	Conchal crest
11	Lacrimal groove ⎭
12	Descending process of lacrimal bone
13	Left ethmoidal labyrinth ⎫
14	Right ethmoidal bulla ⎬ of ethmoid bone
15	Right uncinate process ⎭
16	Orbital process ⎫
17	Ethmoidal crest ⎬ of palatine bone
18	Conchal crest
19	Maxillary process ⎭
20	Posterior end ⎫
21	Ethmoidal process ⎬ of inferior concha
22	Lacrimal process
23	Anterior end ⎭
24	Palatine process of maxilla
25	Horizontal plate of palatine bone

• When articulated, the four bones arranged around the maxilla in B (lacrimal, ethmoid and palatine bones and the inferior nasal concha) reduce the size of the maxillary hiatus (B7) to the size shown in A7 or smaller. In life the size is further reduced by mucous membrane (as in page 128, C21).

• In B and D the ethmoid bone has been tilted upwards to show the right ethmoidal bulla (14) and uncinate process (15). These bony features are not seen in A because they are under cover of the middle nasal concha (2); they are shown on page 32, D61 and 46, respectively, after removal of the concha.

• The roof of each half of the nasal cavity is formed centrally by the cribriform plate of the ethmoid bone (page 30, 28), with anteriorly the nasal bone and the nasal spine of the frontal bone (page 54, A2 and 14), and posteriorly the body of the sphenoid bone overlapped by the ala of the vomer and the sphenoidal process of the palatine bone (page 72, B2 and 11).

• The floor is formed by the palatine process of the maxilla and the horizontal plate of the palatine bone (C24 and 25).

• The medial wall is the nasal septum, whose bony part consists of the perpendicular plate of the ethmoid bone and the vomer (page 30, 27 and 26), with the nasal crests of the maxilla (page 46, D21) and palatine bone (page 48, C13) at the very base, and (in front) the septal cartilage (page 126, A22).

• The lateral wall consists of the medial surface of the maxilla with the large maxillary hiatus (B7) being reduced in size by the overlapping of the lacrimal and ethmoid bones (above), the palatine bone (behind) and the inferior nasal concha (below) (as indicated in B, C and D—see also pages 62 and 63).

• In A the left frontal sinus (unlabelled) is large and extends backwards at its lower end into the crista galli.

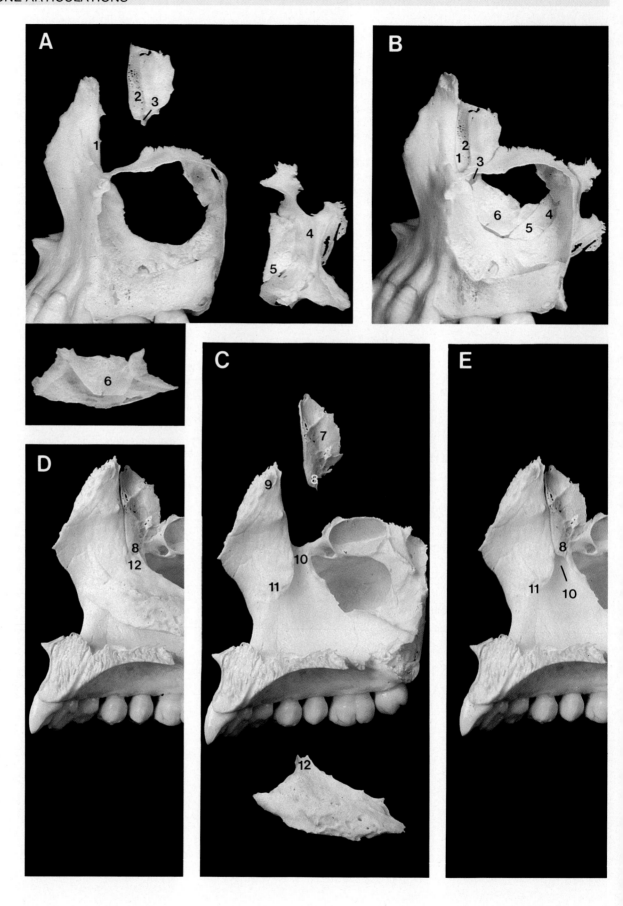

NASAL CAVITY
Maxillary hiatus and nasolacrimal canal

A and B The left maxilla, lacrimal and palatine bones, and the inferior nasal concha, separated and articulated

C The right maxilla, lacrimal bone and inferior nasal concha, separated

D The right maxilla, lacrimal bone and inferior concha articulated

E The right maxilla and lacrimal bone articulated

In A much of the lateral wall and orbital surface of the maxilla have been removed, so that the hiatus can be viewed from the lateral side. In B the hiatus seen in A is shown to be partly filled in by the descending process of the lacrimal bone at the upper anterior corner (3), the maxillary process of the inferior nasal concha below (6), and the maxillary process and perpendicular plate of the palatine bone behind (5 and 4). (The ethmoid bone which covers much of the upper part of the hiatus is not shown.)

In C–E the conversion of the nasolacrimal groove of the maxilla (10) into the nasolacrimal canal is illustrated by its articulation with the lacrimal bone and inferior nasal concha (8 and 12).

---

1 Lacrimal groove of maxilla
2 Lacrimal groove ⎫
3 Descending process ⎬ of lacrimal bone
4 Perpendicular plate ⎫
5 Maxillary process ⎬ of palatine bone
6 Maxillary process of inferior nasal concha
7 Nasal surface ⎫
8 Descending process ⎬ of lacrimal bone
9 Frontal process ⎫
10 Lacrimal groove ⎬ of maxilla
11 Conchal crest ⎭
12 Lacrimal process of inferior nasal concha

• Note that A and B show bones of the left side, with a large hole cut in the lateral wall of the maxilla, so that when articulated in B the lateral sides of the lacrimal and palatine bones and the inferior nasal concha can be seen partly filling the maxillary hiatus (the gap in the medial wall of the maxilla). In C–E the bones are those of the right side, showing their medial surfaces.

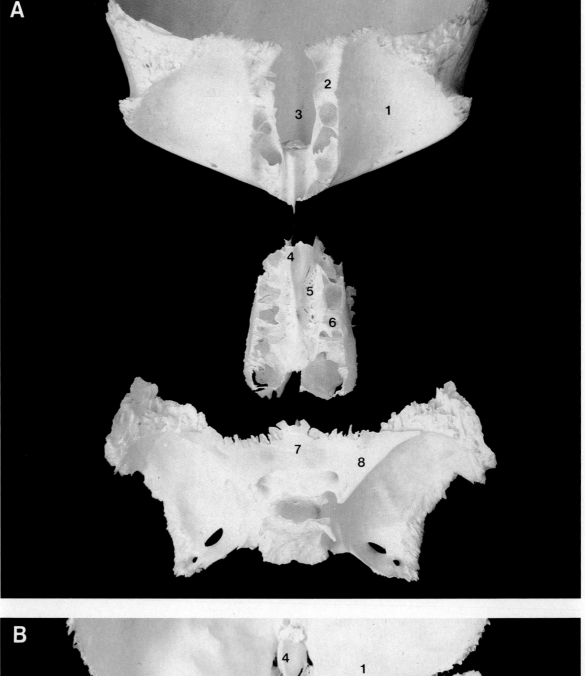

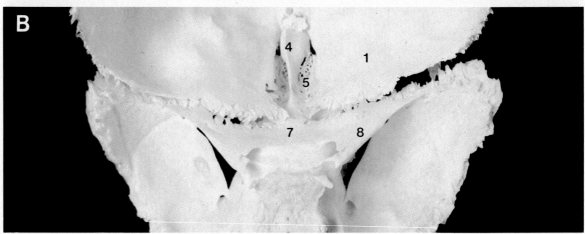

BASE OF THE SKULL
Anterior cranial fossa
A The frontal, ethmoid and sphenoid bones, from above and
behind, with the frontal bone tilted forwards
B The bones articulated
In A the frontal bone has been tilted forwards to show the orbital
(lower) surface of the orbital part (1), whose medial edge (2) forms the
roof of the ethmoidal labyrinth (6). With the bones articulated in B, the
cerebral (upper) surface of the orbital part is seen.

```
1  Orbital part of frontal bone
2  Roof of ethmoidal air cells
3  Ethmoidal notch
4  Crista galli
5  Cribriform plate of ethmoid bone
6  Ethmoidal labyrinth and air cells
7  Jugum of sphenoid bone
8  Lesser wing of sphenoid bone
```

• The anterior cranial fossa is formed by the orbital parts of the frontal
bone (1), the crista galli and cribriform plates of the ethmoid bone (4
and 5), and the jugum and lesser wings of the sphenoid bone (7 and 8).

• For the contents of the anterior cranial fossa see page 169.

• The medial part of the orbital part of the frontal bone (2) forms the
roof of the ethmoidal air cells (6), while the anterior wall of the body of
the sphenoid completes the posterior wall of the ethmoidal labyrinth.

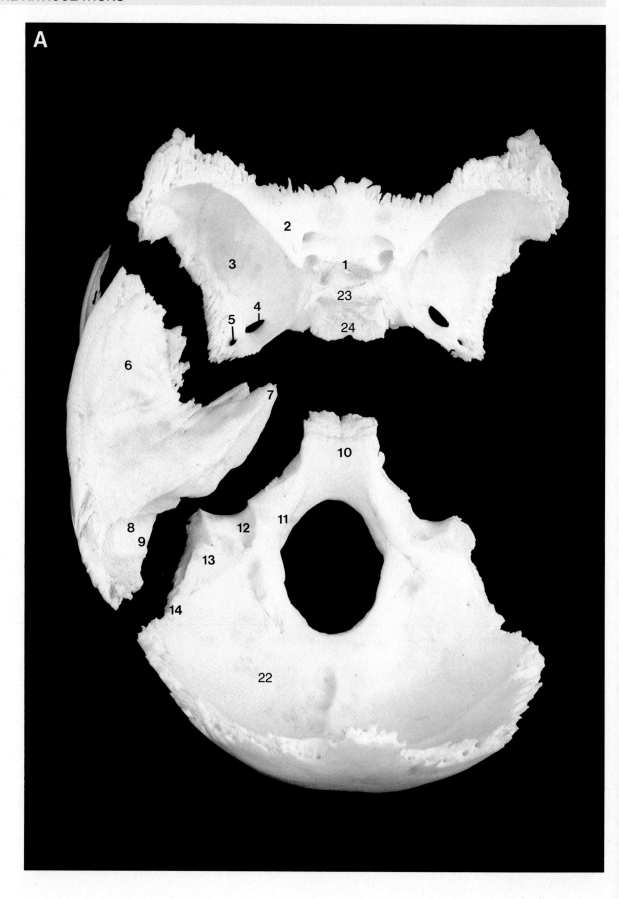

1 Body	
2 Lesser wing	
3 Greater wing	of sphenoid bone
4 Foramen ovale	
5 Foramen spinosum	
6 Squamous part of temporal bone	
7 Apex	
8 Groove for sigmoid sinus	of petrous part of temporal bone
9 Occipital margin	
10 Basilar part	
11 Lateral part	
12 Jugular notch	of occipital bone
13 Groove for sigmoid sinus	
14 Mastoid margin	
15 Foramen lacerum	
16 Sphenopetrosal synchondrosis	
17 Spheno-occipital synchondrosis	
18 Petro-occipital suture and groove for inferior petrosal sinus	
19 Jugular foramen	
20 Occipitomastoid suture	
21 Sphenosquamosal suture	
22 Squamous part of occipital bone	
23 Dorsum sellae	
24 Basisphenoid	

BASE OF THE SKULL
Middle and posterior cranial fossae
A and B The sphenoid, left temporal and occipital bones, from above, separated and articulated

The posterior angle of the greater wing of the sphenoid, containing the foramen spinosum (5), fits into the angle between the squamous and petrous parts of the temporal bone (6 and 7).

• The middle cranial fossa consists of a central part, formed by the body of the sphenoid bone (1), and right and left lateral parts, each formed by the greater wing of the sphenoid (3) and the squamous and petrous parts of the temporal bone (6 and 7).

• The posterior cranial fossa is formed by the basilar, lateral and squamous parts of the occipital bone (10, 11 and 22), the petrous parts of the temporal bones (7-9), a small part of the postero-inferior (mastoid) angles of the parietal bones (not shown here but see page 28, A34 and page 52, B14), and the dorsum sellae (23) and posterior part of the body of the sphenoid bone.

• The gap between the front of the apex of the petrous part of the temporal bone (7) and the sphenoid bone is the foramen lacerum (B15). A very small portion of the basilar part of the occipital bone (10) is at the medial margin of the foramen.

• The gap between the jugular notch of the occipital bone (A12) and the petrous part of the temporal bone forms the jugular foramen (B19).

• The junction between the basilar part of the occipital bone (10, often called the basi-occiput) and the posterior part of the body of the sphenoid bone (24, often called the basisphenoid) is a synchondrosis, which becomes a complete bony union by the age of 25 years.

• For the contents of the middle and posterior cranial fossae see page 169.

• For the contents of the middle and posterior cranial fossae see page 169.

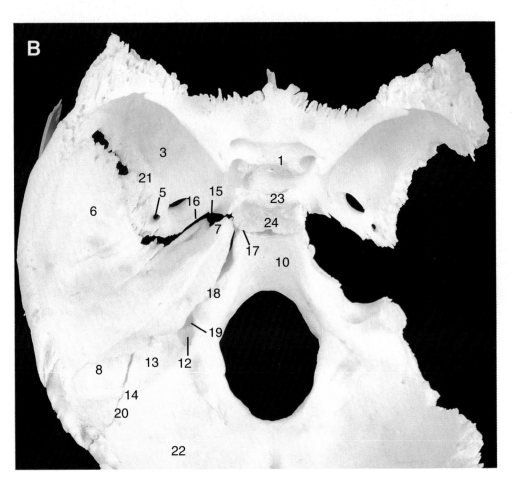

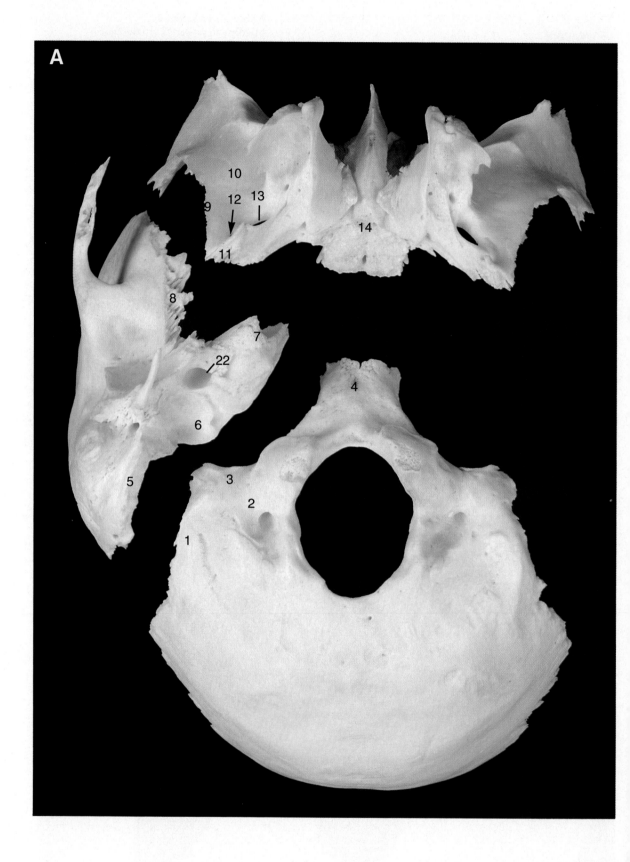

1 Mastoid margin ⎫
2 Lateral part   ⎬ of occipital bone
3 Jugular notch   ⎪
4 Basilar part ⎭
5 Occipital margin ⎫
6 Jugular notch   ⎬ of petrous part of temporal bone
7 Apex ⎭
8 Sphenoidal margin of squamous part of temporal bone
9 Squamous margin ⎫
10 Greater wing   ⎪
11 Spine   ⎬ of sphenoid bone
12 Foramen spinosum ⎪
13 Foramen ovale   ⎪
14 Body ⎭
15 Occipitomastoid suture
16 Jugular foramen
17 Petro-occipital suture
18 Foramen lacerum
19 Spheno-occipital synchondrosis
20 Sphenopetrosal synchondrosis and groove for auditory tube
21 Sphenosquamosal suture
22 Carotid canal

BASE OF THE SKULL
External surface, posterior part
A and B The sphenoid, right temporal and occipital bones, from below, separated and articulated
(Compare with the upper surfaces of these bones in pages 66, A and 67, B and the whole base in pages 24 and 28, A)

• The foramen lacerum (B18) is the gap between the front of the apex of the petrous part of the temporal bone (A and B, 7) and the sphenoid bone; at its medial margin is a small portion of the basilar part of the occipital bone (A and B, 4).
• The jugular foramen (B16) is the gap between the jugular notch of the petrous part of the temporal bone (A6) and the jugular notch of the occipital bone (A3).
• The carotid canal (B22) is within the petrous part of the temporal bone. From its lower opening (as seen here) it turns medially and forwards in the bone to an upper opening in the back part of the foramen lacerum; this upper opening can only be seen when looking very obliquely into the foramen from the front, or when looking 'end-on' at the apex of the petrous temporal (page 50, E44).

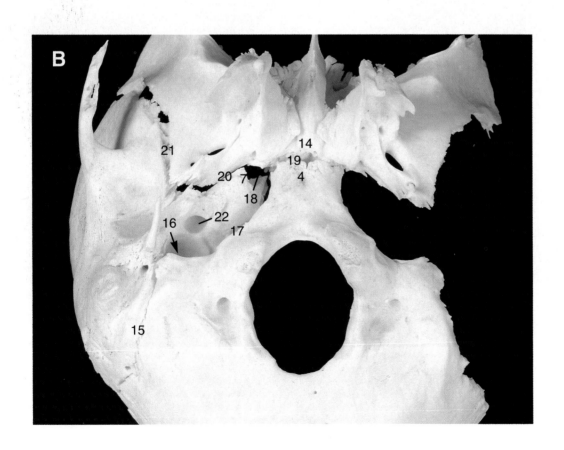

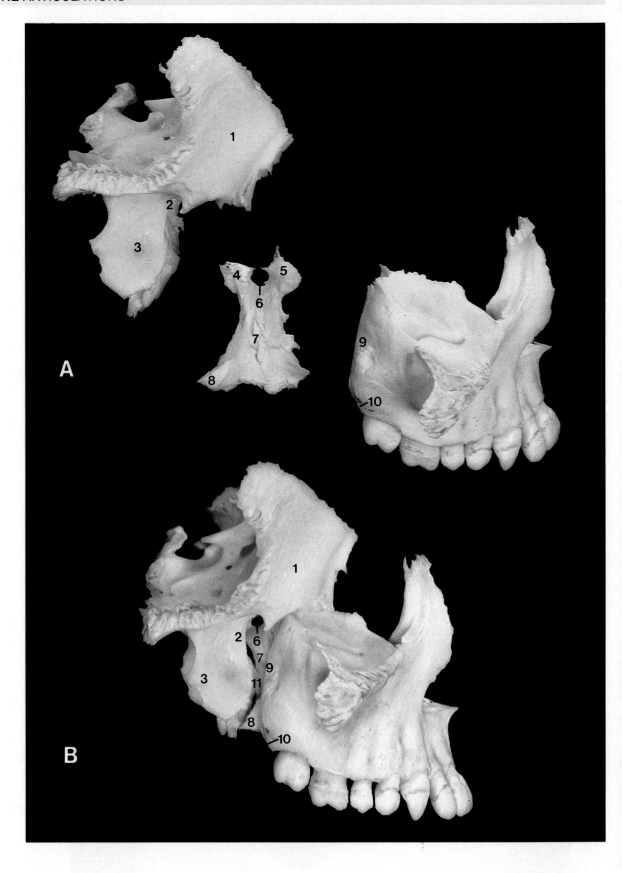

A

B

BASE OF THE SKULL
Right pterygopalatine fossa
A and B The right maxilla and palatine bone and the sphenoid
**   bone, from the right, separated and articulated**
(Compare with page 26, A)

1	Temporal surface of greater wing	}
2	Pterygoid process	} of sphenoid bone
3	Lateral pterygoid plate	}
4	Sphenoidal process	}
5	Orbital process	}
6	Sphenopalatine notch	} of palatine bone
7	Perpendicular plate	}
8	Pyramidal process	}
9	Infratemporal surface	} of maxilla
10	Tuberosity	}
11	Pterygomaxillary fissure	

• The pterygopalatine fossa is the space behind the maxilla and in front of the pterygoid process of the sphenoid bone (see the first note on page 27).

• The anterior wall of the fossa is formed by the infratemporal (posterior) surface of the maxilla (9).

• The posterior wall of the fossa is formed by the pterygoid process of the sphenoid bone (2).

• The medial wall of the fossa is formed by the perpendicular plate of the palatine bone (7). The sphenopalatine notch at the upper end of the plate (6) is converted into the sphenopalatine foramen (as in B6) by the overlying body of the sphenoid bone (hidden in this side view by the greater wing, 1).

• Laterally, the pterygomaxillary fissure (B11) forms the communication between the pterygopalatine fossa and the infratemporal fossa (see also page 26, A4).

• The pyramidal process of the palatine bone (8) articulates with the tuberosity of the maxilla (10) and fills in the triangular gap between the lower ends of the medial and lateral pterygoid plates (page 23, B10).

• For the contents of the pterygopalatine fossa see page 117.

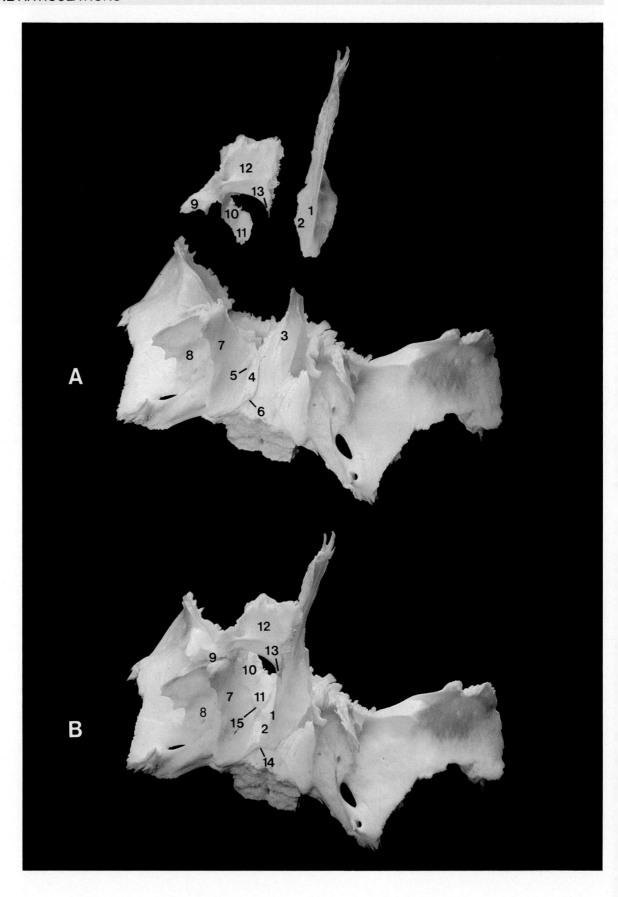

BASE OF THE SKULL
A and B Right posterior nasal aperture
The sphenoid and right palatine bones and the vomer, from the left,
below and behind, separated and articulated
The vomer (1) forms the posterior part of the (midline) nasal septum,
and parts of the palatine and sphenoid bones form the remaining
boundaries of the posterior nasal apertures.

• The posterior nasal aperture is commonly called the choana.

• The posterior border of the vomer (1) separates the two choanae,
forming their medial boundaries.

• The other boundaries are:
   laterally—the medial pterygoid plate of the sphenoid bone (7);
   below—the posterior border of the horizontal plate of the palatine
      bone (12);
   above—the body and vaginal process of the sphenoid bone (4) and
      the ala of the vomer (2).

• A groove on the lower surface of the vaginal process of the sphenoid
bone (A5) is converted into the palatovaginal canal (B15) by
articulation with the upper surface of the sphenoidal process of the
palatine bone (B11).

• The vomerovaginal canal (B14) lies between the upper surface of the
vaginal process of the sphenoid bone (A6) and the ala of the vomer (2).
Anteriorly, the vomerovaginal canal joins the palatovaginal canal
(B15).

• The pyramidal process of the palatine bone (9) fills in the gap between
the lower ends of the medial and lateral pterygoid plates (7 and 8; page
23, B10).

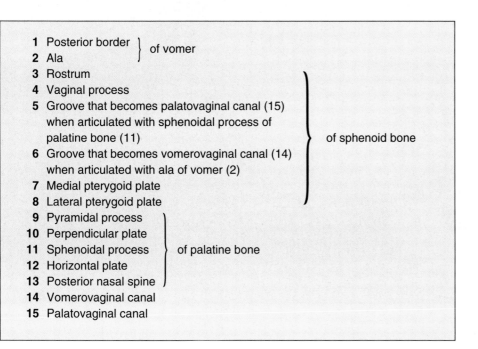

1 Posterior border ⎫ of vomer
2 Ala   ⎭
3 Rostrum
4 Vaginal process
5 Groove that becomes palatovaginal canal (15)
   when articulated with sphenoidal process of
   palatine bone (11)   ⎫ of sphenoid bone
6 Groove that becomes vomerovaginal canal (14)   ⎬
   when articulated with ala of vomer (2)   ⎭
7 Medial pterygoid plate
8 Lateral pterygoid plate
9 Pyramidal process   ⎫
10 Perpendicular plate   ⎪
11 Sphenoidal process   ⎬ of palatine bone
12 Horizontal plate   ⎪
13 Posterior nasal spine ⎭
14 Vomerovaginal canal
15 Palatovaginal canal

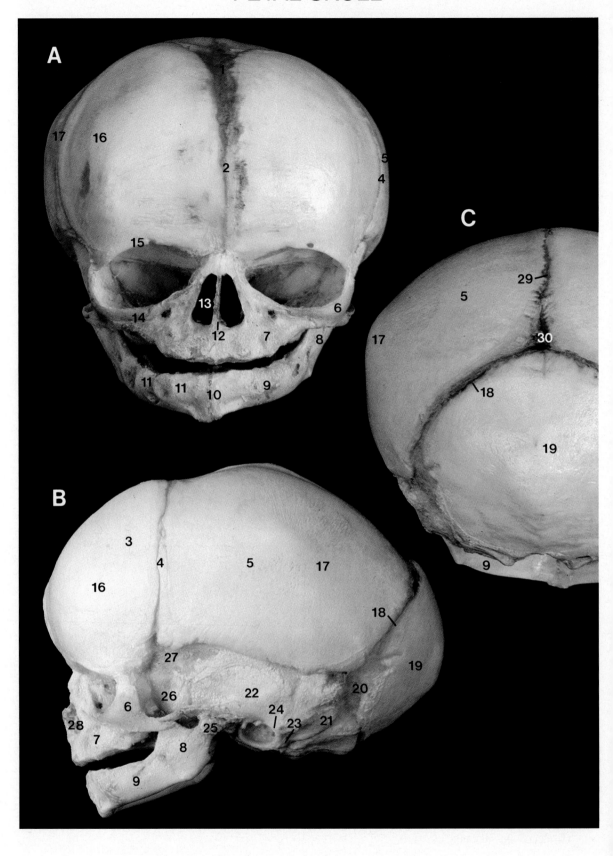

FETAL SKULL
Skull of a full-term fetus
A From the front
B From the left
C From behind (left side)
D From above

Apart from size differences (see notes below) and the lack of erupted teeth, the striking features of the fetal skull compared with the adult are the large sutures (2, 4, 18 and 29) and the fontanelles, the unossified spaces at the four angles of the parietal bone (1, 20, 27 and 30)

• The small sizes of the nasal cavity and maxillary sinuses and the lack of erupted teeth all contribute to the face at birth, forming a relatively smaller proportion of the skull than in the adult. (Compare A with the adult skull on page 10.)

• The posterior and sphenoidal fontanelles (30 and 27) close (become bony) within 3 months of birth, the mastoid fontanelle (20) at 1 year and the anterior fontanelle (1) at about 18 months.

• The mastoid process does not develop until the second year, so that before then the stylomastoid foramen (23) and the emerging facial nerve are relatively near the surface and unprotected. (Compare with the adult skull (page 22, A22 and 23)

1	Anterior fontanelle
2	Frontal (metopic) suture
3	Half (squamous part) of frontal bone
4	Coronal suture
5	Parietal bone
6	Zygomatic bone
7	Maxilla
8	Ramus ⎱ of mandible
9	Body ⎰
10	Symphysis menti
11	Elevations over deciduous teeth
12	Nasal septum
13	Anterior nasal aperture
14	Infra-orbital margin
15	Supra-orbital margin
16	Frontal tuberosity
17	Parietal tuberosity
18	Lambdoid suture
19	Occipital bone
20	Mastoid (posterolateral) fontanelle
21	Petrous part ⎱ of temporal bone
22	Squamous part ⎰
23	Stylomastoid foramen
24	Tympanic ring
25	Condylar process of mandible
26	Greater wing of sphenoid bone
27	Sphenoidal (anterolateral) fontanelle
28	Septal cartilage
29	Sagittal suture
30	Posterior fontanelle

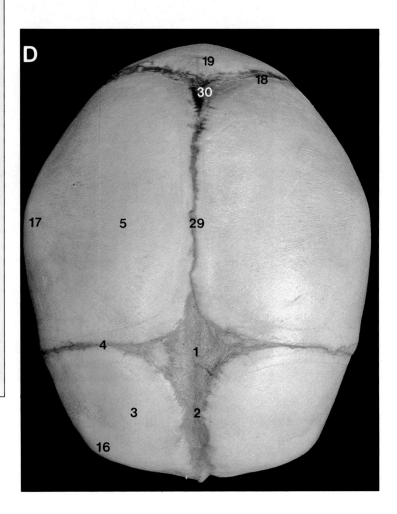

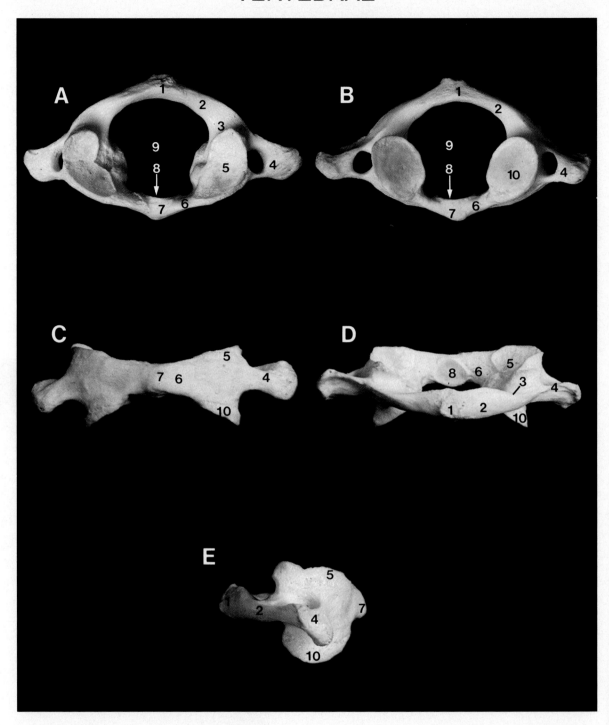

ATLAS (first cervical vertebra)
A From above
B From below
C From the front
D From behind
E From the right
The atlas is unique in having no body; it consists of a lateral mass on each side with upper and lower articular facets (A5; B10), and anterior and posterior arches (A and B, 6 and 2).

---

1 Posterior tubercle
2 Posterior arch
3 Groove for vertebral artery
4 Transverse process and foramen
5 Lateral mass with superior articular facet
6 Anterior arch
7 Anterior tubercle
8 Facet for dens of axis
9 Vertebral foramen
10 Lateral mass with inferior articular facet

• All seven cervical vertebrae have a foramen in their transverse processes (as at A4). This feature alone distinguishes them from the vertebrae of all other parts of the vertebral column. Formerly called the foramen transversarium, it is now properly known as the vertebrarterial foramen.

• The typical cervical vertebrae are the third to the sixth; as an example, the fifth is illustrated on page 80.

• The first cervical vertebra (the atlas, this page), the second (the axis, page 78), and the seventh (page 80), have characteristic features.

• The atlas is the only vertebra that has no body—it has been considered in the past to be represented by the dens of the axis (page 78, A1 and 3; page 79, F16), but see the note on page 79.

• The atlas has no spinous process; instead there is a small posterior tubercle (A1).

• The shapes of the articular facets on the lateral masses of the atlas enable the upper and lower surfaces to be identified:

the superior articular facets are concave and kidney-shaped (A5), for articulation with the occipital condyles of the skull (page 22, A33), forming the atlanto-occipital joints (page 200, B43);
the inferior facets are round and almost flat (B10), for articulation with the superior articular processes of the axis (page 78, C4), forming the lateral atlanto-axial joints (page 200, B41).

• The anterior arch of the atlas (6) is straighter and shorter than the posterior arch (2), thus distinguishing the front and back of the bone. The anterior arch bears on its posterior surface the articular facet for the dens of the axis (A, B and D, 8), forming the median atlanto-axial joint (page 79, F17).

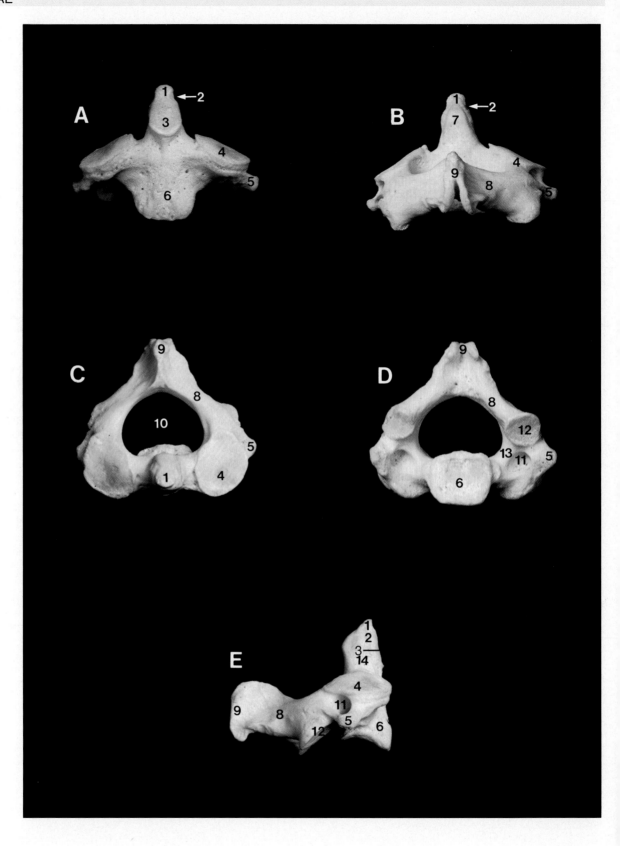

AXIS (second cervical vertebra)
A From the front
B From behind
C From above
D From below
E From the right
F Articulated with the atlas, from above and behind
The axis is unique in having the dens (odontoid process, A and E, 1–3), which projects upwards from the body (6).

• The dens has long been considered to represent the 'missing body' of the atlas, fused to the body of the axis, but studies in comparative anatomy suggest that it is a development in its own right.

• The anterior articular surface of the dens (A and E, 3) forms a synovial joint (the median atlanto-axial joint, F17) with the facet on the posterior surface of the anterior arch of the atlas (page 76, D8).

• The posterior articular surface of the dens (B7) forms a synovial joint (sometimes continuous with the joint cavity of one of the lateral atlanto-occipital joints) with the cartilage-covered anterior surface of the transverse ligament of the atlas.

• The spinous process of the axis is large and often almost rectangular when viewed from the side (E9).

• The surfaces of the superior articular processes are round and almost flat (C4), for articulation with the inferior articular facets of the atlas (page 76, B10), forming the lateral atlanto-axial joints.

1	Apex of dens
2	Impression for alar ligament
3	Anterior articular surface of dens
4	Superior articular process
5	Transverse process
6	Body
7	Posterior articular surface of dens
8	Lamina
9	Bifid spinous process
10	Vertebral foramen
11	Foramen of transverse process
12	Inferior articular process
13	Pedicle
14	Dens
15	Anterior arch
16	Dens of axis
17	Median atlanto-axial joint

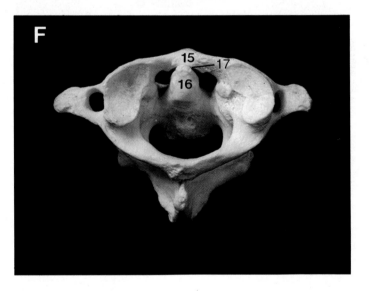

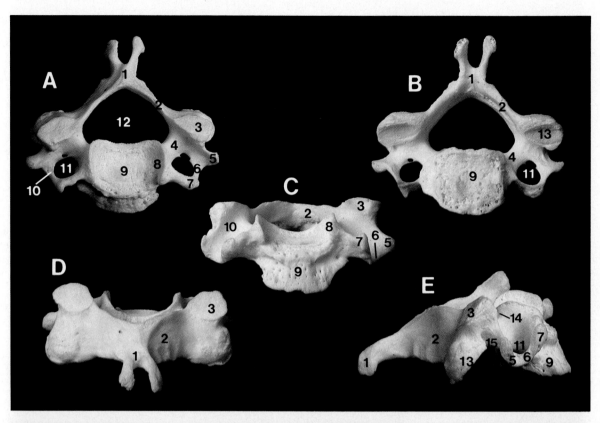

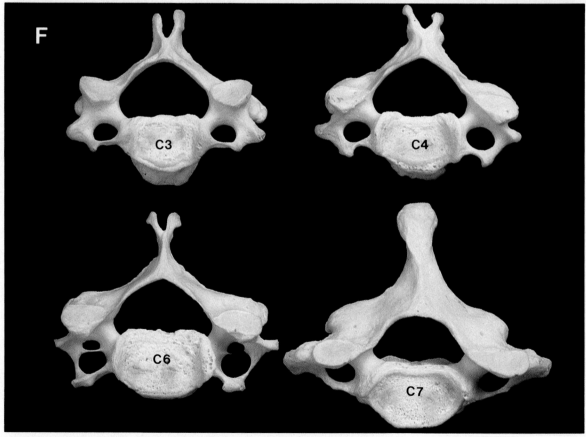

THIRD TO SEVENTH CERVICAL VERTEBRAE

A Fifth cervical vertebra, from above
B From below
C From the front
D From behind
E From the right
F Third, fourth, sixth and seventh vertebrae, from above and
**   numbered C3, C4, C6 and C7, respectively**

The typical cervical vertebrae (third to sixth, exemplified here by the fifth, A–E) have superior articular processes (A and D, 3) that face upwards and backwards, an uncus (posterolateral lip, A and C, 8) at each side of the upper surface of the body, a triangular vertebral foramen (A12), and a bifid spinous process (A, B and D, 1).

```
 1  Bifid spinous process
 2  Lamina
 3  Superior articular process
 4  Pedicle
 5  Posterior tubercle       ⎫
 6  Intertubercular lamella  ⎬ of transverse process
 7  Anterior tubercle        ⎭
 8  Uncus (posterolateral lip) of body
 9  Body
10  Groove for spinal nerve (ventral ramus)
11  Foramen of transverse process
12  Vertebral foramen
13  Inferior articular process
14  Superior ⎫ vertebral notch
15  Inferior ⎭
```

• The spinous process of any vertebra is commonly called the spine.

• The vertebral arch is formed by the two pedicles (A4) and the two laminae (A2).

• The vertebral *foramen* is the space between the arch and body. When vertebrae are articulated to form the vertebral column, the serial vertebral foramina constitute the vertebral *canal*. Do not confuse the vertebral foramen with the *intervertebral* foramen, which is the space between the pedicles of adjacent vertebrae through which the spinal nerves emerge—see the note on page 83 and page 83, D13.

• The seventh cervical vertebra (vertebra prominens, F, C7) has a spinous process that ends in a single tubercle (instead of being bifid).
• The costal (rib) element of a cervical vertebra is represented by the anterior root of the transverse process with the anterior tubercle (A7), the intertubercular lamella (A6) and the anterior part of the posterior tubercle (A5).

• The intertubercular lamella (A and E, 6) is often but erroneously called the costotransverse bar.

• The sixth cervical vertebra shown here (F, C6) has a small bony septum in the foramen of the right transverse process.

81

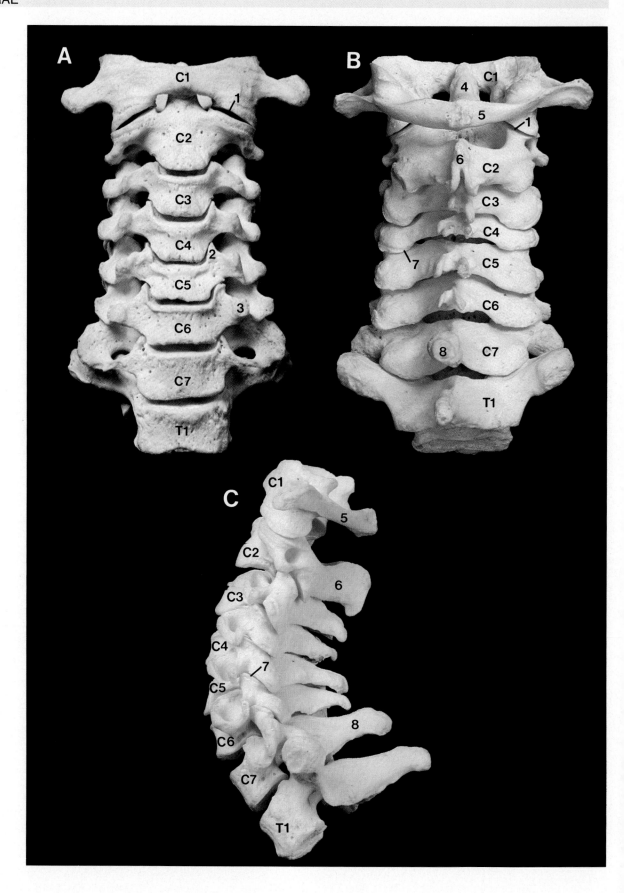

CERVICAL AND FIRST THORACIC VERTEBRAE
Articulated cervical vertebrae and first thoracic vertebra
A Articulated (but without intervertebral discs) and numbered C1-C7 and T1, from the front
B From behind
C From the left
D C4 and C5 vertebrae, from the left and slightly from the front
E First thoracic vertebra, from above
F From the left

1 Lateral atlanto-axial joint
2 Uncus of fifth cervical vertebra
3 Carotid tubercle of sixth cervical vertebra
4 Dens of axis
5 Posterior arch of atlas
6 Spinous process of axis
7 Zygapophysial joint
8 Spinous process of seventh cervical vertebra
9 Body
10 Uncus
11 Pedicle
12 Zygapophysial joint between adjacent inferior and superior articular facets
13 Intervertebral foramen
14 Posterior tubercle ⎫
15 Intertubercular lamella ⎬ of transverse process
16 Anterior tubercle ⎭
17 Spinous process
18 Lamina
19 Superior articular process
20 Transverse process
21 Pedicle
22 Uncus of body
23 Body
24 Vertebral foramen
25 Superior vertebral notch
26 Costal facet of transverse process
27 Inferior articular process
28 Inferior vertebral notch
29 Inferior ⎫ costal facet of body
30 Superior ⎭

The cervical part of the vertebral column with the first thoracic vertebra is illustrated in A-C. The side view in D is shown to emphasize the boundaries of an intervertebral foramen, while E and F give details of the first thoracic vertebra.

• The cervical curvature of the vertebral column has an anterior convexity, as in C (like the lumbar curvature; the thoracic and sacral curvatures are concave anteriorly).

• The spinous process of the seventh cervical vertebra is not bifid like that of typical cervical vertebrae but ends in a rounded tubercle (B and C, 8). Because of the extent of its backward projection it is usually the highest palpable spine in the median furrow at the back of the neck (hence the name vertebra prominens often given to this vertebra).

• The intervertebral foramen (D13) is bounded above and below by the pedicles of adjacent vertebrae (D11), in front by the intervertebral disc and parts of the adjacent vertebral bodies (D9), and behind by the zygapophysial joint (D12).

• Typical thoracic vertebrae (the second to ninth, not illustrated) are characterised by upper and lower articular facets (demifacets) on the sides of the bodies (for joints with the heads of the ribs), an articular facet on the front of each transverse process (for joints with the tubercles of the ribs), a round vertebral foramen, a spinous process that points downwards and backwards, and superior articular processes that are vertical, flat, and face backwards and laterally.

• The first thoracic vertebra differs from a typical thoracic vertebra in having an uncus on each side of the upper surface of the body (E22) and a triangular vertebral foramen (features like typical cervical vertebrae, although the foramen in E24 is rather oval), and a complete (round) superior costal facet (F30) on each side of the body (instead of just a demifacet, half-round).

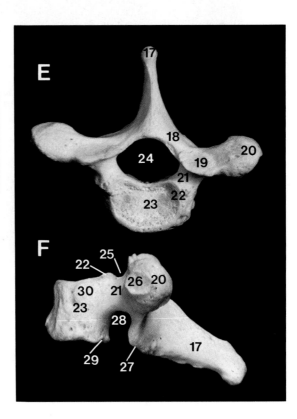

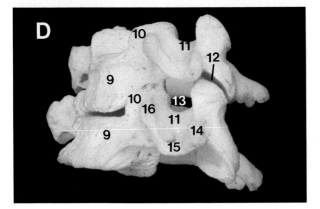

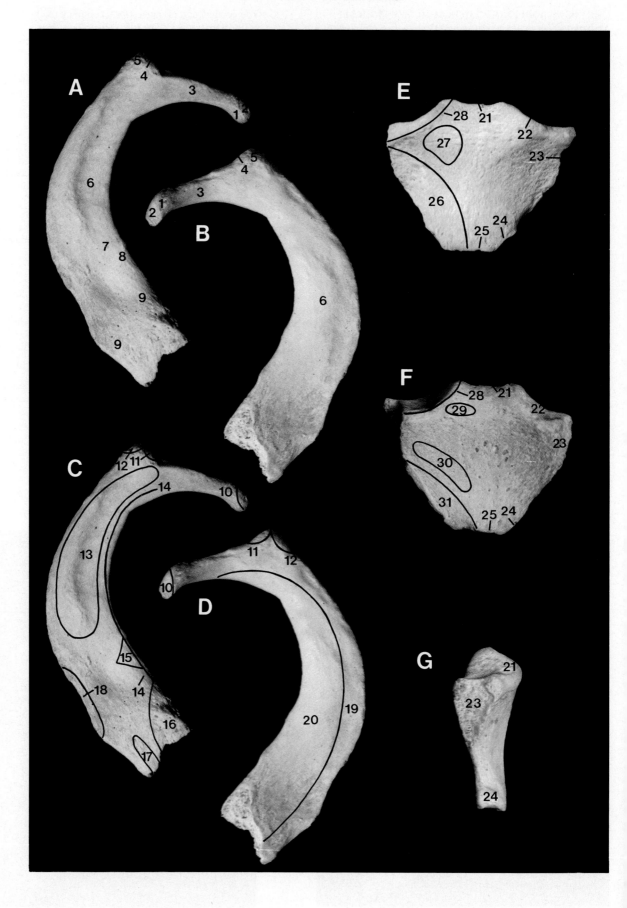

FIRST RIB, right
A From above
B From below
C From above. Attachments
D From below. Attachments
The 12 pairs of ribs form much of the bony framework of the thorax; only the first rib is shown here, since it is part of the thoracic inlet, at the junction of the neck and thorax (page 89).

MANUBRIUM OF THE STERNUM
E From the front, with attachments
F From behind, with attachments
G From the right
The manubrium of the sternum is its upper part, joined to the body of the sternum at the manubriosternal joint (E25), and forming the front part of the thoracic inlet (page 89)

COSTOVERTEBRAL JOINTS
H Left first rib and first thoracic vertebra, articulated, from above
The head of the rib (34) articulates with the upper costal facet on the body of the vertebra (35), forming the joint of the head of the rib. The tubercle of the rib (33) articulates with the costal facet of the transverse process of the vertebra (32), forming the costotransverse joint. These joints collectively form the costovertebral joints .

• The main features of the *first rib* are:

the head (A, 1 and 2)
the neck (A3)
the shaft or body (A6), with the scalene tubercle (A8) on the upper surface
the tubercle (A, 4 and 5), at the back of the junction of the neck and body

• The head of the first rib makes a synovial joint with the upper costal facet on the side of the body of T1 vertebra (H, 34 and 35).

• The tubercle has articular and nonarticular parts. The articular part (A4) makes a synovial joint with the costal facet of the transverse process of T1 vertebra (H, 32 and 33).

• The upper surface of the first rib is characterised by the scalene tubercle (A8), to which scalenus anterior is attached, with a slight groove behind it for the subclavian artery (A7) and a slight groove in front of it for the subclavian vein (A9). There is also a rough area for the attachment of scalenus medius.

• The lower surface of the first rib is relatively smooth (B6) compared with the upper surface, and is largely covered by the pleura (D20).

• The jugular notch at the top of the *manubrium of the sternum* (E21) is a readily visible and palpable landmark in the centre of the lowest part of the neck, and on either side the sternal end of the clavicle at the sternoclavicular joint (page 86, A11) is also easily seen and felt.

• The anterior end of the first rib is joined to the side of the manubrium (E23) by the first costal cartilage (page 89, C23), to form the first sternocostal joint.

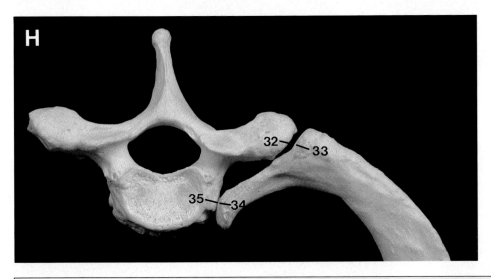

1 Head	**19** Intercostal muscles	
2 Articular surface of head	**20** Area covered by pleura	
3 Neck	**21** Jugular notch	
4 Articular surface of tubercle	**22** Clavicular notch	
5 Tubercle	**23** Notch for first costal cartilage	
6 Body	**24** Notch for upper part of second costal cartilage	
7 Groove for subclavian artery	**25** Surface for manubriosternal joint	
8 Scalene tubercle	**26** Pectoralis major	
9 Groove for subclavian vein	**27** Sternocleidomastoid	
10 Capsule of joint of head	**28** Capsule of sternoclavicular joint	
11 Capsule of costotransverse joint	**29** Sternohyoid	
12 Lateral costotransverse ligament	**30** Sternothyroid	
13 Scalenus medius	**31** Area covered by pleura	
14 Suprapleural membrane	**32** Transverse process and costal facet	} forming costo-
15 Scalenus anterior	**33** Tubercle and articular facet	} transverse joint
16 Costoclavicular ligament	**34** Head and articular surface	} forming joint of head of rib
17 Subclavius	**35** Costal facet of body	
18 Serratus anterior		

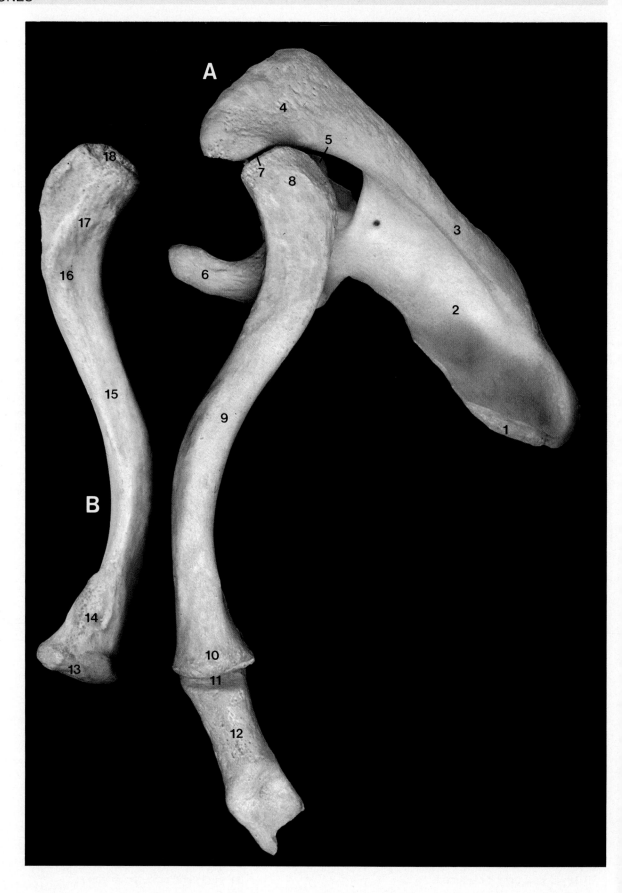

BONES OF SHOULDER GIRDLE
Clavicle and scapula, right
A From above, articulated, with the manubrium of the sternum
B Clavicle, from below

The clavicle and scapula are the bones of the shoulder girdle (pectoral girdle), connecting the upper limb to the axial skeleton. The clavicle forms an obvious landmark at the root of the neck, and is easily palpable throughout its whole length.

1 Superior angle
2 Supraspinous fossa
3 Spine
4 Acromion   } of scapula
5 Upper margin of glenoid cavity
6 Coracoid process
7 Acromioclavicular joint
8 Acromial end }
9 Body   } of clavicle
10 Sternal end }
11 Sternoclavicular joint
12 Jugular notch of manubrium of sternum
13 Sternal articular surface
14 Impression for costoclavicular ligament
15 Groove for subclavius muscle
16 Conoid tubercle
17 Trapezoid line
18 Acromial articular surface

• The main features of the *clavicle* are:

  the bulbous medial (sternal) end (A10)
  the flattened lateral (acromial) end (A8)
  the groove for the subclavius muscle on the middle of the inferior surface (B15)
  rough ligamentous markings near each end of the inferior surface (B, 14, 16 and 17)

• The sternal end (A10) makes the sternoclavicular joint (A11) with the clavicular notch of the manubrium of the sternum (page 84, E22).

• The acromial end (A8) makes the acromioclavicular joint (A7) with the acromion of the scapula (A4).

• The rough marking on the inferior surface near the sternal end (B14) is for the costoclavicular ligament (page 88, B12).

• The rough markings on the inferior surface near the acromial end (the conoid tubercle and the trapezoid line, B16 and 17) are for the conoid and trapezoid parts of the coracoclavicular ligament (page 88, B14 and 15).

• The body of the clavicle is not straight but (when seen from above or below) is somewhat S-shaped; the medial part of the bone is curved forwards, to allow room for the subclavian vessels and the components of the brachial plexus to pass between the neck and arm. The formal description is that the bone has an anterior convexity in its medial two-thirds and an anterior concavity in its lateral one-third.

• The acromion of the *scapula* (4), at the lateral end of the scapular spine (3), is palpable beyond the outer end of the clavicle (8).

• For attachments to the clavicle and scapula see page 88.

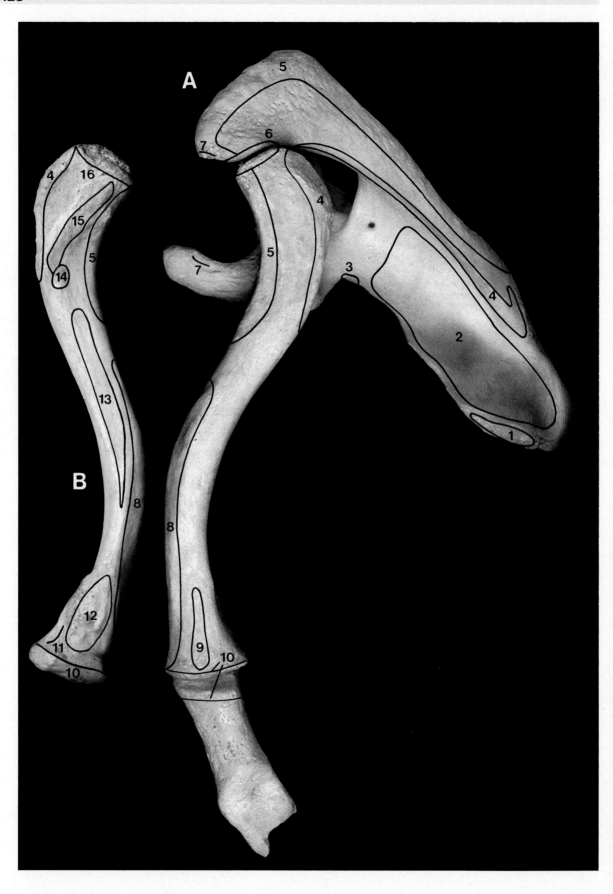

1 Levator scapulae
2 Supraspinatus
3 Inferior belly of omohyoid
4 Trapezius
5 Deltoid
6 Capsule of acromioclavicular joint
7 Coraco-acromial ligament
8 Pectoralis major
9 Sternocleidomastoid
10 Capsule of sternoclavicular joint
11 Sternohyoid
12 Costoclavicular ligament
13 Subclavius
14 Conoid ligament } coracoclavicular
15 Trapezoid ligament } ligament
16 Capsule of acromioclavicular joint
17 Seventh cervical vertebra
18 First thoracic vertebra
19 Head }
20 Neck } of first rib
21 Tubercle }
22 Body }
23 First costal cartilage
24 Sternal end of clavicle
25 Jugular notch of manubrium of sternum

SHOULDER GIRDLE AND UPPER THORACIC SKELETON

Clavicle and scapula and the thoracic inlet

A Right clavicle and scapula, from above, articulated and with the manubrium of the sternum. Attachments

B Right clavicle, from below. Attachments

C Thoracic inlet, in an articulated skeleton, from the front

Of the muscles whose attachments are shown here, deltoid (A5), supraspinatus (A2) and pectoralis major (A8) help to join the upper limb to the shoulder girdle (clavicle and scapula), while trapezius (A4) joins the girdle to the axial skeleton, together with the small subclavius (B13) and the much more important sternocleidomastoid (A9).

In C the bones forming the boundaries of the thoracic inlet are shown: T1 vertebra (C18); the first ribs and costal cartilages (C22 and 23); and the manubrium of the sternum (C25)

• Clinically, the thoracic inlet is sometimes called the thoracic outlet.

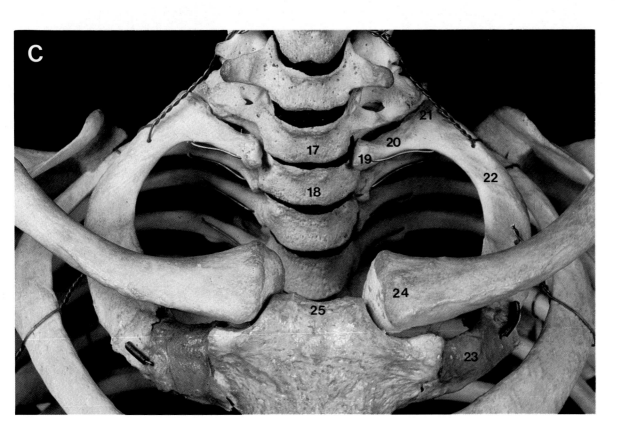

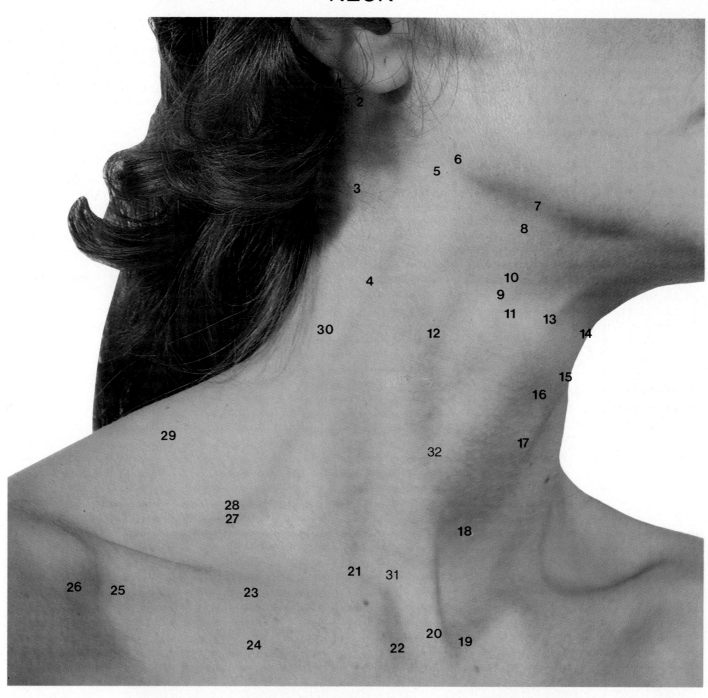

NECK
Surface markings
Some surface markings on the front and right side of the neck
Sternocleidomastoid (3) is the most obvious feature. The external jugular vein (4) courses obliquely downwards over its upper part. The accessory nerve (30) emerges from the posterior border of the junction of the upper and middle thirds of sternocleidomastoid (3). It runs down through the posterior triangle to pass under the anterior border of trapezius about 5 cm above the clavicle and enters the muscle on its deep surface. The upper trunk of the brachial plexus (28) can be felt in the angle between the clavicle (23) and the posterior border of sternocleidomastoid (21). The pulsation of the common carotid artery (carotid pulse, 32) can be felt in the angle between the side of the larynx (15) and the anterior border of sternocleidomastoid (3). The lower end of the internal jugular vein (31) lies behind the gap between the sternal and clavicular heads of the muscle (20 and 21). Compare with the dissections on pages 94–100.

• The hyoid bone (14) is at the level of C3 vertebra.

• The laryngeal prominence (15) is at the upper border of the central part of the thyroid cartilage (page 152, C22), which is at the level of C4 and 5 vertebrae.

• The cricoid cartilage (17) is at the level of C6 vertebra. Confirm these levels in the sagittal section of the neck (page 136, 18, 20 and 11).

• For surface markings on the face see page 110.

 1 Mastoid process
 2 Tip of transverse process of atlas
 3 Sternocleidomastoid
 4 External jugular vein
 5 Lowest part of parotid gland
 6 Angle of mandible
 7 Anterior border of masseter and facial artery
 8 Submandibular gland
 9 Tip of greater horn of hyoid bone
10 Hypoglossal nerve
11 Internal laryngeal nerve
12 Bifurcation of common carotid artery
13 Anterior jugular vein
14 Body of hyoid bone
15 Laryngeal prominence
16 Vocal fold
17 Arch of cricoid cartilage
18 Isthmus of thyroid gland
19 Jugular notch and trachea
20 Sternal head
21 Clavicular head of sternocleidomastoid
22 Sternoclavicular joint and union of internal jugular and subclavian veins to form the brachiocephalic vein
23 Clavicle
24 Pectoralis major
25 Infraclavicular fossa and cephalic vein
26 Deltoid
27 Inferior belly of omohyoid
28 Upper trunk of brachial plexus
29 Trapezius and entry of accessory nerve
30 Accessory nerve emerging from sternocleidomastoid
31 Lower end of internal jugular vein
32 Position for palpation of common carotid pulse

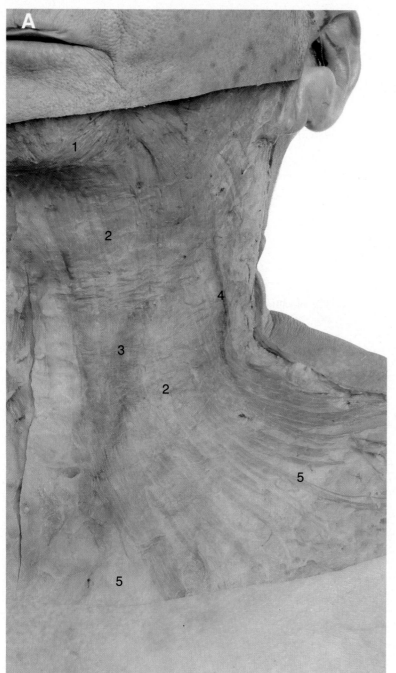

NECK
Superficial dissection I
The left platysma and superficial veins
A Platysma, from the front
B Superficial veins and nerves, from the left.
In A the skin has been removed and platysma has been
dissected out from the subcutaneous tissue. In B platysma has
been removed, to show that the larger superficial veins and
nerves lie deep to the muscle but are superficial to the various
parts of the deep cervical fascia (described in more detail in
this same dissection on pages 94 and 95).

1	Lower border of body of mandible
2	Platysma
3	Anterior jugular vein
4	External jugular vein
5	Clavicle
6	Parotid gland
7	Great auricular nerve
8	Accessory nerve
9	Trapezius
10	Cervical nerves to trapezius
11	Superficial cervical vein
12	Supraclavicular nerves
13	Sternocleidomastoid
14	Transverse cervical nerve
15	Investing layer of deep cervical fascia
16	Submandibular gland

• The lowest of the muscular strands that form platysma (2) are attached to the fascia overlying the upper part of pectoralis major and the medial part of deltoid.

• The upper attachment of the muscle is to the lower border of the mandible (1) , with some fibres blending with adjacent facial muscles and others (below the chin) interdigitating with their fellows of the opposite side.

• The motor nerve supply of platysma is by the cervical branch of the facial nerve (page 96, 6). The muscle can be made to contract visibly by 'forcibly showing the teeth'.

• The larger superficial veins (the anterior and external jugulars, 3 and 4), cutaneous branches of the cervical plexus (as at 7, 12 and 14), and the cervical branch of the facial nerve (page 96, 6) are all deep to the muscle, which is subcutaneous but superficial to the investing layer of the deep cervical fascia (see the notes on page 95).

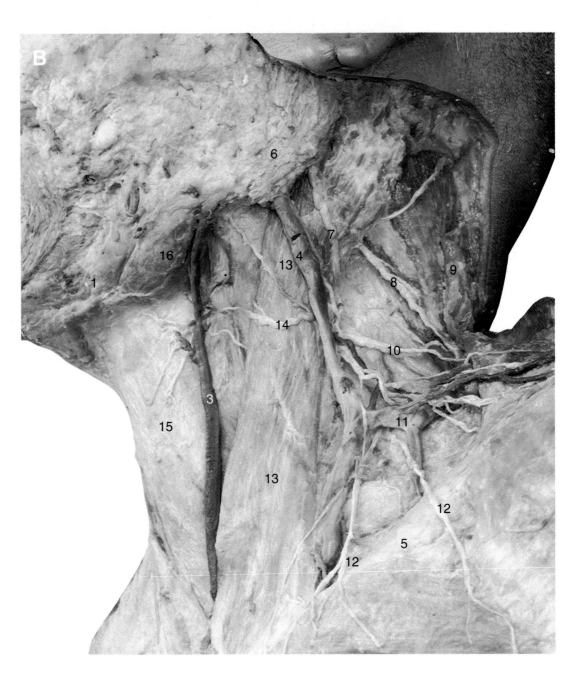

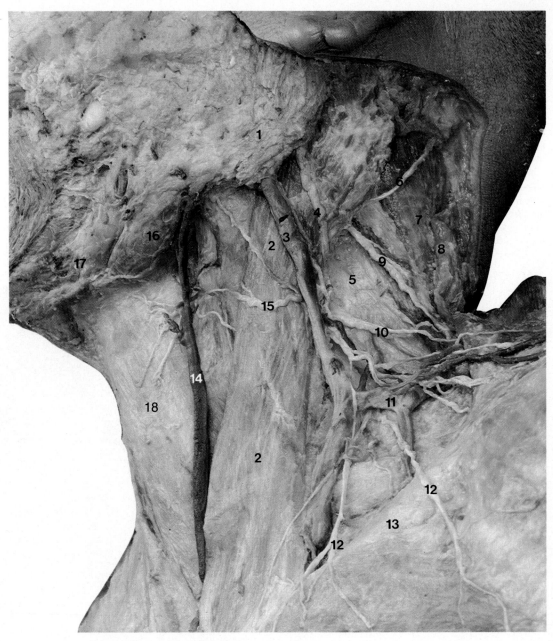

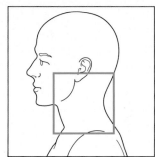

NECK
Superficial dissection II
The left sternocleidomastoid and related structures

Platysma has been removed together with the investing layer of deep cervical fascia posterior to sternocleidomastoid (2), but the fascia (18) remains in place over the front part of the neck (deep to the anterior jugular vein, 14). Of the cutaneous branches of the cervical plexus which emerge behind the posterior border of sternocleidomastoid (2), the transverse cervical nerve (15) runs transversely forwards across the muscle; the great auricular nerve (4) passes upwards, crossing the muscle obliquely; the lesser occipital nerve (6) runs upwards and backwards at the posterior border of the muscle; and the branches of the supraclavicular nerve (12) pass downwards to fan out over the clavicle (13). The accessory nerve (9) leaves the posterior border of sternocleidomastoid (2) and runs down (embedded in the investing layer of deep cervical fascia that forms the roof of the posterior triangle—page 99) to pass under the anterior border of trapezius (8) about 5 cm above the clavicle (13). Branches of cervical nerves (10) also run into trapezius (and into sternocleidomastoid at a higher level, not shown).

1	Parotid gland
2	Sternocleidomastoid
3	External jugular vein
4	Great auricular nerve
5	Prevertebral fascia overlying levator scapulae
6	Lesser occipital nerve
7	Splenius capitis
8	Trapezius
9	Accessory nerve
10	Cervical nerves to trapezius
11	Superficial cervical vein
12	Supraclavicular nerves
13	Clavicle
14	Anterior jugular vein
15	Transverse cervical nerve
16	Submandibular gland
17	Lower border of mandible
18	Investing layer of deep cervical fascia

• The nerve commonly known in English as the accessory nerve or *spinal part* of the accessory nerve (9) is in official anatomical nomenclature the nervus externus of the truncus nervi accessorii. The cells of origin are in the upper five or six segments of the cervical part of the spinal cord, and the fibres are motor to sternocleidomastoid and trapezius. Both muscles receive some fibres from the cervical plexus (as at 10, and see the note on page 99), but these are usually afferent only. (The *cranial part* of the accessory nerve is derived from the nucleus ambiguus in the medulla oblongata of the brainstem and joins the vagus nerve to supply muscles of the larynx and soft palate (page 217)).

• The deep cervical fascia consists of:

> the investing layer
> the pretracheal layer
> the prevertebral layer
> the carotid sheath

• The investing layer (18) surrounds the neck like a subcutaneous stocking. It forms the roof of the anterior and posterior triangles (page 97); it splits to enclose sternocleidomastoid and trapezius, and forms capsules for the parotid and submandibular glands.

• The pretracheal layer forms a sheath for the thyroid gland (page 104).

• The prevertebral layer forms the floor of the posterior traingle (5), lying in front of the vertebral column and prevertebral muscles (page 108).

• The carotid sheath is formed by condensations of the prevertebral and pretracheal layers enclosing the internal jugular vein, common and internal carotid arteries, vagus nerve and the ansa cervicalis with its superior and inferior roots (page 100). Immediately below the base of the skull the last four cranial nerves (glossopharyngeal, vagus, accessory and hypoglossal) run a very short course through the uppermost part of the sheath.

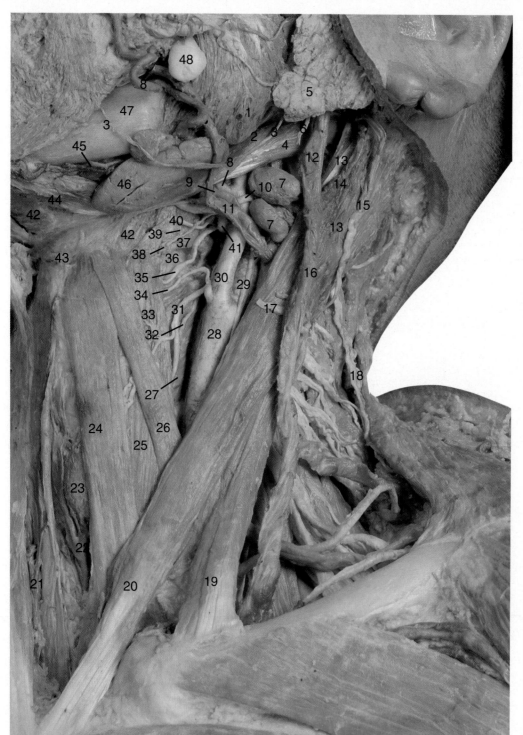

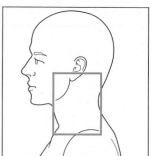

NECK
Superficial dissection III
The left anterior triangle, from the left

All skin and fascia and contained superficial structures have been removed. The labelling in this illustration has largely concentrated on the structures in front of sterno-cleidomastoid (13); those behind it are shown on page 98, A. The upper part of the common carotid artery (28), and the lower parts of the internal and external carotid arteries (29 and 30), are seen at the anterior border of sternocleidomastoid (13). The submandibular gland (46) is below the body of the mandible (47), and the lower pole of the parotid gland (5) projects behind the angle of the mandible (1). The isthmus of the thyroid gland (23) is in the midline of the lower neck, with the lateral lobe under cover of sternohyoid (24) and sternothyroid (25).

1 Masseter and angle of mandible
2 Stylohyoid
3 Marginal mandibular branch of facial nerve
4 Posterior belly of digastric
5 Parotid gland (lower pole)
6 Cervical branch of facial nerve
7 Jugulodigastric lymph nodes
8 Facial artery
9 Lingual vein
10 Hypoglossal nerve
11 Facial vein
12 Posterior branch of retromandibular vein
13 Sternocleidomastoid
14 Posterior auricular vein
15 Great auricular nerve
16 External jugular vein
17 Transverse cervical nerve
18 Accessory nerve
19 Clavicular head ⎱ of sternocleidomastoid
20 Sternal head ⎰
21 Anterior jugular vein
22 Inferior thyroid vein
23 Isthmus of thyroid gland
24 Sternohyoid
25 Sternothyroid
26 Superior belly of omohyoid
27 Inferior constrictor of pharynx
28 Common carotid artery
29 Internal carotid artery and superior root of ansa cervicalis
30 External carotid artery
31 Superior thyroid artery
32 External laryngeal nerve
33 Thyrohyoid
34 Superior laryngeal artery
35 Internal laryngeal nerve
36 Thyrohyoid membrane
37 Greater horn of hyoid bone
38 Nerve to thyrohyoid
39 Hyoglossus
40 Suprahyoid artery
41 Lingual artery
42 Mylohyoid
43 Body of hyoid bone
44 Anterior belly of digastric
45 Submental artery and vein
46 Submandibular gland
47 Body of mandible
48 Buccal fat pad

• The division of the neck into triangles (see the notes) is simply a descriptive means of sorting out a complicated region into a number of smaller 'packages', related to muscular landmarks that are easy to identify, and each containing specific structures.

• While the bifurcation of the common carotid artery (28) is seen in the carotid triangle (see notes), the internal jugular vein is more posterior and covered by sternocleidomastoid (13); it is only seen when the muscle is displaced or removed (as on page100, 14). The jugular venous pulse, which under certain conditions can be observed in the lower neck, is due to pulsation transmitted through the overlying muscle and not to direct vision of the vein itself.

• Triangles of the neck:
    Anterior triangle, subdivided into
        Submental triangle
        Digastric triangle
        Muscular triangle
        Carotid triangle
    Posterior triangle (see pages 98 and 99)

• Anterior triangle
Boundaries: anterior border of sternocleidomastoid (20), lower border of the mandible (47) and the midline.

• Submental triangle
Boundaries: anterior belly of digastric (44), body of hyoid bone (43) and the midline.
Floor: mylohyoid (42, below 44).
Contents: anterior jugular vein (page 94, 14) and submental lymph nodes.

• Digastric triangle
Boundaries: the two bellies of digastric (44 and 4) and the lower border of the mandible (47).
Floor: mylohyoid, hyoglossus and middle constrictor (page 144, 23, 26 and 28).
Contents: submandibular gland (46) and lymph nodes, and the lower part of the parotid gland posteriorly (5);
facial artery (8) and vein (11) and submental vessels (45), and the carotid sheath posteriorly (under cover of 4);
hypoglossal nerve (page 102, A14), mylohyoid nerve (page 102, A6) and vessels, stylopharyngeus and the glossopharyngeal nerve (page 116, C49).

• Muscular triangle
Boundaries: Anterior border of sternocleidomastoid (20), superior belly of omohyoid (26) and the midline.
Floor: sternohyoid (24) and sternothyroid (25).
Contents (beneath the floor): thyroid gland, larynx, trachea, oesophagus.

• Carotid triangle
Boundaries: anterior border of sternocleidomastoid (20), posterior belly of digastric (4) and superior belly of omohyoid (26).
Floor: thyrohyoid (33), hyoglossus (39), middle constrictor (unlabelled, above 37) and inferior constrictor (27).
Contents: bifurcation of the common carotid artery (28);
superior thyroid (31), lingual (41), facial (8), occipital and ascending pharyngeal branches (page 116, C52 and 50) of the external carotid artery (30);
hypoglossal nerve (10) and its two branches—nerve to thyrohyoid (38) and superior root of ansa cervicalis (29);
internal and external laryngeal nerves (35 and 32).

• For notes on the submandibular gland see page 141.

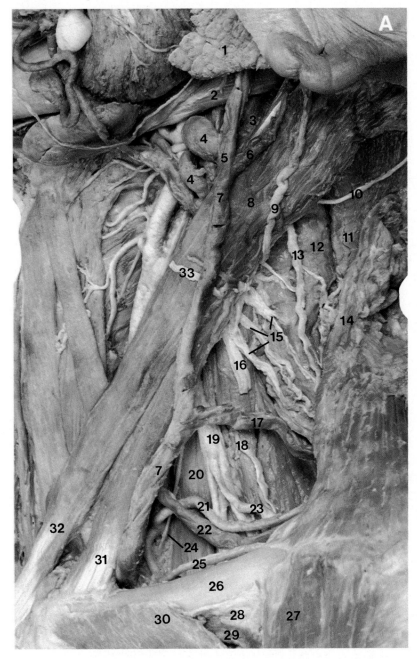

A

1 Parotid gland
2 Posterior belly of digastric
3 Internal jugular vein
4 Jugulodigastric lymph nodes
5 Posterior branch of retromandibular vein
6 Posterior auricular vein
7 External jugular vein
8 Sternocleidomastoid
9 Great auricular nerve
10 Lesser occipital nerve
11 Splenius capitis
12 Levator scapulae
13 Accessory nerve
14 Trapezius
15 Cervical nerves to trapezius
16 Supraclavicular nerve
17 Superficial cervical vein
18 Dorsal scapular nerve and scalenus
   medius
19 Upper trunk of brachial plexus
20 Scalenus anterior
21 Superficial cervical artery
22 Inferior belly of omohyoid
23 Suprascapular nerve
24 Phrenic nerve
25 Suprascapular artery
26 Clavicle
27 Deltoid
28 Clavipectoral fascia
29 Cephalic vein
30 Pectoralis major
31 Clavicular head } of sternocleidomastoid
32 Sternal head
33 Transverse cervical nerve
34 Occipital vein
35 Occipital belly of occipitofrontalis
36 Greater occipital nerve
37 Occipital artery
38 Semispinalis capitis
39 Third occipital nerve

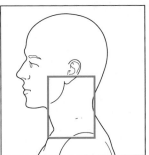

NECK
Superficial dissection IV
The left posterior triangle
A From the left
B The upper part of the triangle, from behind

The dissection in A is the labelled posterior part of the illustration shown on page 96. The most important structure near the middle of the triangle is the accessory nerve (13). In the lower part of the triangle the upper trunk of the brachial plexus (19) gives off the suprascapular nerve (23), with the superficial cervical and suprascapular arteries (21 and 25) running laterally below it. In B the apex of the posterior triangle is shown, with the occipital artery (37) at the very top of the triangle (see notes) and parts of semispinalis (38) and splenius (11) in the floor.

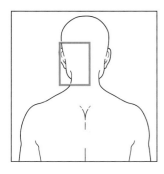

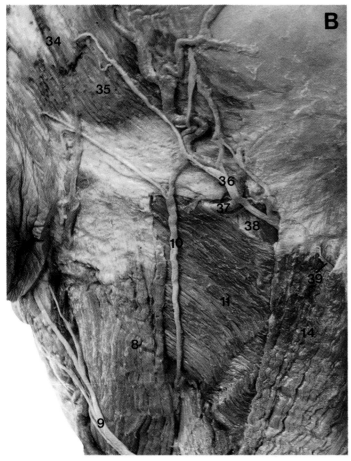

• The posterior triangle:
  Boundaries: posterior border of sternocleidomastoid (A8); anterior border of trapezius (A14); middle third of clavicle (A26).
  Roof: investing layer of deep cervical fascia (here removed), with accessory nerve (A13) embedded in it.
  Contents: arteries—occipital (B37); superficial cervical (A21); suprascapular (A25); subclavian (here just out of sight in A below origin of 21 and 25, behind tip of leaderline 24).
    veins—external jugular (lower part of A7); superficial cervical (A17), suprascapular (removed).
    nerves—branches of cervical plexus (great auricular, A9; lesser occipital, A10; transverse cervical, A33; supraclavicular, A16; muscular, A15); trunks of brachial plexus (as at A19; others hidden by sternocleidomastoid); branches of upper trunk—nerve to subclavius (removed) and suprascapular (A23); dorsal scapular nerve (A18, from uppermost root of plexus); accessory (A13, embedded in fascia of roof).
    muscle—inferior belly of omohyoid (A22)
    lymph nodes and fat (especially in lower part, removed)
  Floor: prevertebral layer of deep cervical fascia (page 94, 5), covering semispinalis capitis (B38); splenius capitis (A and B, 11); levator scapulae (A12); scalenus medius (A18); scalenus anterior (A20, easily seen here but usually hidden by sternocleidomastoid).

• The highest structure in the posterior triangle is the occipital artery (B37), right up in the top corner on semispinalis capitis (38) and between sternocleidomastoid (8) and trapezius (14).

• The subclavian artery is classified as one of the contents of the lower part of the triangle (in A it is unlabelled, behind the tip of the leaderline 24), but because of the downward slope of the first rib the subclavian vein is usually too low to be in the triangle (although it can just be seen on page 100, 42).

• Do not confuse the accessory nerve (13) entering trapezius (14) with the branches of the cervical plexus to the muscle (15): the accessory nerve emerges from *within* sternocleidomastoid (8), whereas the cervical plexus branches emerge from *behind* the muscle.

• In the lower part of the triangle, the suprascapular nerve (23), from the upper trunk of the brachial plexus (19), is a prominent nerve running just above the clavicle near the superficial cervical and suprascapular arteries (21 and 25). The dorsal scapular nerve (18) is smaller and emerges from scalenus medius.

• The inferior belly of omohyoid (22) may be smaller than in this specimen and may be mistaken for a vessel or nerve

• The vessels commonly known as the superficial cervical artery (21) and vein (page 94, 11) are properly called transverse cervical, and are seen in the lower part of the posterior triangle. Note that the transverse cervical *nerve* (33) is at a much higher level and passes forwards over the anterior triangle.

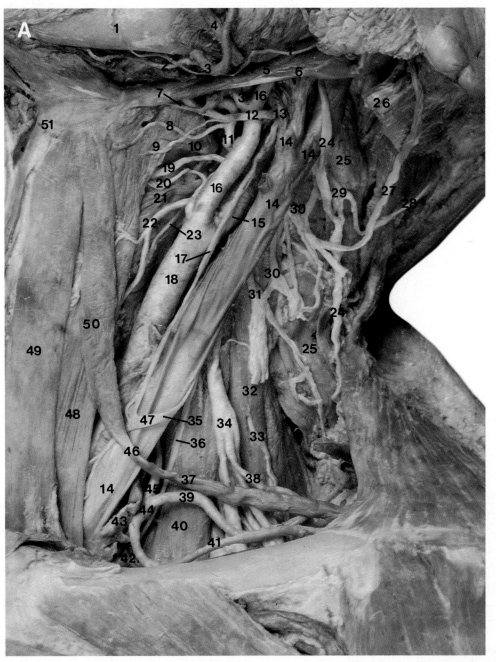

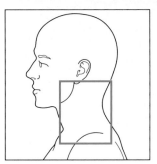

NECK
Deep dissection I
Great vessels and nerves and the thyroid gland
A Vessels and nerves of the left side, from the left
B Thyroid gland, from the front

In A the removal of most of sterno-cleidomastoid (26) and its overlying cutaneous nerves displays the internal jugular vein (14) and adjacent structures. The vein lies posterolateral to the carotid vessels (18, 16 and 15); in this specimen the upper end of the vein is double, with the accessory nerve (24) passing between the two parts. The superior thyroid, lingual and facial arteries (22, 11 and 3) pass forward from the external carotid artery (16). The superior and inferior roots of the ansa cervicalis (17 and 35) embrace the lower part of the internal jugular vein (14) to form the ansa itself (47), which here lies just above the tendon of omohyoid (46). The phrenic nerve (36) runs obliquely down over the surface of scalenus anterior (40). The thyrocervical trunk (44) gives origin to the inferior thyroid, superficial cervical and supra-scapular arteries (45, 39 and 41), and the thoracic duct (43) curls down to enter the junction of the internal jugular and subclavian veins (14 and 42).

In B parts of the left strap muscles (48 and 49) have been removed to display the left lateral lobe of the thyroid gland (54). The inferior thyroid vein (57) is here an unusually large single vessel whose upper end overlies the isthmus of the gland.

• The hypoglossal nerve (12) passes forwards *above* the tip of the greater horn of the hyoid bone (10), while the internal laryngeal nerve (19) passes downwards and forwards *below* the bone.

• The common carotid artery (18) usually divides into the internal and external carotids (15 and 16) at about the level of the upper border of the thyroid cartilage (C4 vertebra).

• The external carotid artery (16) can be distinguished easily from the internal carotid (15) because it gives off a number of branches. The internal carotid gives no branches in the neck.

1	Marginal mandibular branch of facial nerve	29	Second ⎫
2	Submental artery	30	Third ⎬ cervical nerve ventral rami
3	Facial artery	31	Fourth ⎭
4	Facial vein	32	Scalenus medius
5	Stylohyoid	33	Dorsal scapular nerve
6	Posterior belly of digastric	34	Upper trunk of brachial plexus
7	Vena comitans of hypoglossal nerve	35	Inferior root of ansa cervicalis
8	Suprahyoid artery and hyoglossus	36	Phrenic nerve
9	Thyrohyoid (and nerve in A)	37	Inferior belly of omohyoid
10	Greater horn of hyoid bone	38	Suprascapular nerve
11	Lingual artery	39	Superficial cervical artery
12	Hypoglossal nerve	40	Scalenus anterior
13	Lingual vein	41	Suprascapular artery
14	Internal jugular vein (double at upper end in A)	42	Subclavian vein
15	Internal carotid artery and carotid sinus	43	Thoracic duct
16	External carotid artery	44	Thyrocervical trunk
17	Superior root of ansa cervicalis	45	Inferior thyroid artery
18	Common carotid artery	46	Omohyoid tendon
19	Internal laryngeal nerve and thyrohyoid membrane	47	Ansa cervicalis
20	Superior laryngeal artery	48	Sternothyroid
21	Inferior constrictor of pharynx	49	Sternohyoid
22	Superior thyroid artery	50	Superior belly of omohyoid
23	External laryngeal nerve	51	Hyoid bone
24	Accessory nerve	52	Laryngeal prominence (Adam's apple)
25	Levator scapulae	53	Cricothyroid
26	Sternocleidomastoid	54	Lateral lobe of thyroid gland
27	Great auricular nerve	55	Middle thyroid vein
28	Lesser occipital nerve	56	Trachea
		57	Inferior thyroid vein
		58	Isthmus of thyroid gland

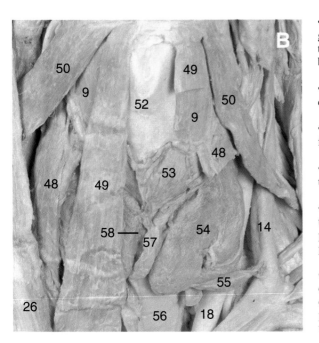

• The superior root (17) of the ansa cervicalis (47) runs down from the hypoglossal nerve (12) between the carotid and internal jugular vessels (18 and 14); the inferior root (35, from the cervical plexus) emerges from behind the posterior border of the vein.

• The superior thyroid artery (22) runs downwards from the beginning of the external carotid artery (16), and has the external laryngeal nerve (23) immediately behind it.

• The superior laryngeal artery (20, a branch of the superior thryoid, 22) runs forwards below the internal laryngeal nerve (19).

• The tendon of omohyoid (46) lies over the internal jugular vein (14)—a guide to the position of the vein in operations on the lower neck.

• The carotid *sinus* is a *baroreceptor* (pressure receptor) at the commencement of the internal carotid artery (within its wall); it receives nerve fibres from the glossopharyngeal and vagus nerves and is concerned with monitoring changes in blood pressure.

• The carotid *body* is a *chemoreceptor* behind or between the bifurcation of the common carotid artery. An oval body a few millimeters long, it contains glomus cells within a connective tissue capsule; it receives nerve fibres from the glossopharyngeal and vagus nerves and is concerned with monitoring oxygen levels in the blood.

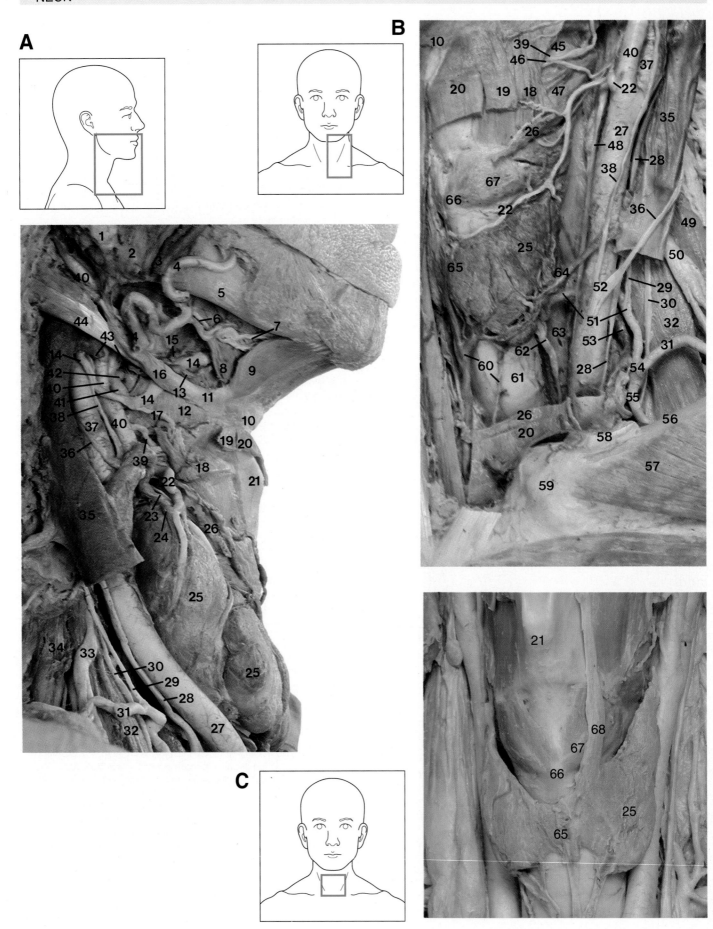

NECK
Deep dissection II
The great vessels and the thyroid gland
A From the right
B From the front and left
C From the front

In the upper part of A, the submandibular gland has been removed to show the facial artery (4) curling upwards over the body of the mandible (5) on to the face, with the facial vein (3, cut end) just behind it. Lower down, with the lower part of the internal jugular vein (35) removed, the vagus nerve (28) is revealed passing down between the vein and the common carotid artery (27). The thyroid gland (25) is here larger than normal, and is displayed by removing all but the uppermost ends of sternohyoid (20), omohyoid (19) and sternothyroid (26).

In contrast with A, the thyroid gland in B (25 and 65) is of normal size and has again been displayed by removing most of the three 'strap' muscles (19, 20 and 26). The gap between the cut ends of the internal jugular vein (35) shows the phrenic nerve (30) running down over scalenus anterior (32); the thyrocervical trunk (54, from the underlying subclavian artery) giving rise to the three arteries —inferior thyroid (51), superficial cervical (31) and suprascapular (55); and the end of the thoracic duct (53), emerging from behind the common carotid artery (27) to run into the junction of the internal jugular and subclavian veins (see page 106, A14). In C the gland has a pyramidal lobe and levator muscle (68).

• The *thyroid gland*, consisting of a central isthmus (B65) and two lateral lobes (B25), is enclosed in a connective tissue capsule derived from the pretracheal fascia, which attaches it to the larynx (hence the gland moves with the larynx during swallowing).

It extends from the level of C5 vertebra to T1 vertebra.

The isthmus of the gland (B and C, 65) overlies the second and third tracheal rings, with an anastomosis between the superior thyroid arteries of each side along its upper border (B22) and inferior thyroid veins leaving its lower border (B60).

The occasional pyramidal lobe (C68), usually on the left side, represents part of the remains of the embryonic thyroglossal duct (page 139).

Important relations of the lateral lobes include:

laterally—sternothyroid (which limits upward extension of the gland), sternohyoid, omohyoid and sternocleidomastoid (page101, B48, 49, 50 and 26).

medially—lower larynx and upper trachea in front of the lower pharynx and upper oesophagus (page 102, B61 and 63), cricothyroid (page 102, B67), inferior constrictor of the pharynx (page 154, A17), external and recurrent laryngeal nerves (page 154, A16 and 23).

posterolaterally—common carotid artery within the carotid sheath (C27), parathyroid glands (page 105, B41, 44 and 47), inferior thyroid artery (B51), thoracic duct (on the left, page 102, B53).

• The external laryngeal nerve lies just behind the superior thryoid artery as the artery approaches the upper pole of the lateral lobe (page 104, A5 and 4). Ligation of the artery during thyroidectomy is usually carried out at the very tip of the pole, to avoid damaging the nerve.

• The recurrent laryngeal nerve (B62) (which enters the larynx by passing under the lower border of the inferior constrictor of the pharynx, immediately behind the cricothyroid joint, page154, B23) lies either anterior or posterior to the inferior thyroid artery as the artery arches medially behind the lower part of the lateral lobe (B51). Ligation of the artery is usually carried out well away from the gland.

• For laryngeal nerve injuries see page 157.

1 Parotid gland	**24** Superior thyroid vein	**47** Inferior constrictor of pharynx
2 Masseter	**25** Lateral lobe of thyroid gland	**48** Sympathetic trunk
3 Facial vein	**26** Sternothyroid	**49** Scalenus medius
4 Facial artery	**27** Common carotid artery	**50** Upper trunk of brachial plexus
5 Body of mandible	**28** Vagus nerve	**51** Inferior thyroid artery
6 Nerve to mylohyoid	**29** Ascending cervical artery	**52** Ansa cervicalis
7 Submental artery	**30** Phrenic nerve	**53** Thoracic duct
8 Mylohyoid	**31** Superficial cervical artery	**54** Thyrocervical trunk
9 Anterior belly of digastric	**32** Scalenus anterior	**55** Suprascapular artery
10 Body of hyoid bone	**33** Ventral ramus of fifth cervical nerve	**56** Clavicle
11 Digastric tendon	**34** Scalenus medius	**57** Pectoralis major
12 Hyoglossus	**35** Internal jugular vein	**58** Sternocleidomastoid
13 Vena comitans of hypoglossal nerve	**36** Inferior root of ansa cervicalis	**59** Capsule of sternoclavicular joint
14 Hypoglossal nerve	**37** Internal carotid artery	**60** Inferior thyroid veins
15 A tributary of **13**	**38** Superior root of ansa cervicalis	**61** Trachea
16 Stylohyoid	**39** Internal laryngeal nerve	**62** Recurrent laryngeal nerve
17 Nerve to thyrohyoid	**40** External carotid artery	**63** Oesophagus
18 Thyrohyoid	**41** Linguofacial trunk	**64** Middle thyroid vein
19 Superior belly of omohyoid	**42** Lingual artery	**65** Isthmus of thyroid gland
20 Sternohyoid	**43** Lingual vein	**66** Arch of cricoid cartilage
21 Laryngeal prominence	**44** Posterior belly of digastric	**67** Cricothyroid
22 Superior thyroid artery	**45** Thyrohyoid membrane	**68** Pyramidal lobe of thyroid gland and levator muscle
23 External laryngeal nerve	**46** Superior laryngeal artery	

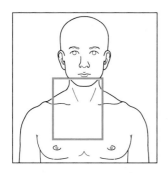

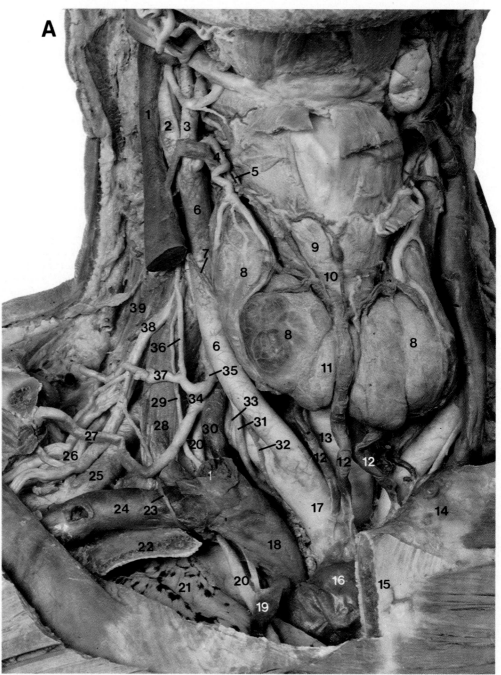

A

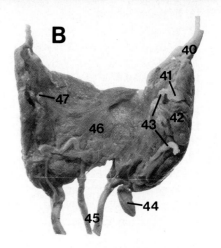

B

1 Internal jugular vein
2 Internal carotid artery
3 External carotid artery
4 Superior thyroid artery and vein
5 External laryngeal nerve
6 Common carotid artery
7 Middle thyroid vein
8 Lateral lobe of thyroid gland
9 Cricothyroid
10 Arch of cricoid cartilage
11 Isthmus of thyroid gland
12 Inferior thyroid veins
13 Trachea
14 Capsule of sternoclavicular joint
15 Manubrium of sternum
16 Left brachiocephalic vein
17 Brachiocephalic artery
18 Right brachiocephalic vein
19 Internal thoracic vein
20 Internal thoracic artery
21 Lung
22 First rib
23 Accessory phrenic nerve
24 Subclavian vein
25 Subclavian artery
26 Brachial plexus
27 Suprascapular artery
28 Scalenus anterior
29 Phrenic nerve
30 Vertebral vein
31 Vagus nerve
32 Jugular lymphatic trunk
33 Ansa subclavia
34 Thyrocervical trunk
35 Inferior thyroid artery
36 Ascending cervical artery
37 Superficial cervical artery
38 Ventral ramus of fifth cervical nerve
39 Scalenus medius
40 Superior thyroid artery and vein
41 Right superior parathyroid gland
42 Posterior border of right lateral lobe of thyroid gland
43 Branches of inferior thyroid artery
44 Right inferior parathyroid gland
45 Inferior thyroid veins
46 Isthmus of thyroid gland
47 Left superior parathyroid gland

NECK
Deep dissection III
The thyroid gland, parathyroid glands and the root of the neck
A The central and right side of the neck
B An isolated thyroid gland, from behind

In A, part of the right clavicle, first rib (22) and manubrium of the sternum (15) have been removed, together with the lower part of the internal jugular vein (1) and infrahyoid muscles. In this specimen the thyroid gland is enlarged; compare with the normal size in B. The superior thryoid artery (4) approaches the front of the upper part of the lateral lobe (8), with the external laryngeal nerve (5) immediately behind it. The inferior thyroid artery (35) runs up behind the lower part of the lobe. The superior and middle thyroid veins (4 and 7) drain laterally to the internal jugular vein (1), but the inferior thyroid veins (12) run downwards in front of the trachea (13) to reach the left brachiocephalic vein (16). The subclavian vein (24) passes medially over the first rib (22) in front of scalenus anterior (28) to be joined by the internal jugular vein (1) to form the right brachiocephalic vein (18). The subclavian artery (25) is at a higher level behind scalenus anterior (28). The vertebral vein (30) and artery are deeply placed medial to scalenus anterior.

In B, the view of the thyroid gland from behind shows three visible parathyroid glands (41, 44 and 47).

• On the front of scalenus anterior (28), do not confuse the phrenic nerve (29) with the ascending cervical artery (36, here a branch of the superficial cervical artery, 37, but usually coming from the inferior thyroid, 35). Compare with page 106, A5 and 6.

• The typical number of *parathyroid glands* is four (in 90% of individuals) but there may be more or less; in B, there are three (B41, 44 and 47).

The glands usually lie between the posterior surface of the lateral lobes of the thyroid gland and the thin capsule of the gland (which is inside the fascial sheath, derived from the pretracheal fascia).

The superior gland usually lies approximately level with the upper border of the thyroid isthmus (B41 and 47), and the inferior gland behind the lower pole of the lateral lobe (in B44 it is below the lower pole).

The blood supply of both superior and inferior parathyroid glands is from the inferior thyroid artery (A35). If the glands are difficult to identify, following small branches of this artery should lead to the glands.

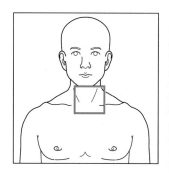

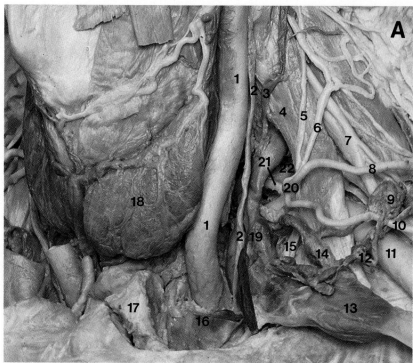

A

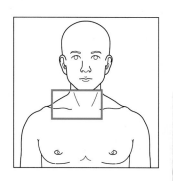

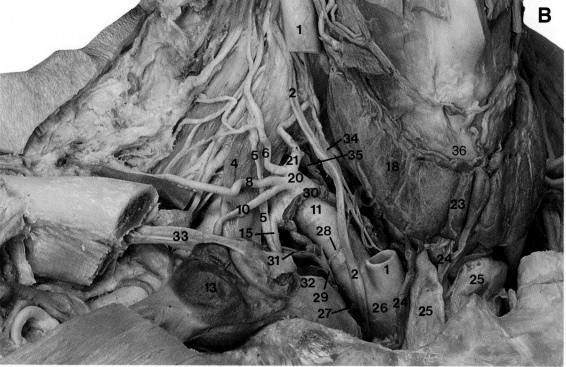

B

NECK
Deep dissection IV
The thyroid gland, thymus and the root of the neck
A Left side, from the front and the left
B Right side, from the front and the right

In A, on the left side, the clavicle has been removed at the sterno-clavicular joint (17), and so has the internal jugular vein at its junction with the subclavian vein (13) to form the brachiocephalic vein (16). The vertebral vein (19) is seen joining the subclavian (13), and the thoracic duct (14) here runs into the subclavian vein, a little more laterally than usual (see page 100, 43). A lymph node (9) and a small lymphatic trunk (12) have been preserved.

In B, on the right side, the dissection is similar to that in A (and to page 104, A) but part of the common carotid artery (1) has been removed. The mediastinal lymphatic trunk (30) is seen curling over the subclavian artery (11) to join the subclavian lymphatic trunk (31) to form the right lymphatic duct (29) which (like the thoracic duct on the left side, page108, 37) joins the junction of the internal jugular and subclavian veins (32 and 13). The recurrent laryngeal branch (27) of the vagus nerve (2) has just begun to hook underneath the subclavian artery (11).

1	Common carotid artery
2	Vagus nerve
3	Ascending cervical vein
4	Scalenus anterior
5	Phrenic nerve
6	Ascending cervical artery
7	Upper trunk of brachial plexus
8	Superficial cervical artery
9	A lower deep cervical lymph node
10	Suprascapular artery
11	Subclavian artery
12	A subclavian lymph trunk
13	Subclavian vein
14	Thoracic duct
15	Internal thoracic artery
16	Brachiocephalic vein
17	Disc of sternoclavicular joint
18	Lateral lobe of thyroid gland
19	Vertebral vein
20	Thyrocervical trunk
21	Inferior thyroid artery
22	Vertebral artery
23	Isthmus of thyroid gland
24	Inferior thyroid veins
25	Lobes of persistent thymus gland
26	Brachiocephalic artery
27	Recurrent laryngeal nerve
28	Ansa subclavia
29	Right lymphatic duct
30	Mediastinal lymphatic trunk
31	Subclavian lymphatic trunk
32	Cut end of internal jugular vein
33	Suprascapular vein
34	Sympathetic trunk and middle cervical ganglion
35	Tracheal branch of inferior thyroid artery
36	Cricoid cartilage

• At the level of C6 vertebra:
the cricoid cartilage (B36)
the larynx continues as the trachea
the pharynx continues as the oesophagus
the middle cervical ganglion (B34)
the vertebral artery (A and B, 22) enters the foramen of the transverse process of C6 vertebra
the inferior thyroid artery (B21) arches medially

• The sympathetic nervous system in the neck consists of the sympathetic trunk with the superior, middle and inferior cervical sympathetic ganglia and their branches.

• The rather elongated *superior cervical ganglion* (page 108, 19) lies at the level of the second and third vertebrae between longus capitis (behind) and the internal carotid artery (page 108, 5), which is within the carotid sheath (in front). It gives off from its upper end the internal carotid nerve, which constitutes the cephalic part of the sympathetic nervous system and enters the cranial cavity with the internal carotid artery. Other branches include grey rami communicantes to the upper four cervical nerves, a cardiac branch and branches to cervical viscera and vessels and the carotid body.

• The *middle cervical ganglion* (B34, the smallest of the three) is at the level of the sixth cervical vertebra, usually in front of the inferior thyroid artery and always in front of the vertebral artery. It gives grey rami communicantes to the fifth and sixth cervical nerves, forms the ansa subclavia (B28), and gives a cardiac branch and branches to cervical viscera and vessels.

• The *inferior cervical ganglion* (page 108, 53) lies in front of the neck of the first rib and behind the vertebral artery; it is frequently fused with the first thoracic sympathetic ganglion to form the cervicothoracic (stellate) ganglion. It gives grey rami communicantes to the seventh and eighth cervical nerves (and to the first thoracic nerve if fused), a cardiac branch and branches to adjacent vessels.

• The middle cervical ganglion (B34) lies in front of the vertebral artery; the inferior cervical ganglion lies behind it (page 108, 53 and 39).

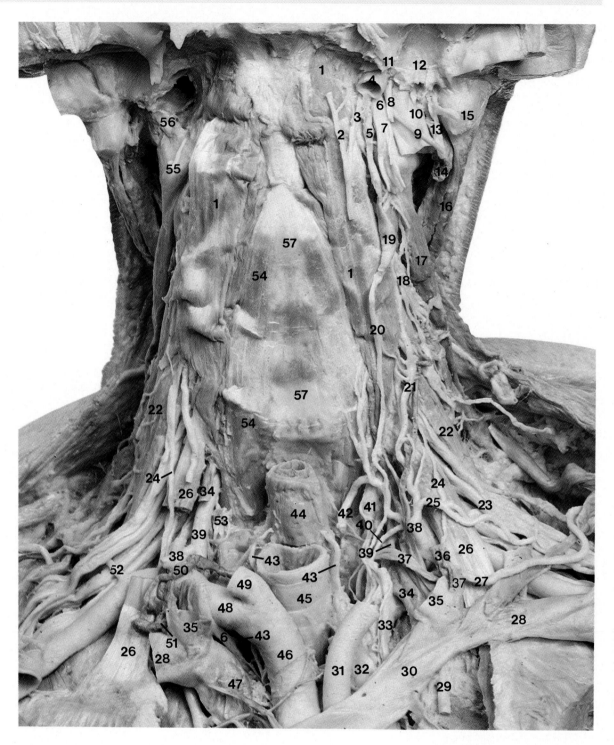

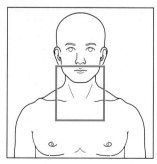

NECK
Deep dissection V
The prevertebral muscles

All the viscera and some major vessels have been removed except for the lower ends of the trachea (45), oesophagus (44), internal jugular veins (35), and the left and right common carotid arteries (31 and 49). Longus capitis (1) and longus colli (54) are the more medial prevertebral muscles, with levator scapulae (17), scalenus medius (22) and scalenus anterior (26) more laterally. The internal carotid nerve (5) extends up from the superior cervical ganglion (19), which is joined by a long length of sympathetic trunk (20) to the middle cervical ganglion (41). The inferior thyroid artery (42) arches medially from the thyrocervical trunk (38), and at a lower level the thoracic duct (37) arches laterally in front of the vertebral vessels (34 and 39). The origin of the right recurrent laryngeal nerve (43) from the vagus (6) is seen just below the right subclavian artery (48).

• In the lowest part of the neck the thoracic duct lies behind the left margin of the oesophagus. It ascends to arch laterally (37) at the level of C7 vertebra, passing behind the common carotid artery and internal jugular vein (31 and 35, here cut just below the duct) and in front of the vertebral artery and vein (39 and 34), and enters the junction of the internal jugular and subclavian veins (35 and 28). The right lymphatic duct (51) pursues a similar course on the right side.

• The recurrent laryngeal nerves (43) run up on each side in the groove between the trachea and oesophagus. The right nerve arises in the lower part of the neck from the vagus (6) and hooks under the right subclavian artery (48); the left nerve arises in the thorax and hooks under the arch of the aorta.

1	Longus capitis	30	Left brachiocephalic vein
2	Ascending pharyngeal artery	31	Left common carotid artery
3	Meningeal branch of ascending pharyngeal artery	32	Left subclavian artery
		33	Vagus nerve
4	Internal carotid artery	34	Vertebral vein
5	Internal carotid nerve	35	Internal jugular vein
6	Vagus nerve	36	Jugular lymphatic trunk
7	Inferior vagal ganglion	37	Thoracic duct
8	Glossopharyngeal nerve	38	Thyrocervical trunk
9	Accessory nerve (spinal root)	39	Vertebral artery
10	Internal jugular vein	40	A large oesophageal branch of inferior thyroid artery
11	Spine of sphenoid bone		
12	Tympanic part of temporal bone	41	Middle cervical ganglion
13	Occipital artery	42	Inferior thyroid artery
14	Posterior belly of digastric	43	Recurrent laryngeal nerve
15	Mastoid process	44	Oesophagus
16	Sternocleidomastoid	45	Trachea
17	Levator scapulae	46	Brachiocephalic artery
18	Ventral ramus of third cervical nerve	47	Right brachiocephalic vein
19	Superior cervical ganglion	48	Right subclavian artery
20	Sympathetic trunk	49	Right common carotid artery
21	Ascending cervical artery and vein	50	Mediastinal lymphatic trunk
22	Scalenus medius	51	Right lymphatic duct
23	Upper trunk of brachial plexus	52	Dorsal scapular artery
24	Phrenic nerve	53	Inferior cervical ganglion
25	Superficial cervical artery	54	Longus colli
26	Scalenus anterior	55	Transverse process of atlas
27	Suprascapular artery	56	Rectus capitis lateralis
28	Subclavian vein	57	Anterior longitudinal ligament
29	Internal thoracic artery		

FACE

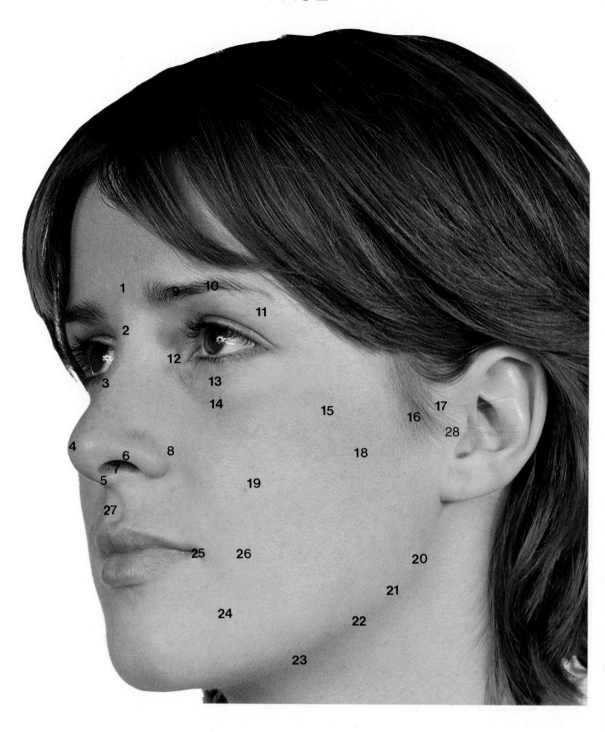

FACE
Surface markings
Some surface markings of the front and left side
Among the more important surface markings on the face are those for the pulses of the superficial temporal artery (17), in front of the tragus of the ear (28) and behind the head of the mandible (16), and the facial artery (22), where it passes on to the face from the neck at the anterior border of the masseter muscle and 2.5 cm in front of the angle of the mandible (20). The parotid duct (18 and 19) lies under the middle third of a line drawn between the tragus of the ear (28) and the midpoint of the philtrum (27), the rectangular area between the two ridges below the nose and above the upper lip.

1	Glabella
2	Root
3	Dorsum
4	Apex
5	Septum	of nose
6	Ala
7	Anterior naris
8	Alar groove
9	Frontal notch and supratrochlear nerve and artery
10	Supra-orbital notch (or foramen), nerve and artery
11	Lateral part of supra-orbital margin
12	Medial palpebral ligament and lacrimal sac
13	Infra-orbital margin
14	Infra-orbital foramen, nerve and vessels
15	Zygomatic arch
16	Head of mandible
17	Auriculotemporal nerve and superficial temporal artery
18	Parotid duct emerging from gland
19	Parotid duct turning medially at anterior border of masseter
20	Angle of mandible
21	Lower border of ramus
22	Anterior border of masseter and facial artery and vein
23	Lower border of body of mandible
24	Mental foramen, nerve and artery
25	Lateral angle of mouth
26	Modiolus
27	Philtrum
28	Tragus of ear

• The supra-orbital, infra-orbital and mental foramina (10, 14 and 24) lie in approximately the same vertical plane, in line with the pupil when looking straight ahead and viewed from the front. Compare with page 10, 6, 12 and 16.

• The medial end of the eyebrow is level with the supra-orbital margin (as at 9), but the lateral end is above the margin (above 11).

• For further details of the eye see page 118, and of the ear see page 148.

• The anterior naris (7) is commonly called the nostril.

• The muscles of the face (including buccinator) and platysma are all supplied by the facial nerve (page 113).

• Facial nerve paralysis (Bell's palsy):
  The lower eyelid droops (but not the upper lid, which is supplied by the oculomotor nerve), and the cornea may become damaged by dryness because the eye cannot be closed properly
  The angle of the mouth droops, with dribbling of saliva, and it is not possible to 'show the teeth' on the affected side
  Whistling is not possible, and food collects between the teeth and the cheek (due to paralysis of the buccinator)

• The facial paralysis may be accompanied by the following additional features depending on the site of the damage. If the damage:
  is in the pons (where the facial nerve fibres overlie the abducent nucleus) there may be paralysis of the lateral rectus
  is in the cerebellopontine angle or internal acoustic meatus where the facial and vestibulocochlear nerves lie close together, there may be deafness
  involves the nerve to stapedius, there may be hyperacusis (extreme sensitivity to sound) due to loss of the dampening effect on the vibration of the stapes
  involves the chorda tympani, there may be loss of taste sensation from the anterior two-thirds of the tongue (the unilateral loss of submandibular and sublingual secretion will not be noticed)

• The above notes on facial nerve paralysis refere to 'infranuclear paralysis', i.e. damage to the axons derived from the facial nerve nucleus in the pons.

• Supranuclear paralysis refers to paralysis due to interruption of the pathway from the cerebral cortex to the facial nerve nucleus, i.e. damage to corticonuclear fibres. The axons from the cell bodies of the upper part of the facial nerve nucleus (in the pons) supply the forehead muscle (frontal belly of occipitofrontalis) and receive corticonuclear fibres from the cerebral cortex of both sides, i.e. there are two sources of corticonuclear supply. The lower part of the facial nerve nucleus supplying the lower facial muscles and platysma receives corticonuclear fibres from the opposite cerebral cortex only, i.e. only one source of corticonuclear supply. Therefore, unilateral supranuclear lesions (e.g. from haemorrhage in the internal capsule involving corticonuclear fibres) causes paralysis of the lower facial muscles of the opposite (contralateral) side but does not affect movement of the forehead on that side, because the neurons supplying the forehead muscle still have an intact corticonuclear supply from the same (ipsilateral) side.

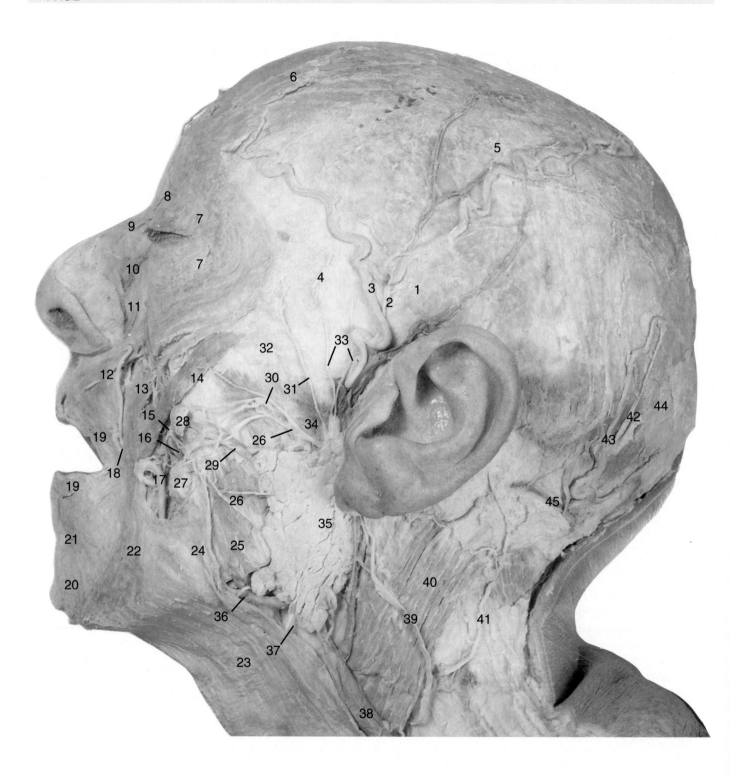

FACE
Superficial dissection
The left parotid gland, facial nerve and muscles

Skin and subcutaneous tissues have been removed to display the superficial structures of the face. Five groups of branches of the facial nerve fan out from below the anterior border of the parotid gland (35): temporal (33), zygomatic (31), buccal (26), marginal mandibular (36) and cervical (37). The facial artery and vein (17 and 16) lie deep to platysma (23), risorius (24), and zygomaticus major and minor (14 and 13).

1 Temporoparietalis
2 Auriculotemporal nerve
3 Superficial temporal artery
4 Zygomaticotemporal nerve piercing temporalis fascia
5 Epicranial aponeurosis (galea aponeurotica)
6 Frontal belly of occipitofrontalis
7 Orbicularis oculi
8 Depressor supercilii
9 Procerus
10 Nasalis
11 Levator labii superioris alaeque nasi
12 Levator labii superioris
13 Zygomaticus minor
14 Zygomaticus major
15 Levator anguli oris
16 Facial vein
17 Facial artery
18 Superior labial artery
19 Orbicularis oris
20 Mentalis
21 Depressor labii inferioris
22 Depressor anguli oris
23 Platysma
24 Risorius
25 Masseter
26 Buccal branches of facial nerve
27 Buccal fat pad
28 Accessory parotid gland
29 Parotid duct
30 Transverse facial artery
31 Zygomatic branch of facial nerve
32 Zygomatic arch
33 Temporal branches of facial nerve
34 Deep part of parotid gland
35 Superficial part of parotid gland
36 Marginal mandibular branch of facial nerve
37 Cervical branch of facial nerve
38 External jugular vein
39 Great auricular nerve
40 Sternocleidomastoid
41 Lesser occipital nerve
42 Greater occipital nerve
43 Occipital artery
44 Occipital belly of occipitofrontalis
45 Occipital vein

• The marginal mandibular branch of the facial nerve (36) usually runs near the lower border of the mandible (to supply facial muscles near the mouth), but it may dip below the mandible (as on page 96, 3) and overlie the submandibular gland. The nerve may be at risk in incisions to expose the gland unless the cut is made 2 cm below the mandible.

• The *parotid gland* (35) spills over into the irregular space bounded in front by the ramus of the mandible (page 14, 30, with the attachments of masseter laterally and the medial pterygoid medially), behind by the mastoid process (page 14, 13, with the attachments of sternocleidomastoid laterally and the posterior belly of digastric medially), and medially by the styloid process (page 14, 18, with its three attached muscles—stylohyoid, styloglossus and stylopharyngeus). It is enclosed in a capsule derived from the investing layer of the deep cervical fascia.
    Embedded within the gland are:
        the various facial branches of the facial nerve (33, 31, 26, 36 and 37)
        the retromandibular vein (page 140, C64 and 65)
        the upper end of the external carotid artery (page 140, C62) and the beginning of its two terminal branches (superficial temporal, 3, and maxillary, page 140, 62)
        lymph nodes
        filaments from the auriculotemporal nerve (2)

The pathway for parotid gland secretion: from the inferior salivary nucleus in the pons by the glossopharyngeal nerve and its tympanic branch, the tympanic plexus and the lesser petrosal nerve to the otic ganglion (synapse), and then to the gland by filaments of the auriculotemporal nerve.
    For the parotid gland in transverse section and a medial view, see page 140.

• The main part of the epicranius muscle (a term rarely used) consists of the frontal and occipital bellies of occipitofrontalis (6 and 44, commonly called occipitalis and frontalis), united centrally by the epicranial aponeurosis (galea aponeurotica, 5). Temporoparietalis (1), which is also classified as part of epicranius, is the name given to muscle fibres (if present) at the side of the scalp between frontalis and the auricular muscles (usually small and unimportant and not illustrated here).

• The occipital belly of occipitofrontalis (see also page 99) has a bony attachment to the supreme nuchal line (page 18, A1) and the mastoid process; the frontal belly has no bony attachment.

A

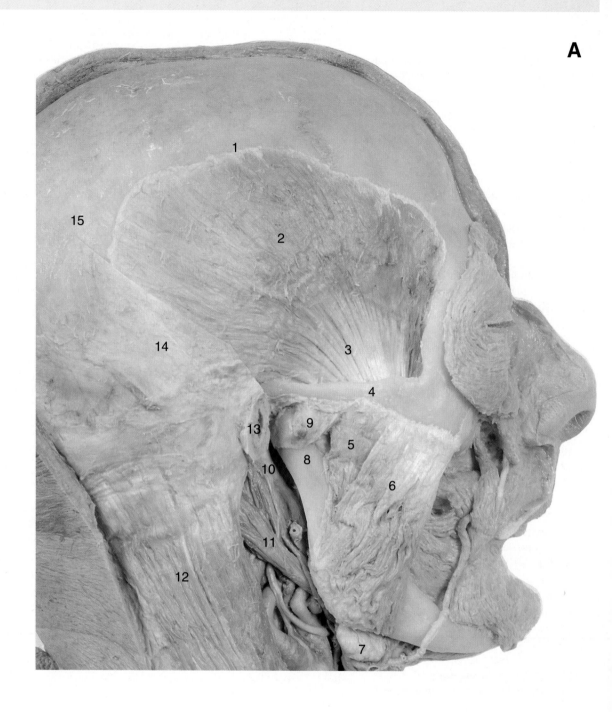

1 Inferior temporal line
2 Temporalis muscle
3 Temporalis tendon
4 Zygomatic arch
5 Middle layer ⎫ of masseter
6 Superficial layer ⎭
7 Submandibular gland
8 Neck of mandible
9 Lateral ligament of temporomandibular joint
10 Styloid process
11 Posterior belly of digastric
12 Sternocleidomastoid
13 Cartilage of external acoustic meatus
14 Temporalis fascia
15 Superior temporal line
16 Coronoid process ⎫ of mandible
17 Ramus ⎭
18 Medial pterygoid
19 Cut edge of mucous membrane of mouth
20 Angle of mandible

FACE
Deep dissection I
The right temporalis and masseter muscles and the temporomandibular joint
A Muscles and joint, from the right
B Temporalis insertion, from the right and front

In A, the parotid gland, facial muscles and all vessels and nerves have been removed, together with part of the temporalis fascia (14). The capsule of the temporomandibular joint is displayed (9), below the zygomatic arch (4) and in front of the external acoustic meatus (13). The posterior belly of digastric is seen between the ramus of the mandible (17) and sternocleidomastoid (12), and the styloid process (10) is more deeply placed.

In B, part of the zygomatic arch (4) and the whole of the masseter have been removed to show the extensive attachment of the tendon of temporalis (3) to the front of the ramus of the mandible (17).

• Although superficially placed, temporalis and masseter are classified (with the medial and lateral pterygoids) as muscles of mastication, not muscles of the face.

• Temporalis (2) arises from the floor of the temporal fossa and from the overlying temporalis fascia (14), which passes from the superior temporal line to the zygomatic arch. The attachment of the muscle is limited above by the inferior temporal line.

The insertion of temporalis is to the apex, anterior and posterior borders and medial surface of the coronoid process (16), and extends down the anterior border of the ramus (17) almost as far as the third molar tooth.

• Masseter consists of three overlapping layers:

superficial (6), arising from the zygomatic process of the maxilla and the anterior two-thirds of the lower border of the zygomatic arch
middle, arising from the deep surface of the anterior two-thirds of the arch and the lower border of the posterior third
deep, from the deep surface of the arch

The layers fuse anteriorly and are inserted into the lateral surface of the angle, ramus and coronoid process of the mandible (20, 17 and 16).

• Both temporalis and masseter, together with the medial and lateral pterygoid muscles (the 'muscles of mastication' group), are supplied by the mandibular branch of the trigeminal nerve.

• In trigeminal nerve paralysis, there is paralysis of the muscles of mastication with eventual hollowing above and below the zygomatic arch due to wasting of temporalis and masseter.

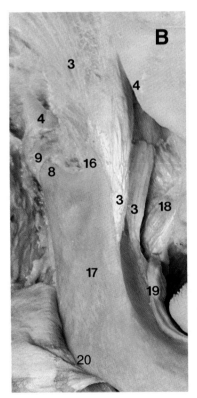

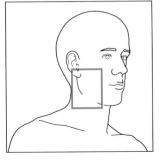

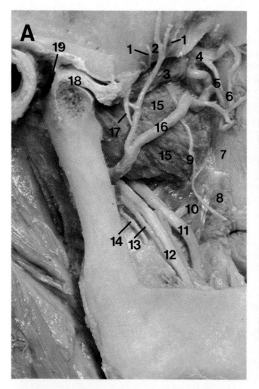

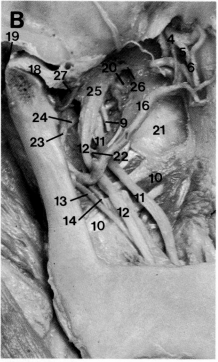

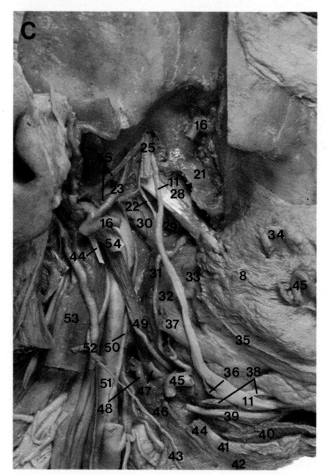

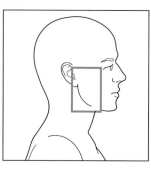

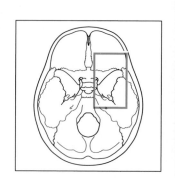

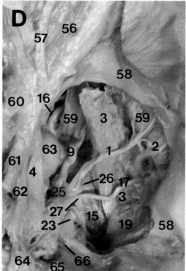

FACE

Deep dissection II

The right infratemporal fossa and temporomandibular joint

A After removal of temporalis, the zygomatic arch, masseter and part of the mandible

B After removal of the lateral pterygoid

C After removal of the mandible and some adjacent neck structures

D From above, after removal of part of the floor of the middle cranial fossa

In A the removal of much of the ramus of the mandible displays the two pterygoid muscles and associated structures. The maxillary artery (16) runs obliquely upwards across the lateral pterygoid (15), and the lingual and inferior alveolar nerves (11 and 12) pass obliquely downwards over the medial pterygoid (10). Farther forward the buccal nerve (9) emerges between the two heads of the lateral pterygoid (3 and 15).

In B after removing the lateral pterygoid, the mandibular nerve (25) is seen just after emerging from the foramen ovale, with the chorda tympani (22) joining the back of the lingual nerve (11), as also seen more clearly in C, after removal of the whole mandible and the medial pterygoid.

The view in D looks down on the temporomandibular joint (19) from above after removing the floor of the lateral part of the middle cranial fossa. It shows temporal and masseteric nerves (1 and 17), running laterally above the upper head of the lateral pterygoid (3), with the buccal nerve (9) and the nerve to the lateral pterygoid (26) passing below this head; i.e. *between* the two heads (3 and 15).

• The boundaries of the infratemporal fossa (see pages 22, A and 30):
  roof—the infratemporal surface of the greater wing of the sphenoid bone (bounded laterally by the infratemporal crest, page 22, A15), containing the foramen ovale and spinosum (page 22, A44 and 43), a small part of the squamous part of the temporal bone in front of the articular tubercle (page 22, A17), and laterally the gap between the zygomatic arch (page 22, A16) and the side of the skull (forming the communication between the temporal and infratemporal fossae)
  medially—the lateral pterygoid plate (pages 22, A14 and 26, A2)
  laterally—the ramus of the mandible (page 14, 30)
  in front—the infratemporal (posterior) surface of the maxilla (page 26, A5)
  behind—the styloid process and tympanic part of the temporal bone (page 14, 18 and 14)

• The contents of the infratemporal fossa:
  the temporalis muscle and its insertion into the coronoid process (page 115, B3 and 16)
  the medial and lateral pterygoid muscles (A10 and 15)
  the pterygoid plexus of veins
  the maxillary artery and its branches (B16)

the mandibular nerve and its branches (B25)
the chorda tympani (C22)

• In C the maxillary artery (upper 16) is seen passing through the pterygomaxillary fissure (page 26, A4) in front of the lateral pterygoid plate (21) to enter the pterygopalatine fossa. For the boundaries of the fossa see page 71.

• The contents of the pterygopalatine fossa:
  the maxillary artery (C, upper 16)
  the maxillary nerve (page 142, A2)
  the pterygopalatine ganglion (page142, A4)

• The medial and lateral pterygoid muscles both have an origin from the respective sides of the *lateral* pterygoid plate (page 24, 3, 4 and 6).

• The lateral pterygoid helps to *open* the mouth by pulling the head of the mandible forwards on to the articular tubercle in front of the mandibular fossa (page 22, A17). The other muscles of the mastication group (medial pterygoid, temporalis and masseter) help to *close* it.

1	Deep temporal nerve	35	Mucoperiosteum of mandible
2	Deep temporal artery	36	Submandibular ganglion
3	Upper head of lateral pterygoid	37	Styloglossus
4	Maxillary nerve	38	Submandibular duct
5	Posterior superior alveolar nerve	39	Hypoglossal nerve
6	Posterior superior alveolar artery	40	Mylohyoid
7	Infratemporal surface of maxilla	41	Tendon of digastric
8	Buccinator	42	Hyoid bone
9	Buccal nerve	43	Thyrohyoid and nerve
10	Medial pterygoid	44	Stylohyoid
11	Lingual nerve	45	Facial artery
12	Inferior alveolar nerve	46	Hyoglossus
13	Inferior alveolar artery	47	Stylohyoid ligament
14	Nerve to mylohyoid	48	Lingual artery
15	Lower head of lateral pterygoid	49	Stylopharyngeus and glossopharyngeal nerve
16	Maxillary artery	50	Ascending pharyngeal artery
17	Masseteric nerve	51	Internal carotid artery
18	Articular disc and head of mandible } of temporo-mandibular joint	52	Hypoglossal nerve hooking round occipital artery and sternocleidomastoid branch
19	Capsule	53	Internal jugular vein
20	Nerve to medial pterygoid	54	Styloid process
21	Lateral pterygoid plate	55	Roots of auriculotemporal nerve
22	Chorda tympani	56	Posterior part of orbit
23	Middle meningeal artery	57	Frontal nerve
24	Accessory meningeal artery	58	Floor of lateral part of middle cranial fossa
25	Mandibular nerve	59	Temporalis
26	Nerve to lateral pterygoid	60	Optic nerve
27	Auriculotemporal nerve	61	Oculomotor nerve
28	Tensor veli palatini	62	Ophthalmic nerve
29	Levator veli palatini	63	Sphenoidal sinus
30	Pharyngobasilar fascia	64	Trigeminal nerve and ganglion
31	Ascending palatine artery	65	Petrous part of temporal bone
32	Superior constrictor of pharynx	66	Greater petrosal nerve
33	Pterygomandibular raphe		
34	Parotid duct		

A

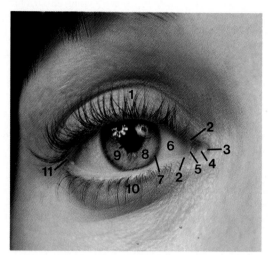

B

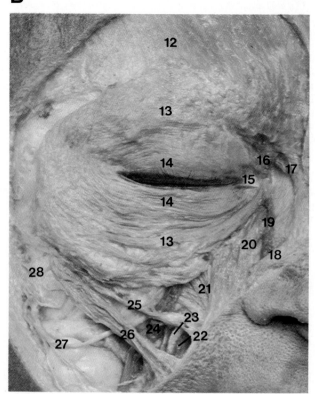

C

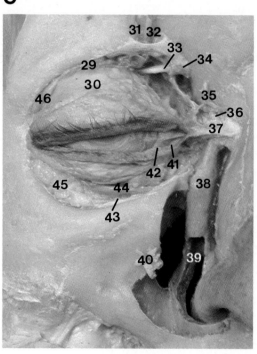

D

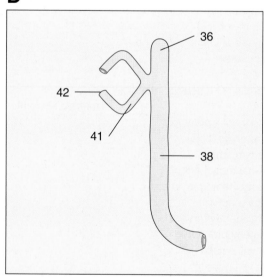

1 Upper eyelid
2 Lacrimal papilla
3 Medial angle (inner canthus)
4 Lacrimal caruncle
5 Plica semilunaris
6 Sclera with overlying conjunctiva
7 Sclerocorneal junction (limbus)
8 Iris
9 Pupil
10 Lower eyelid
11 Lateral angle (outer canthus)
12 Frontal belly of occipitofrontalis
13 Orbital part ⎫
14 Palpebral part ⎭ of orbicularis oculi
15 Medial palpebral ligament
16 Depressor supercilii
17 Procerus
18 Nasalis
19 Angular vein
20 Levator labii superioris alaeque nasi
21 Levator labii superioris
22 Levator anguli oris
23 Facial artery
24 Facial vein
25 Zygomaticus minor
26 Zygomaticus major
27 Buccal ⎫
28 Zygomatic ⎭ branches of facial nerve
29 Muscle fibres ⎫
30 Aponeurosis ⎭ of levator palpebrae superioris
31 Supra-orbital nerve
32 Supra-orbital artery
33 Tendon of superior oblique
34 Trochlea
35 Dorsal nasal artery
36 Lacrimal sac (upper extremity)
37 Medial palpebral ligament
38 Nasolacrimal duct
39 Opening of nasolacrimal duct (anterior wall removed) in inferior meatus of nose
40 Infra-orbital nerve
41 Lower lacrimal canaliculus
42 Lower lacrimal papilla and punctum
43 Cut edge of orbital septum and periosteum
44 Inferior oblique
45 Orbital fat pad
46 Lacrimal gland

EYE AND LACRIMAL APPARATUS
The right eye
A Surface features
B The orbicularis oculi muscle
C The nasolacrimal duct
D Diagram of the lacrimal passages

When looking straight ahead, as in A, the lower eyelid (10) is approximately level with the sclerocorneal junction (7), but the upper eyelid (1) is below the junction.

In B, skin and subcutaneous tissue have been removed to show orbicularis oculi (13 and 14), with the angular vein (19) beginning near the medial palpebral ligament (15).

In C, the facial muscles and part of the skull have been dissected away to display the nasolacrimal duct (38) opening into the inferior meatus of the nose (39; compare with page 128, B17).

• The lacrimal apparatus consists of:
the lacrimal gland (C46; page 120, A1)
the upper and lower lacrimal puncta (C and D, 42) opening into the lacrimal canaliculi (C and D, 41)
the lacrimal sac (C and D, 36) into which the canaliculi drain
the nasolacrimal duct (C and D, 38), continuing downwards from the lacrimal sac and opening into the inferior meatus of the nose (page128, B17)

• Some connective tissues of the eye and orbit:
Orbital septum—a thin sheet of tissue continuous with the periosteum at the orbital margin (C43), blending in the upper eyelid with the superficial lamella of the aponeurosis of levator palpebrae superioris (C30), and in the lower eyelid with the anterior surface of the tarsus.
Lacrimal fascia—stretches between the anterior and posterior lacrimal crests, behind the medial palpebral ligament (C37) and covering the lacrimal sac (C36), being pierced by the lacrimal canaliculi (C41).
Fascial sheath of the eyeball (Tenon's capsule)—envelops the eyeball from the optic nerve to the sclerocorneal junction. It is pierced by the ciliary vessels and nerves and the tendons of the eyeball muscles, being reflected on to each muscle as a sheath.
Medial and lateral check ligaments—expansions of the sheaths of the medial and lateral rectus muscles, attached to the posterior lacrimal crest (medial) and marginal tubercle (lateral) (page 32, A26 and 9).
Suspensory ligament of the eyeball—the lower part of the sheath of the eyeball, between the medial and lateral check ligaments.
Medial palpebral ligament (B15; C37)—from the medial ends of the two tarsi to the anterior lacrimal crest (page 32, A23) and the adjoining part of the frontal process of the maxilla. It lies in front of the lacrimal sac (C36) with the lacrimal fascia intervening.
Lateral palpebral ligament—from the lateral ends of the two tarsi to the marginal tubercle (page 32, A9) where it is attached in front of the lateral check ligament and behind the lateral palpebral raphe. It is a less well-defined structure than the medial palpebral ligament.
Lateral palpebral raphe—formed by the interlacing fibres of the palpebral part of orbicularis oculi (B14).

• The angular vein (19, the name given to the uppermost end of the facial vein) lies *in front of* the medial palpebral ligament (B15, C37), and may cause haemorrhage during incisions to divide the ligament to expose the lacrimal sac (C36) which is *behind* the ligament.

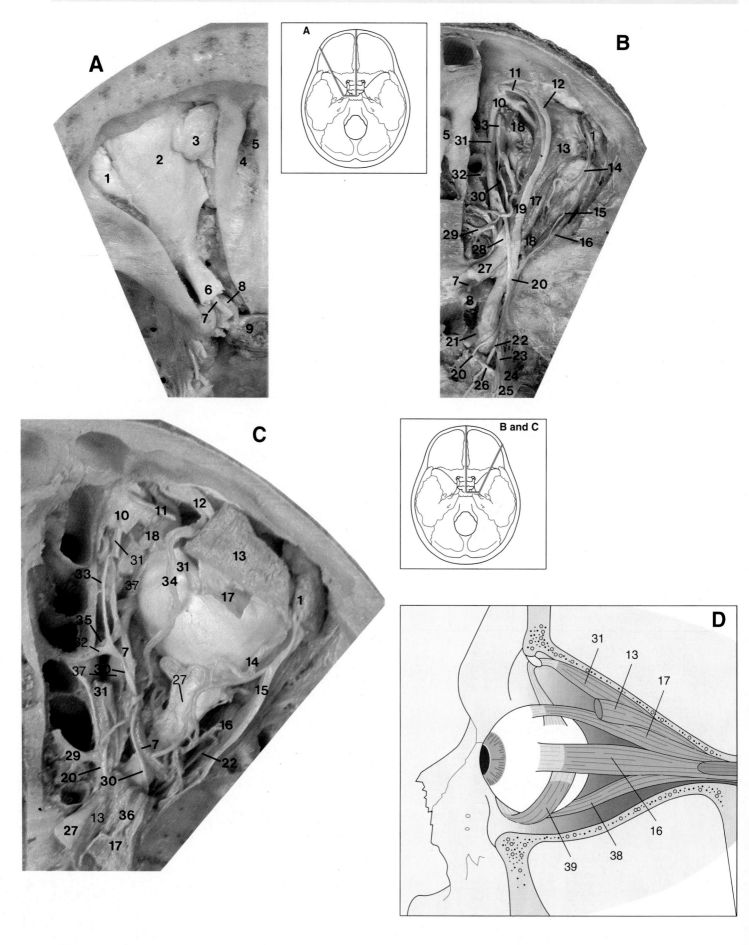

ORBIT AND EYE
Orbital contents I
The orbits from above, and the extraocular muscles
A The left orbit, after removal of the roof
B Superficial dissection of the right orbit
C Dissection of the right orbit (enlarged)
D Diagram of the left extraocular muscles, from the left

A is the view looking down from the anterior cranial fossa after removing bone of part of the floor of the fossa, i.e. the roof of the orbit. The orbital contents are embedded in a mass of orbital fat (2), with the lacrimal gland (1) at the anterolateral corner.

In B the contents of the orbit are shown from above after removal of the orbital fat. The frontal nerve (19) lies on top of levator palpebrae superioris (13), which in turn overlaps most of the superior rectus (17). The superior oblique (31), high on the medial wall with its nerve, the trochlear (20), and its tendon hooking through the trochlea (10), obscures the medial rectus, which is lower down and only seen when the superior oblique is removed (as in C37). The lateral rectus (16) lies along the lateral wall with the lacrimal nerve (15) above it, running to the gland (1) with the lacrimal artery (14).

In C (magnified), parts of levator palpebrae superioris (13) and the superior rectus (17) have been removed and reflected to show the optic nerve (27) being crossed superficially by the nasociliary nerve (30) and the ophthalmic artery (7). About halfway along the medial side of the orbit, the nasociliary nerve (30) gives off the anterior ethmoidal nerve (32) and then continues forwards as the infratrochlear nerve (33). At the bottom of the picture, the superior branch of the oculomotor nerve (36) is on the under surface of the proximal reflected part of the superior rectus (17), and on the lateral side the abducent nerve (22) enters the deep surface of the lateral rectus (16).

The diagram in D shows the extraocular muscles from the left side (the medial rectus is obscured by the eye and the lateral rectus).

• The supra-orbital artery, which normally arises from the ophthalmic artery near the back of the orbit, as in C34, was absent in B.
• Nerve supplies of the eye and eye muscles:
    Motor to eye muscles:
        Lateral rectus (C16) by the abducent nerve (C22)
        Superior oblique (B31) by the trochlear nerve (B20)
        All other muscles by the oculomotor nerve: superior rectus (B and C, 17) by the superior branch (C36, which also supplies levator palpebrae superioris, B and C, 13), and inferior rectus, inferior oblique and medial rectus by the inferior branch (page 122, A19, 17, 18 and 15)
    Sensory:
        To the cornea: long and short ciliary nerves (page 122, A28)
        To the conjunctiva: lacrimal, supra-orbital, supratrochlear, infratrochlear and infra-orbital (the same nerves that supply the skin of the eyelids)

• Individual eye muscles turn the eye as follows:
    Lateral rectus: out
    Medial rectus: in
    Superior rectus: up and in
    Inferior rectus: down and in
    Superior oblique: out, and down when turned in
    Inferior oblique: out, and up when turned in
• The superior and inferior recti not only turn the eye upwards or downwards, respectively, but also assist the medial rectus in turning it inwards. This is because the insertions of the superior and inferior recti on the eye lie medial to the vertical axis.
• The superior and inferior oblique muscles not only turn the eye downwards or upwards, respectively, but also outwards. This is because their insertions lie lateral to the vertical axis. However, it must be noted that the *depressor* action of the *superior* oblique and the *elevator* action of the *inferior* oblique can only occur when the eye is turned in.
• Levator palpebrae superioris contains some smooth muscle fibres which receive a sympathetic nerve supply.
• Apart from the six muscles that move the eye (the four recti and two obliques) and the levator palpebrae superioris, there is an eighth muscle within the orbit, the orbitalis. It consists of smooth muscle that bridges over the infra-orbital groove and inferior orbital fissure (page 32, A15 and 11), and although large in some animals it is an unimportant vestigial structure in the human orbit.
• Lesions of the motor nerves to the eye muscles all give varying degrees of diplopia (double vision) and strabismus (squint).
    Oculomotor nerve paralysis:
        The upper eyelid droops (ptosis), closing the eye, due to paralysis of levator labii superioris (the part of the levator supplied by sympathetic fibres is not sufficient to keep the eye open).
        When the upper eyelid is lifted up, the eye is seen to be looking outwards and slightly downwards, due the unopposed action of the lateral rectus (abducent nerve) and superior oblique (trochlear nerve).
        The eye cannot look straight upwards or downwards or inwards, due to paralysis of the superior, inferior and medial recti.
        The pupil is dilated and does not react to light or on accommodation, due to interruption of the parasympathetic fibres from the Edinger–Westphal nucleus that run in the oculomotor nerve to the ciliary ganglion and which normally act to constrict the pupil.
    Trochlear nerve paralysis:
        There is a weakness when looking downwards with the eye turned in, due to paralysis of the superior oblique.
    Abducent nerve paralysis:
        The eye cannot look outwards, due to paralysis of the lateral rectus, and is deviated inwards by the unopposed action of the medial, superior and inferior recti (oculomotor nerve).

1	Lacrimal gland	15	Lacrimal nerve	29	Posterior ethmoidal artery
2	Orbital fat	16	Lateral rectus	30	Nasociliary nerve
3	Ethmoidal air cell	17	Superior rectus	31	Superior oblique
4	Cribriform plate of ethmoid bone	18	Superior ophthalmic vein	32	Anterior ethmoidal nerve
5	Crista galli	19	Frontal nerve	33	Infratrochlear nerve
6	Dural sheath of optic nerve	20	Trochlear nerve	34	Supra-orbital artery
7	Ophthalmic artery	21	Oculomotor nerve	35	Anterior ethmoidal artery
8	Internal carotid artery	22	Abducent nerve	36	Superior branch of oculomotor nerve
9	Pituitary gland	23	Ophthalmic nerve	37	Medial rectus
10	Trochlea	24	Trigeminal ganglion	38	Inferior rectus
11	Supratrochlear nerve	25	Trigeminal nerve	39	Inferior oblique
12	Supra-orbital nerve	26	Petrosphenoidal ligament		
13	Levator palpebrae superioris	27	Optic nerve		
14	Lacrimal artery	28	Common tendinous ring		

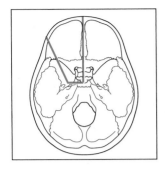

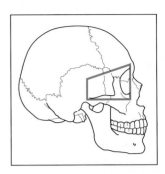

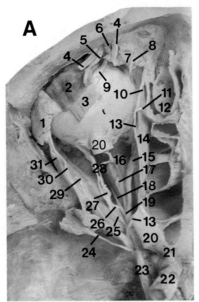

A

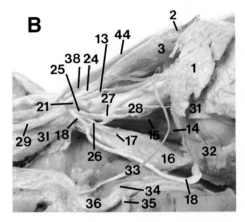

B

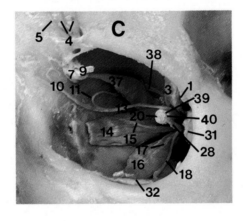

C

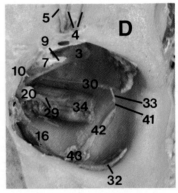

D

ORBIT AND EYE
Orbital contents II
The ciliary ganglion and dissection from the front
A The left orbit and ciliary ganglion, from above
B The right orbit and ciliary ganglion, from the right
C The left orbit, from the front and the left
D The left orbit, from the front and the right

In A removal of the superior oblique (seen high on the lateral wall; C37) enables the lateral rectus to be seen (31), with its nerve, the abducent (29). Removal of much of the optic nerve (20) displays the inferior rectus (16) with its nerve (17) and the nerves to the medial rectus (15) and inferior oblique (18); these three nerves are all branches of the inferior branch of the oculomotor nerve (19).

In B with the lateral wall of the orbit removed, the ciliary ganglion (27) is shown, lying lateral to the optic nerve (20) near the back of the orbit.

The views in C and D show muscles and nerves in relation to the orbital walls after removal of the eye. In C note the extension of the subarachnoid space (39) and the dural sheath (40) round the optic nerve (20). In B the zygomatic branch of the maxillary nerve has been removed, and the communicating branch (33) with the lacrimal nerve (30) has arisen directly from the maxillary nerve (36).

• Ciliary nerves:
  The short ciliary nerves (A and B, 28, eight to ten in number) are branches from the ciliary ganglion (B27) that contain postganglionic parasympathetic fibres for the pupillary and ciliary muscles. They also contain afferent fibres from the eye, including the cornea.
  The long ciliary nerves (two or three in number, here removed) are branches of the nasociliary nerve (A and B, 13) and contain afferent fibres from the eye, including the cornea.

• Ciliary arteries (here removed to display the more important nerves):
  The *anterior* ciliary arteries (variable in number) are so named because they arise near the front of the orbit from muscular branches of the ophthalmic artery, and run to the front of the eyeball along the tendon of the rectus muscles.
  The *posterior* ciliary arteries are so named because they arise near the back of the orbit.
  The *short posterior* ciliary arteries (about seven in number) run from the ophthalmic artery along the outside of the dural sheath of the optic nerve and divide into further branches before piercing the sclera near the nerve.

The *long posterior* ciliary arteries (usually two) pass from the ophthalmic artery to pierce the sclera on either side of the optic nerve.

• The four parasympathetic ganglia in the head and neck:
  The ciliary ganglion (B27), lying at the back of the orbit on the lateral side of the optic nerve about 8 mm in front of the opening of the optic canal;
  The pterygopalatine ganglion (page 142, A4) in the pterygopalatine fossa below the maxillary nerve;
  The otic ganglion (page 142., A11) on the medial side of the mandibular nerve just below the foramen ovale.
  The submandibular ganglion (page 142, A40) below the lingual nerve on the outer surface of hyoglossus.

• The pupillary light reflexes:
  The direct pupillary light reflex—shining a light into one eye causes the pupil of that eye to constrict.
  The indirect (consensual) pupillary light reflex—shining a light into one eye causes the pupil of the opposite eye to constrict.
The pathway for the pupillary light reflexes: from the retina by the optic nerve, chiasma and tract to the pretectal nucleus (synapse) at the level of the superior colliculus, then to the Edinger–Westphal part of the oculomotor nucleus and by the inferior division of the oculomotor nerve and the branch to the inferior oblique to reach the ciliary ganglion (synapse), and then by short ciliary nerves to the sphincter pupillae. The pupils of both eyes constrict because (a) some fibres cross in the optic chiasma, and (b) fibres from the pretectal nucleus pass to the Edinger–Westphal nuclei of both sides.

• The accommodation–convergence (near) reflex: for looking at near objects the eye is focussed by adjustment of the lens by the ciliary muscles (accommodation), the pupil constricts, and the eyes converge by contraction of both medial rectus muscles. These combined reflexes are sometimes collectively called the near reflex.
  The probable pathways for the near reflex:
  For accomodation: from the visual cortex by the posterior limb of the internal capsule to the Edinger–Westphal nucleus (*not* via the pretectal nucleus) and so to the ciliary ganglion, sphincter pupillae and ciliary muscle as for the pupillary light reflexes.
  For convergence: from the visual cortex by association fibres to the frontal eye field (middle frontal gyrus) (synapse), then by the anterior limb of the internal capsule to those cell bodies of the oculomotor nucleus that supply the medial rectus.

1 Lacrimal gland	17 Nerve to inferior rectus	30 Lacrimal nerve
2 Levator palpebrae superioris	18 Nerve to inferior oblique	31 Lateral rectus
3 Superior rectus	19 Inferior branch of oculomotor nerve	32 Inferior oblique
4 Supra-orbital nerve	20 Optic nerve	33 Communication between **30** and **36** (in B) or **42** (in D)
5 Supra-orbital artery	21 Ophthalmic artery	34 Infra-orbital nerve
6 Superior ophthalmic vein	22 Internal carotid artery	35 Infra-orbital artery
7 Trochlea	23 Oculomotor nerve	36 Maxillary nerve
8 Supratrochlear nerve	24 Superior branch of oculomotor nerve	37 Superior oblique
9 Tendon of superior oblique	25 Nasociliary root of ciliary ganglion	38 Trochlear nerve
10 Infratrochlear nerve	26 Oculomotor (parasympathetic) root of ciliary ganglion	39 Subarachnoid space
11 Anterior ethmoidal nerve	27 Ciliary ganglion	40 Dural sheath of optic nerve
12 Ethmoidal air cell	28 Short ciliary nerves	41 Zygomatico-orbital foramen
13 Nasociliary nerve	29 Abducent nerve	42 Zygomatic nerve
14 Medial rectus		43 Inferior orbital fissure
15 Nerve to medial rectus		44 Frontal nerve
16 Inferior rectus		

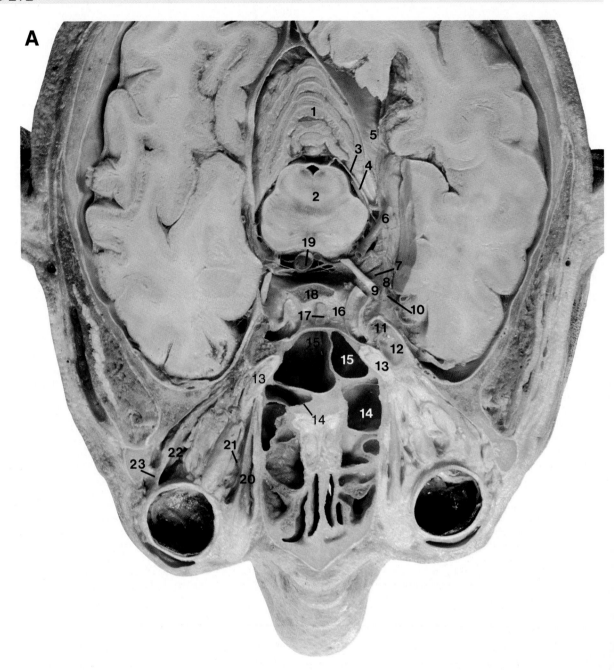

A

1
5
3
4
2
6
19
7
8
18
9
17   16   10
11
12
15   15   13
13
14   14
22
23   21
20

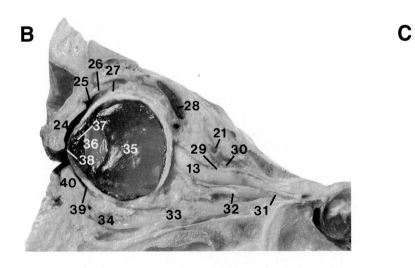

B

26   27
25   28
24   37
36   35
38   21
29   30
13
40   32   31
39   33
34

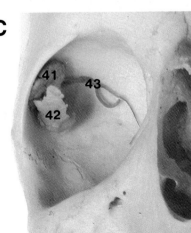

C

41   43
42

ORBIT AND EYE
Orbital contents III
The eyes in section and the lacrimal gland

A Transverse section through the orbits and the nasal and cranial cavities, from above

B Sagittal section through the right orbit, from the left

C An isolated right lacrimal gland, replaced within the orbit, from the left and below

D The anterior half of an eye sectioned through the equator, from behind (enlarged)

E The section in D with the lens removed and placed at the side (enlarged)

In A the section has passed through the eyes just above the optic nerves (13) which, at the back of the orbits, lie immediately adjacent to the sphenoidal sinuses (15) and the most posterior ethmoidal air cells (14).

In B the vertically-sectioned eye shows the extent of the conjunctival fornices (25 and 39) with the lids almost closed (24 and 40).

In C the right lacrimal gland has been dissected free from all other structures apart from the lacrimal artery and nerve (43), to emphasise its position in the upper outer corner of the front of the orbit.

In D and E (enlarged) the eye has been sectioned through the equator, i.e. in the coronal plane, and the front half is viewed from behind. In D the lens (49) is in place, and in E it has been removed and placed at one side to show the margin of the pupil (51) and the posterior surface of the cornea (52).

• The *lacrimal gland* has an upper (larger) orbital part (C41) and a lower (smaller) palpebral part (C42), continuous with each other round the lateral (concave) border of the aponeurosis of levator palpebrae superioris.

The orbital part lies in the lacrimal fossa of the frontal bone (page 38, B13), above the levator (page 120, A1).

The palpebral part lies below the levator and extends into the lateral part of the upper eyelid (page 118, C46).

About 12 small ducts open into the superior conjunctival fornix (B25)—those from the orbital part passing through the palpebral part.

The pathway for lacrimal gland secretion: from the superior salivary nucleus by the nervus intermedius part of the facial nerve, greater petrosal nerve and nerve of the pterygoid canal to the pterygoplalatine ganglion (synapse), and then to the gland by the maxillary nerve, its zygomatic branch and the communication with the lacrimal nerve.

• The tarsi are plates of dense fibrous tissue within each eyelid.

1 Cerebellum	**17** Pituitary stalk	**35** Vitreous humour
2 Junction of pons and midbrain	**18** Dorsum sellae	**36** Lens
3 Trochlear nerve	**19** Basilar artery	**37** Anterior chamber
4 Superior cerebellar artery	**20** Medial rectus	**38** Cornea
5 Tentorium cerebelli	**21** Ophthalmic artery	**39** Inferior conjunctival fornix
6 Posterior cerebral artery	**22** Lateral rectus	**40** Inferior tarsus in lower eyelid
7 Attached margin of tentorium cerebelli	**23** Lateral check ligament	**41** Orbital part ⎫ of lacrimal gland
	24 Superior tarsus in upper eyelid	**42** Palpebral part ⎭
8 Roof of cavernous sinus	**25** Superior conjunctival fornix	**43** Lacrimal artery and nerve
9 Oculomotor nerve	**26** Levator palpebrae superioris	**44** Retina (optic part)
10 Free margin of tentorium cerebelli	**27** Tendon of superior rectus	**45** Choroid
11 Anterior clinoid process	**28** Superior ophthalmic vein	**46** Sclera
12 Extension of posterior ethmoidal air cell into lesser wing of sphenoid bone	**29** Dural sheath of optic nerve	**47** Ora serrata
	30 Nasociliary nerve	**48** Ciliary part of retina
13 Optic nerve	**31** Central artery of retina	**49** Posterior surface of lens
14 Posterior ethmoidal air cell	**32** Inferior ophthalmic vein	**50** Ciliary processes
15 Sphenoidal sinus	**33** Inferior rectus	**51** Margin of pupil
16 Diaphragma sellae	**34** Inferior oblique	**52** Posterior surface of cornea

D

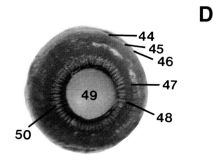

E

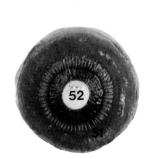
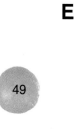

NOSE AND PARANASAL SINUSES

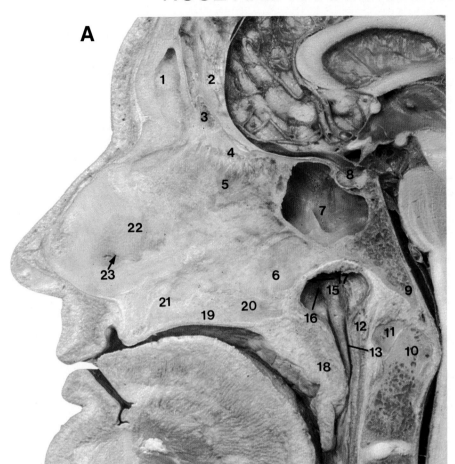

A

NASAL CAVITY
The nasal cartilages and the nasal cavity
A The nasal septum, from the left
B The skeleton of the external nose
C The lateral wall of the left nasal cavity and
   nasopharynx
D As C, with a supreme nasal concha

In A the nasal septum is intact, while in C it has been removed to show the lateral wall of the nasal cavity with the conchae (44, 42 and 40), each with an underlying meatus (43, 41 and 39). The specimen in D shows the occasional supreme concha and meatus (46 and 47). The upper bony and lower cartilaginous parts of the external nose are illustrated in B.

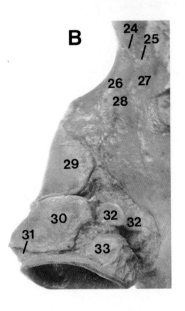

B

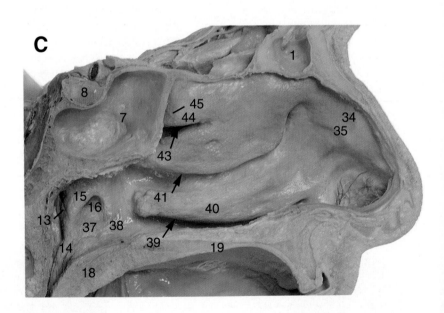

C

• The nose consists of the external nose (on the face) and the nasal cavity. The cavity is divided into right and left halves by the nasal septum, and each half contains olfactory, vestibular and respiratory parts, depending on the type of mucous membrane present. The olfactory part occupies the area over the superior concha on the lateral wall, and the adjacent parts of the roof and of the septum level with the superior concha; it contains olfactory nerve endings as well as fibres for ordinary sensation. The vestibular part is the small area just inside the nostril, and is lined by hairy skin. The large remaining area is the respiratory part, lined by respiratory mucous membrane with pseudostratified columnar ciliated epithelium and mucous glands.

• The main parts of the skeleton of the external nose are the nasal bone (B26), and the lateral, greater and lesser nasal cartilages (B29, 30 and 32).

• The main parts of the nasal septum are the vomer (A6) and the perpendicular plate of the ethmoid (A5), both of bone, and the septal cartilage (A22).

• The nasal conchae are on the lateral wall of the cavity. The superior and middle nasal conchae are part of the ethmoid bone (page 40, C12 and 10); the inferior nasal concha is a separate bone (page 48, G–J).

1 Frontal sinus	16 Opening of auditory tube	32 Lesser alar cartilages
2 Falx cerebri	17 Right choana (posterior nasal aperture)	33 Fibrofattty tissue
3 Crista galli		34 Atrium
4 Cribriform plate of ethmoid bone and filaments of olfactory nerve	18 Soft palate	35 Agger nasi
	19 Hard palate	36 Vestibule
5 Perpendicular plate of ethmoid bone	20 Nasal crest of palatine bone	37 Levator elevation
	21 Nasal crest of maxilla	38 Salpingopalatal fold
6 Vomer	22 Septal cartilage	39 Inferior meatus
7 Sphenoidal sinus	23 Vomeronasal organ	40 Inferior nasal concha
8 Pituitary gland	24 Frontonasal suture	41 Middle meatus
9 Anterior margin of foramen magnum	25 Frontomaxillary suture	42 Middle nasal concha
	26 Nasal bone	43 Superior meatus
10 Dens of axis	27 Frontal process of maxilla	44 Superior nasal concha
11 Anterior arch of atlas	28 Nasomaxillary suture	45 Spheno-ethmoidal recess
12 Pharyngeal tonsil	29 Lateral nasal cartilage	46 Supreme nasal concha
13 Pharyngeal recess	30 Greater nasal cartilage	47 Supreme meatus
14 Salpingopharyngeal fold	31 Septal process (medial crus) of greater nasal cartilage	
15 Tubal elevation		

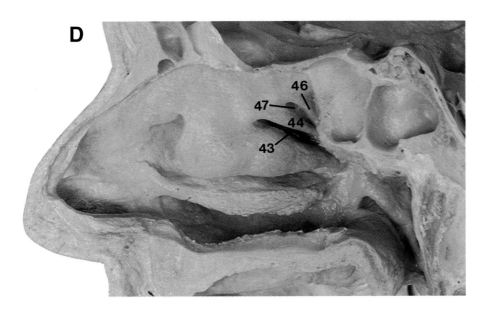

D

NASAL CAVITY
The walls of the nasal cavity
A The left lateral wall
B The left lateral wall and semilunar hiatus
C The left lateral wall and apertures of sinuses
D The right lateral wall and nasal nerves

In cutting the section in A the superior nasal concha and the upper part of the middle concha have been shaved off. The opening of the maxillary sinus (4) is unusually low and large.

In B the middle concha has been removed to show the semilunar hiatus (12) bounded above by the ethmoidal bulla (11) and below by the ridge caused by the uncinate process of the ethmoid bone (14) (compare with page 32, D61 and 46). Removal of the front part of the inferior concha (5) reveals the opening of the nasolacrimal duct (17).

In C parts of all three nasal conchae have been removed to show an ethmoidal air cell aperture (24), the frontonasal duct (19) and the nasolacrimal duct (20).

In D mucous membrane high on the lateral wall has been dissected away to show filaments of the olfactory nerve (25) and the anterior ethmoidal nerve (32). Some bone at the back of the lateral wall has been removed to display the pterygopalatine ganglion (27), seen in the pterygopalatine fossa by looking through the sphenopalatine foramen (26), with the greater palatine nerve (29) running down from the ganglion, and other nasal nerves passing forwards (28 and 30).

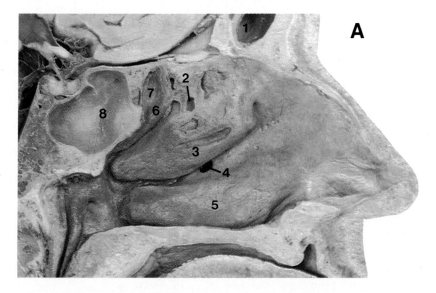

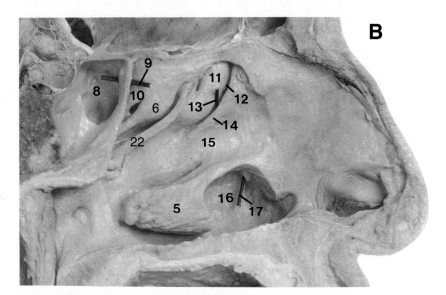

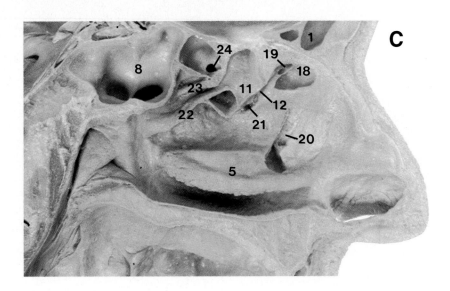

1 Frontal sinus
2 A middle ethmoidal air cell
3 Middle nasal concha
4 Unusually low aperture of maxillary sinus
5 Inferior nasal concha
6 Superior nasal concha
7 Spheno-ethmoidal recess
8 Sphenoidal sinus
9 Bristle in aperture of sphenoidal sinus
10 Supreme nasal concha
11 Ethmoidal bulla
12 Semilunar hiatus
13 Bristle in aperture of maxillary sinus
14 Mucous membrane overlying uncinate process of ethmoid bone
15 Middle meatus
16 Inferior meatus
17 Bristle in opening of nasolacrimal duct
18 An anterior ethmoidal air cell
19 Frontonasal duct
20 Lower end of nasolacrimal duct
21 Aperture of maxillary sinus
22 Base of middle nasal concha
23 Base of superior nasal concha
24 Aperture of a posterior ethmoidal air cell
25 Olfactory nerve filaments
26 Sphenopalatine artery and foramen
27 Pterygopalatine ganglion
28 A lateral posterior superior nasal nerve
29 Greater palatine nerve and canal
30 A posterior inferior nasal nerve
31 Vestibule of nose
32 Anterior ethmoidal nerve

• For details of the sinuses see pages 130–133.
• Drainage of the sinuses:
  Frontal sinus—into the middle meatus by the frontonasal duct (C19)
  Ethmoidal sinus—anterior ethmoidal air cells into the frontonasal duct or the infundibulum (the upward anterior continuation of the semilunar hiatus, B12); middle ethmoidal air cells on or above the ethmoidal bulla in the middle meatus (B11); and posterior ethmoidal air cells into the superior meatus (C24)
  Sphenoidal sinus—into the spheno-ethmoidal recess (B9 and A7)
  Maxillary sinus—into the semilunar hiatus in the middle meatus (B13 and C21)
• Drainage into the meatuses:
  Superior meatus—posterior ethmoidal air cells (C24)
  Middle meatus—frontal sinus (C1 and 19), anterior and middle ethmoidal air cells (A2), and the maxillary sinus (C21)
  Inferior meatus—nasolacrimal duct (C20)
  Spheno-ethmoidal recess—sphenoidal sinus (B8)

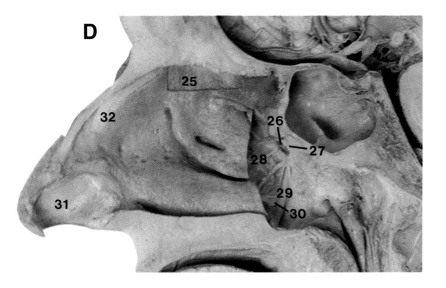

D

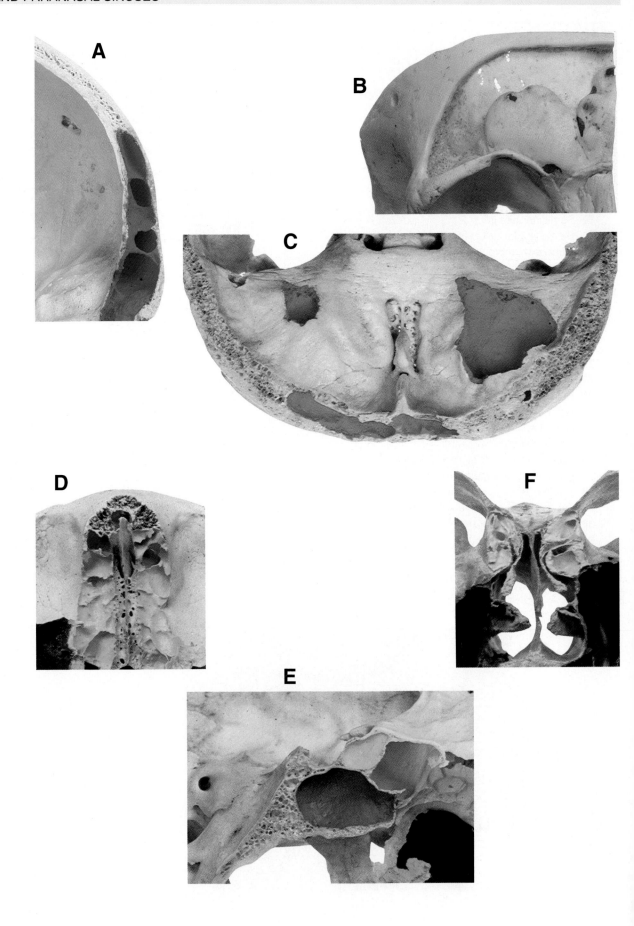

PARANASAL SINUSES

The frontal and ethmoidal sinuses, in sections of parts of the skull
A A large left frontal sinus in sagittal section, from the right
B A right frontal sinus dissected out of the diplöe, from the front
C Large frontal sinuses opened from above
D The roof of the ethmoidal sinuses, from below
E A midline sagittal section through the base of the skull, with
   unusually large left posterior ethmoidal air cells
F The ethmoidal sinuses in coronal section, from the front

In A the frontal sinus has extended far up into the squamous part of the frontal bone

In B the front of the skull and diplöe have been dissected away to show the bony wall of a sinus.

In C parts of the floor of the anterior cranial fossa have been removed to show frontal sinuses extending far back in the orbital part of the frontal bone (over the roof of the orbit).

In D the cribriform plates of the ethmoid bone (in the roof of the nose, with many foramina) are seen adjacent to air cells of the ethmoidal sinuses, whose roofs are formed by the orbital parts of the frontal bone (compare with page 38, B19). In the left sinus some anterior ethmoidal air cells lie in front of the lowest part of the frontal sinus (red).

In E, a midline sagittal section, two large posterior ethmoidal air cells overlap the left sphenoidal sinus (blue).

In F, a coronal section through the centre of the nasal and orbital cavities and looking from the front towards the back of the skull, the middle nasal conchae (brown) on each side overlaps the bulging ethmoidal air cell that forms the ethmoidal bulla (compare with page 40, F13)

Red:	**frontal sinus**
Yellow:	**ethmoidal sinus**
Dark blue:	**sphenoidal sinus**
Green:	**maxillary sinus**
Brown:	**middle nasal concha**
Light blue:	**inferior nasal concha**

• There are four pairs of *paranasal air sinuses*: frontal, ethmoidal, sphenoidal and maxillary. The two of each pair (left and right) are rarely symmetrical and vary greatly in size and shape.

• The *frontal sinus* lies in the lower part of the squamous part of the frontal bone (as in B), and may extend higher into the squamous part (as in A) and back into the orbital part of the bone (as in C). It drains into the middle meatus by the frontonasal duct (page 128, C19).

The *ethmoidal sinus* occupies the body of the ethmoid bone (ethmoidal labyrinth, page 40, A1). It is divided by bony septa into a number of ethmoidal air cells (three to eighteen). The posterior ethmoidal air cells drain into the superior meatus (page 128, C24), and the middle and anterior air cells into the middle meatus (see notes on page 129). The thin lateral wall of the ethmoidal labyrinth (page 40, E8) forms part of the medial wall of the orbit (page 59, D and E, 20). The medial wall of the labyrinth has the superior and middle nasal conchae projecting from it (page 40, C and D, 10 and 12).

• For the sphenoidal and maxillary sinuses see pages 132 and 133.

• For a summary of the drainage of the sinuses see page 129.

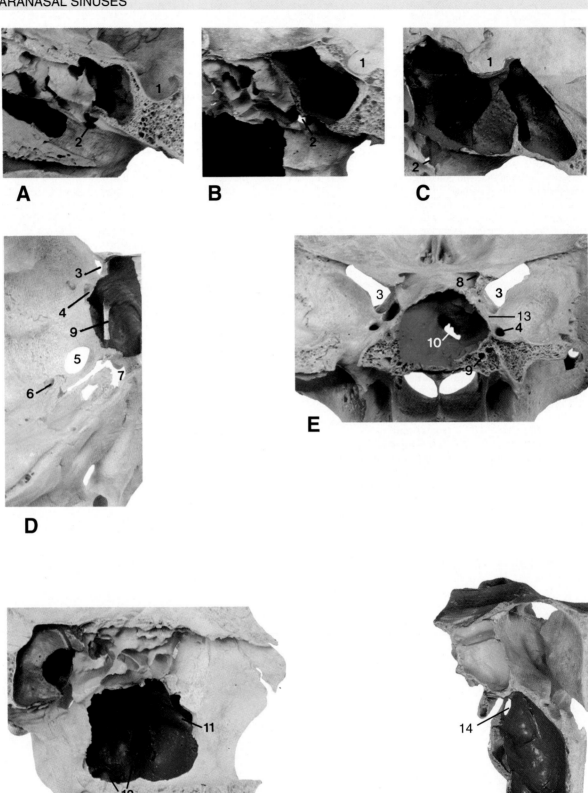

PARANASAL SINUSES
The sphenoidal and maxillary sinuses, in sections of parts of the skull

A A small right sphenoidal sinus, in a midline sagittal section, from the left

B A medium-sized right sphenoidal sinus, sectioned as in A

C A large right sphenoidal sinus, sectioned as in A

D The floor of the left sphenoidal sinus, from above

E Sphenoidal sinuses in coronal section, from behind

F A left maxillary sinus, from the right with the medial wall removed

G A left maxillary sinus in coronal section, from the front

H A left maxillary sinus in coronal section, from behind

J A small right maxillary sinus in coronal section, from the front

Small sphenoidal sinuses (as in A) usually lie in front of the pituitary fossa (1), with larger ones extending below the fossa (as in B) and even backwards into the basisphenoid (as in C). In D a large left sinus has been opened up from above and part of the floor dissected away to show the pterygoid canal (9), which lies below the floor; compare with the section of the right sinus in E. In the coronal section in E there is a large right sinus with its aperture visible at the front (10), and a very small left sinus, seen level with the medial end of the superior orbital fissure (3). In F the maxillary sinus shows indentations of the bony wall produced by the roots of molar teeth (12), and by the infra-orbital canal (11) whose relation to the roof of the sinus is shown in the coronal section H. In G and H the sinus extends into the alveolar process of the maxilla (15), but the smaller sinus in J has not done so. The section in G shows the aperture of the sinus, high up on the medial wall (14).

Yellow:	ethmoidal sinus
Dark blue:	sphenoidal sinus
Green:	maxillary sinus
Brown:	middle nasal concha
Light blue:	inferior nasal concha

1	Pituitary fossa
2	Sphenopalatine foramen
3	Superior orbital fissure
4	Foramen rotundum
5	Foramen ovale
6	Foramen spinosum
7	Foramen lacerum
8	Optic canal
9	Pterygoid canal
10	Aperture of sphenoidal sinus
11	Projection of infra-orbital canal
12	Elevation over molar tooth
13	Carotid groove
14	Aperture of maxillary sinus
15	Alveolar process of maxilla

• The *sphenoidal sinuses* (left and right) occupy the body of the sphenoid bone (page 42, A14). Although adjacent they do not normally communicate with one another. Large sinuses may be indented by the pituitary gland in the pituitary fossa (C1; page 28, A14; page 158, 50); by the optic nerve in the optic canal (E8; page 28, A19; page 168, 4); by the internal carotid artery in the carotid groove (E8; page 28, A17; page 166, C38); by the maxillary nerve in the foramen rotundum (E4; page 29, B50; page 142, A2); and by the pterygoid canal with its nerve (D9; page 42, A18; page 142, A6). Each sinus drains into the spheno-ethmoidal recess of its own side (page 128, B9).

• The *maxillary sinus* occupies the body of the maxilla (page 46, C25); a large sinus may extend into the zygomatic and alveolar processes. Its medial wall forms much of the lateral wall of the nasal cavity (page 62). The roof is indented by the infra-orbital canal (F and H, 11), and the floor by some molar tooth roots (F12), and even by premolar or canine roots, especially if the sinus invades the alveolar process (as in G and H). The sinus drains into the semilunar hiatus of the middle meatus (page 128, C21), by an aperture which is high in the medial wall of the sinus (G14).

• Infection in the frontal or ethmoidal sinuses may become transferred to the maxillary sinus, because they all drain into the semilunar hiatus (page 128, C12) and infected fluid from the first two can gravitate into the maxillary aperture (page 128, C21).

• For a summary of the drainage of the sinuses see page 129.

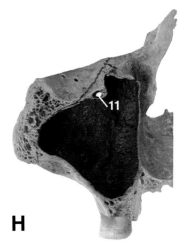

H

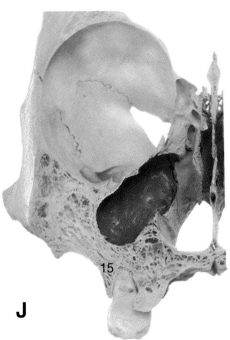

J

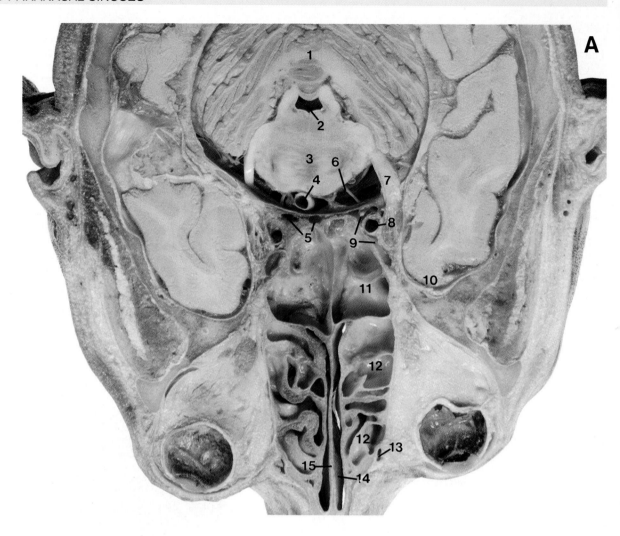

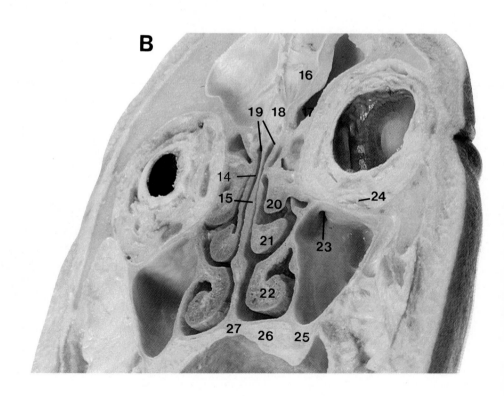

1 Cerebellum
2 Upper part of fourth ventricle
3 Pons
4 Basilar artery
5 Basilar sinus
6 Abducent nerve
7 Trigeminal nerve
8 Internal carotid artery
9 Cavernous sinus
10 Temporal pole
11 Sphenoidal sinus
12 Ethmoidal air cells
13 Nasolacrimal duct
14 Nasal cavity
15 Nasal septum
16 Dura mater of anterior wall of anterior cranial fossa
17 Frontal sinus
18 Crista galli
19 Roof of nasal cavity
20 Superior ⎫
21 Middle   ⎬ nasal concha
22 Inferior ⎭
23 Aperture of maxillary sinus
24 Infra-orbital nerve
25 Alveolar process ⎫
               ⎬ of maxilla
26 Palatine process ⎭
27 Hard palate
28 Olfactory nerve filaments
29 Nasopalatine nerve
30 Incisive canal
31 Anterior ethmoidal nerve

PARANASAL SINUSES AND NASAL SEPTUM
Transverse and coronal sections and nerves of the nasal septum
A Transverse section of the head, at the level of the palpebral fissures, from above
B Oblique coronal section of the head, at the level of the eyes, from the right, behind and below
C Nerves of the left side of the nasal septum

The sections in A and B illustrate the narrowness of the roof (B19) and upper parts of the nasal cavities on either side of the septum (A and B, 14 and 15). The slightly oblique coronal section in B has been orientated so that, looking forwards from below and behind, the aperture of the right maxillary sinus (23) can be seen high up on the medial wall of the sinus.

In C parts of the mucous membrane of the septum have been removed to show the principal nerves: olfactory (28), anterior ethmoidal (31) and nasopalatine (29).

• The narrowness of the roof and upper part of the nasal cavity (A14; B14 and 19), only a millimeter or two wide, should be compared with the floor (B26) which is over a centimeter wide.

• Nerves of the nasal septum:
  Olfactory—over an area opposite the superior nasal concha (C28)
  Anterior ethmoidal—to the anterior part (C31)
  Medial posterior superior nasal—to a small area of the posterior part
  Nasopalatine—to the posterior part (C29)

• Nerves of the lateral wall of the nose:
  Olfactory—over the superior nasal concha (and the narrow roof also) (page 129, D25)
  Infra-orbital—to the skin of the vestibule (page 129, D31)
  Anterior ethmoidal—to the anterior part (page 129, D32)
  Nasal branch of the anterior superior nasal—to a small part of the inferior meatus
  Lateral posterior superior nasal—to the upper posterior part (page 129, D28)
  Posterior inferior nasal—to the lower posterior part (page 129, D30)

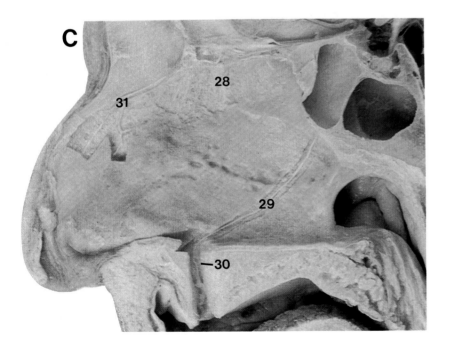

C

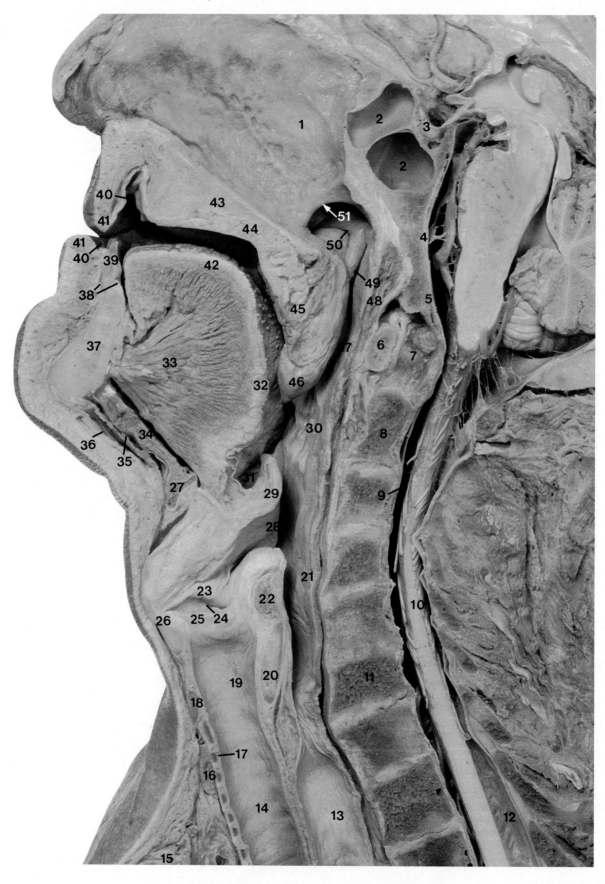

MOUTH, PALATE, PHARYNX AND LARYNX
A sagittal section through the head and neck, from the left

The section is just to the left of the midline (showing the whole of the dens of the axis, 7), and the head is tilted slightly backwards (extended). The hard palate (43) forms the floor of the nose and roof of the mouth, and is on approximately the same level as the foramen magnum (5). The soft palate (45) with the uvula at its lower end (46) hangs down from the back of the hard palate (43). The geniohyoid and mylohyoid muscles (34 and 35) form the floor of the mouth. The opening of the auditory tube (50) is in the nasal part of the pharynx, behind the choana (51), with the pharyngeal tonsil (48) on the posterior wall. Behind the tongue (32) the mouth opens into the oral part of the pharynx (30). Below and behind the epiglottis (29) the larynx opens into the laryngeal part of the pharynx (28 and 21).

• The *mouth* or oral cavity consists of the vestibule (40) and the oral cavity proper.

• The vestibule of the mouth is the narrow space bounded on the outer side by the lips and cheeks, and inside by the gingivae (gums) and teeth.

• The oral cavity proper is bounded at each side and in front by the alveolar arches with the teeth and gingivae; at the back it communicates with the oral part of the pharynx (30) by the oropharyngeal isthmus which lies between the palatoglossal arches (page 138, B22). The (palatine) tonsils, which lie behind the palatoglossal arches (page 138, B21), are therefore in the oral part of the pharynx, not in the mouth.

• The *pharynx* extends from the base of the skull (5) to the level of C6 vertebra (11), a distance of about 12 cm.

• The nasal part (nasopharynx, 47) extends as far down as the lower border of the soft palate (45 and 46). It contains the opening of the auditory tube and the pharyngeal recess laterally (50 and 49), the pharyngeal tonsil on the posterior wall (48), and opens anteriorly into the nasal cavity through the posterior nasal apertures (choanae, 51)

• The oral part (oropharynx, 30), between the soft palate (45 and 46) and the upper border of the epiglottis (29), contains the palatine tonsil and the palatopharyngeal arch in its lateral wall (here obscured by 46), and opens anteriorly into the mouth through the oropharyngeal isthmus (palatoglossal arches).

• The laryngeal part (laryngopharynx, 21) extends from the upper border of the epiglottis (29) to the lower border of the cricoid cartilage (20, level with C6 vertebra, 11), and is continuous below with the oesophagus (13). The larynx projects backwards into the laryngo-pharynx, with a piriform recess on either side (page 156, A4).

• *Muscles of the tongue*
 Extrinsic muscles (attached to structures outside the tongue): genioglossus (the largest), hyoglossus, styloglossus, and palatoglossus. They can alter the shape of the tongue and move it bodily.
 Intrinsic muscles (within the tongue): longitudinal (superior and inferior), transverse and vertical. They can alter the shape of the tongue without moving it bodily.

• *Muscles of the soft palate*
Palatoglossus, palatopharyngeus, tensor veli palatini, levator veli palatini and the muscle of the uvula.

• *Muscles of the pharynx*
Three constrictors and three others: superior, middle and inferior constrictors, palatopharyngeus, stylopharyngeus and salpingopharyngeus.

• *Ligaments or membranes associated with the pharynx*:
Pharyngeal raphe, stylohyoid ligament, pterygomandibular raphe.

• *Layers of the pharynx*:
Mucous membrane, submucous layer (including the pharyngobasilar fascia at the upper end), muscular layer, and buccopharyngeal fascia.

• *Gaps associated with the constrictors and the structures passing through the gaps*:
 Above the superior constrictor—auditory tube and ascending palatine artery (piercing pharyngobasilar fascia).
 Between superior and middle constrictors—stylopharyngeus passing down between the constrictors, and the lingual and glossopharyngeal nerves.
 Between middle and inferior constrictors—internal laryngeal nerve and superior laryngeal vessels (piercing thyrohyoid membrane).
 Below inferior constrictor: recurrent laryngeal nerve and inferior laryngeal vessels.

• The hyoid bone (27) lies at the level of C3 vertebra.

• The thyroid cartilage (26) lies at the level of C4 and C5 vertebrae.

• The cricoid cartilage (18 and 20) lies at the level of C6 vertebra (11).

• The isthmus of the thyroid gland (16) overlies tracheal rings 2-4 (17).

• When enlarged the lymphoid tissue of the pharyngeal tonsil (48) is known as the adenoids.

• The piriform recesses are often called the piriform fossae.

1 Nasal septum	18 Arch of cricoid cartilage	35 Mylohyoid
2 Sphenoidal sinus	19 Lower part of larynx	36 Platysma
3 Pituitary gland	20 Lamina of cricoid cartilage	37 Body of mandible
4 Clivus	21 Laryngeal part of pharynx	38 Gingiva
5 Anterior margin of foramen magnum	22 Transverse arytenoid muscle	39 Left lower central incisor tooth
6 Anterior arch of atlas	23 Vestibular fold	40 Vestibule of mouth
7 Dens of axis	24 Ventricle of larynx	41 Lip
8 Body of axis	25 Vocal fold (vocal cord)	42 Presulcal part of dorsum of tongue
9 Spinal subarachnoid space	26 Lamina of thyroid cartilage	43 Hard palate
10 Spinal cord	27 Body of hyoid bone	44 Palatal glands in mucoperiosteum
11 Body of sixth cervical vertebra	28 Aryepiglottic fold and inlet of larynx	45 Soft palate
12 Subarachnoid septum	29 Epiglottis and epiglottic cartilage	46 Uvula
13 Oesophagus	30 Oral part of pharynx	47 Nasal part of pharynx
14 Trachea	31 Vallecula	48 Pharyngeal tonsil
15 Jugular notch of manubrium of sternum	32 Postsulcal part of dorsum of tongue	49 Pharyngeal recess
16 Isthmus of thyroid gland	33 Genioglossus	50 Opening of auditory tube
17 Second tracheal ring	34 Geniohyoid	51 Posterior nasal aperture (choana)

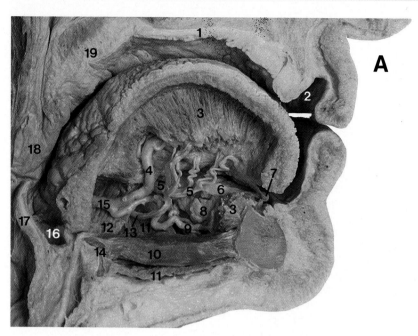

A

TONGUE AND FLOOR OF MOUTH
Dissections of the tongue and surface features
A **Deep dissection of the left half of the tongue, from the right**
B **The left half of the mouth with the tongue removed, from the right**
C **The tongue from above, with the inlet (aditus) of the larynx**

In A and B left-sided structures are viewed from the right. In A much of the tongue musculature has been removed to show the lingual artery (15) dividing into its two tortuous main branches (the deep lingual and sublingual arteries, 4 and 9), and branches of the lingual and hypoglossal nerves (5 and 13).

With the whole tongue removed in B, the lingual nerve (5) is seen coming down from above to hook under the submandibular duct (6). Lower down, the lingual artery (15) and hypoglossal nerve (13) are separated by the (cut end of) hyoglossus (12); as viewed from its own side, the nerve runs superficial to the muscle and the artery deep to it (compare with page 144, A25 and 29).

Looking down on the tongue in C, the V-shaped line of vallate papillae (47) lie just in front of the sulcus terminalis (46). The valleculae (16) are in front of the epiglottis (17), and behind it is the laryngeal inlet with a view (at a lower level) of the vestibular and vocal folds (41 and 40). For details of the larynx see pages 154–157.

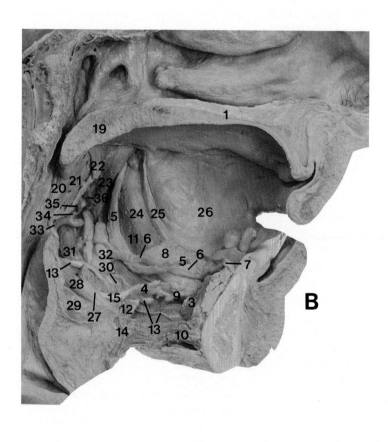

B

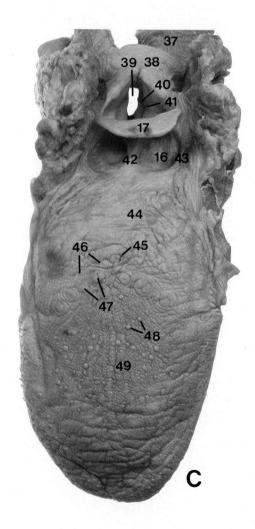

C

1 Hard palate
2 Vestibule of mouth
3 Genioglossus (anterior part)
4 Deep lingual artery
5 Lingual nerve
6 Submandibular duct
7 Orifice of submandibular duct on sublingual papilla
8 Sublingual gland
9 Sublingual artery
10 Geniohyoid
11 Mylohyoid
12 Hyoglossus
13 Hypoglossal nerve
14 Body of hyoid bone
15 Lingual artery
16 Vallecula
17 Epiglottis
18 Oral part of pharynx
19 Soft palate
20 Palatopharyngeal arch
21 Tonsil
22 Upper end of palatoglossal arch
23 Medial pterygoid
24 Upper border of body of edentulous mandible
25 Cut edge of mucous membrane
26 Mucous membrane overlying buccinator
27 Lower end of stylohyoid ligament
28 Middle constrictor of pharynx
29 Greater horn of hyoid bone
30 Vena comitans of hypoglossal nerve
31 Stylohyoid
32 Deep part of submandibular gland
33 Facial artery
34 Ascending palatine artery
35 External palatine (paratonsillar) vein
36 Styloglossus
37 Posterior wall of pharynx
38 Posterior wall of larynx
39 Rima of glottis
40 Vocal fold
41 Vestibular fold
42 Median glosso-epiglottic fold
43 Lateral glosso-epiglottic fold
44 Postsulcal part of dorsum of tongue
45 Foramen caecum
46 Sulcus terminalis
47 Vallate papillae
48 Fungiform papillae
49 Presulcal part of dorsum of tongue

• All the muscles of the tongue (page 137) are supplied by the hypoglossal nerve (A and B, 13), except palatoglossus, which is supplied by the pharyngeal plexus.

• The mucous membrane of the presulcal part (anterior two-thirds) of the tongue (C49) is supplied by the lingual nerve (ordinary sensation) with chorda tympani (facial nerve) fibres (which joined the lingual nerve in the infratemporal fossa) supplying taste buds.

• The mucous membrane of the postsulcal part (posterior one-third) of the tongue (C44) (but including the vallate papillae, C47, which lie in front of the sulcus terminalis, C46) is supplied by the glossopharyngeal nerve (ordinary sensation and taste).

• The mucous membrane of the part of the tongue that forms the front wall of the vallecula (C16) is supplied (like that of the rest of the vallecula) by the internal laryngeal branch of the vagus nerve.

• The cell bodies of the taste fibres in the chorda tympani are in the genicular ganglion of the facial nerve; of those in the glossopharyngeal nerve, in the glossopharyngeal ganglia; and of those in the internal laryngeal nerve (for taste buds in the palate) in the inferior vagal ganglion. The central fibres from all these ganglia converge to synapse with the cell bodies of the nucleus of the tractus solitarius.

• The *sublingual gland* (B8) lies beneath the mucous membrane of the floor of the mouth, contacting the sublingual fossa of the mandible (above the mylohyoid line—page 34, C23; page 140, D70). Important relations include:
 above—mucous membrane of the floor of the mouth (B25)
 below—mylohyoid (B11)
 in front—sublingual gland of the opposite side
 behind—deep part of the submandibular gland (B32)
 laterally—sublingual fossa of the mandible (above the mylohyoid line (page 34, C23)
 medially—genioglossus (page 140, B52) with the lingual nerve and the submandibular duct intervening (B5 and 6)

• Up to 20 small sublingual ducts open separately in the floor of the mouth on the summit of the sublingual fold (page 140, B56), but some of them may open instead into the submandibular duct (page 140, B48).

• The pathway for submandibular and sublingual gland secretion: from the superior salivary nucleus by the nervus intermedius part of the facial nerve, chorda tympani and lingual nerve to the submandibular ganglion (synapse) and then to the glands by lingual nerve filaments.

• For notes on the parotid gland see page 113 and on the submandibular gland see page 141.

• The foramen caecum (C45) marks the position of the upper end of the thyroglossal duct and the thyroid diverticulum, the embryonic outgrowth from which the thyroid gland develops.

• The pyramidal lobe of the thyroid gland (page 102, C68) represents a differentiation of part of the remains of the thyroglossal duct. A fibrous or fibromuscular band may connect the lobe or isthmus to the hyoid bone; if muscular, it constitutes the levator of the thyroid gland. Parts of the duct may persist to form thyroglossal cysts or aberrant masses of thyroid tissue: for example, a lingual thyroid within the tongue.

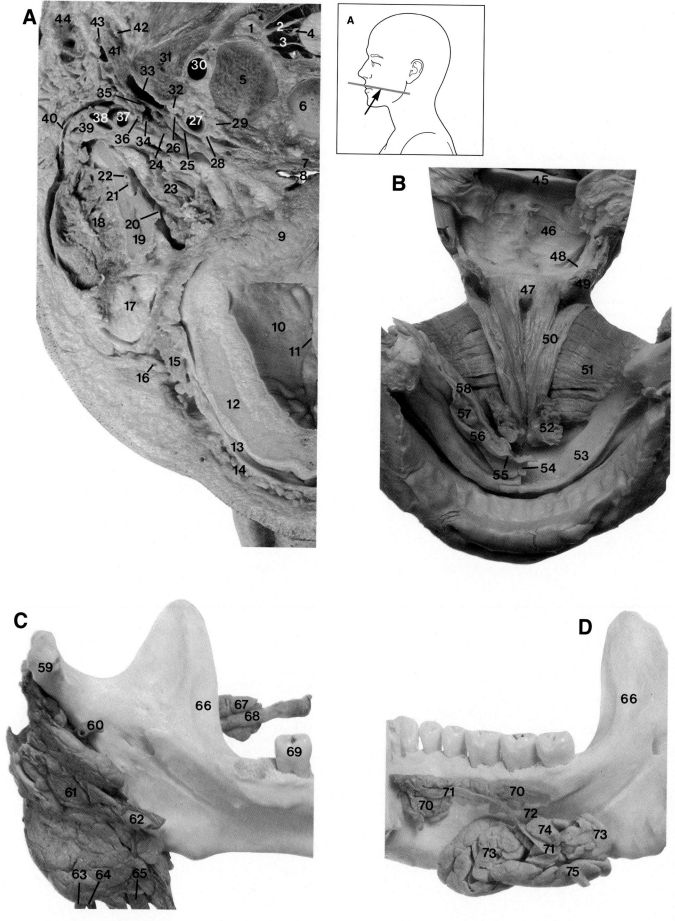

MOUTH AND SALIVARY GLANDS

The roof and floor of the mouth and the salivary glands

A A transverse section of the left half of the head, from below
B The floor of the mouth after removal of the tongue, from above
C The left parotid gland and the mandible, from the medial side
D The right sublingual and submandibular glands and the mandible, from the medial side

In A the section has passed through the alveolar process of the maxilla (12) and about halfway up the ramus of the mandible (19), at the level of the opening of the mandibular foramen containing the inferior alveolar nerve and artery (21 and 22). The lingual nerve (20) is outside the foramen and 1 cm in front of it. The parotid gland (39), C-shaped in horizontal section, clasps the ramus of the mandible (19), which has the masseter on its outer side (18), and the medial pterygoid on the inner side (23).

In B the tongue has been removed so that the floor of the mouth (mylohyoid, 51, and geniohyoid, 50) can be viewed from above

In C and D, isolated salivary glands (61, 73 and 70) have been laid in their proper positions in relation to the mandible.

• The *submandibular gland* has a large superficial and a small deep part (D73 and 74), continuous round the posterior border of mylohyoid.

The superficial part lies in the digastric triangle (page 96, 46). Important relations include:

below—skin, platysma, investing layer of deep cervical fascia, facial vein, cervical branch of the facial nerve, submandibular lymph nodes
laterally—submandibular fossa of the mandible (below the mylohyoid line, page 34, C22), insertion of medial pterygoid, facial artery
medially—mylohyoid muscle, nerve and vessels, lingual nerve and submandibular ganglion, hypoglossal nerve, deep lingual vein, hyoglossus

The deep part of the gland lies on hyoglossus (page 144, A26) with the lingual nerve above, and the hypoglossal nerve and submandibular duct below (page 144, A7, 25 and 21). For secretion see page 139.

• The submandibular duct is 5 cm long. It emerges from the superficial part of the gland (D71) near the posterior border of mylohyoid and passes forward between mylohyoid and hyoglossus and then between the sublingual gland and genioglossus. It opens in the floor of the mouth on the sublingual papilla (B55) at the side of the frenulum of the tongue (B54).

1	Dorsal root ganglion	38	Retromandibular vein
2	Dorsal root (of second cervical nerve)	39	Parotid gland
3	Ventral root	40	A zygomatic branch of facial nerve
4	Spinal root of accessory nerve	41	Posterior belly of digastric
5	Lateral mass of atlas	42	Accessory nerve (spinal part)
6	Dens of axis	43	Occipital artery
7	Superior constrictor of pharynx	44	Sternocleidomastoid
8	Nasal part of pharynx	45	Epiglottis
9	Soft palate	46	Vallecula
10	Hard palate	47	Body (of hyoid bone)
11	Palatal raphe	48	Greater horn
12	Alveolar process of maxilla	49	Hyoglossus
13	Vestibule of mouth	50	Geniohyoid
14	Labial glands	51	Mylohyoid
15	Buccinator	52	Genioglossus
16	Facial artery	53	Edentulous body of mandible
17	Buccal fat pad	54	Frenulum of tongue
18	Masseter	55	Sublingual papilla
19	Ramus of mandible	56	Sublingual fold
20	Lingual nerve	57	Sublingual gland
21	Inferior alveolar nerve	58	Submandibular duct
22	Inferior alveolar artery	59	Condylar process of mandible
23	Medial pterygoid	60	Maxillary artery
24	Styloglossus	61	Parotid gland
25	Stylopharyngeus	62	External carotid artery
26	Glossopharyngeal nerve	63	Great auricular nerve
27	Internal carotid artery	64	Posterior division (of retromandibular vein)
28	Hypoglossal nerve	65	Anterior division
29	Superior cervical sympathetic ganglion	66	Ramus of mandible
30	Vertebral artery	67	Accessory parotid gland
31	Transverse process of atlas	68	Parotid duct
32	Vagus nerve	69	Lower seond molar tooth
33	Internal jugular vein	70	Sublingual gland
34	Stylohyoid ligament	71	Submandibular duct
35	Stylohyoid	72	Mylohyoid line of body of mandible
36	Posterior auricular artery	73	Superficial part (of submandibular gland)
37	External carotid artery	74	Deep part
		75	Facial artery

141

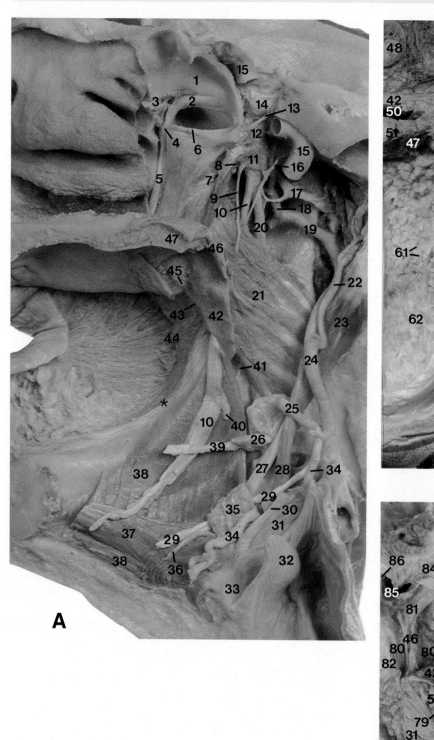

A

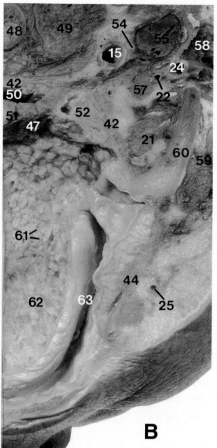

B

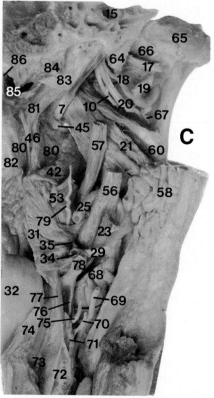

C

MOUTH AND PALATE IN SECTIONS
The inside of the mouth and adjacent structures
A The right half of the mouth, from the left
B Transverse section of the left half of the roof of the mouth, from below
C The right half of the soft palate, from behind

To understand these rather complicated but instructive specimens, they may be considered to give different views of the medial pterygoid muscle (21) and adjacent structures. In A the right muscle is seen from the medial side, with parts of the skull removed to show the trigeminal ganglion (14) with the maxillary and mandibular nerves (2 and 12) branching from it. The pterygopalatine ganglion (4) is attached to the maxillary nerve (2), the otic ganglion (11) to the mandibular nerve (12), and the submandibular ganglion (40) to the lingual nerve (10). The asterisk (*) indicates the position of the lower third molar tooth.

In B the transverse section is below the hard palate (62) and is viewed from below looking upwards. The left ramus of the mandible (60) has the medial pterygoid (21) on its medial side.

The dissection in C is viewed from behind, looking forwards. On the right of the picture the posterior border of the right ramus of the mandible (60), with the medial pterygoid (21) on its medial side, has been exposed by removing most of the parotid gland (58); on the left is seen the posterior surface of the epiglottis (32). Stylohyoid (56) passes downwards and forwards to split round the digastric (23), with styloglossus (57) more anteriorly. The glossopharyngeal nerve (79) winds round stylopharyngeus (53). Palatopharyngeus (46) runs down from the palatine aponeurosis (80), with levator veli palatini (81) approaching the aponeurosis from above, lateral to the auditory tube (83).

• All the muscles of the palate (page 137) are supplied by the pharyngeal plexus, except tensor veli palatini which is supplied by the nerve to the medial pterygoid (mandibular nerve).

• The mucous membrane of the palate is supplied by the nasopalatine, greater and lesser palatine and glossopharyngeal nerves.

• The surface of the tonsil is pitted by downgrowths of the epithelium to form the tonsillar crypts.

• A deep crypt-like structure near the upper pole of the tonsil is the intratonsillar cleft, and represents the proximal end of the embryonic second pharyngeal pouch.

• The mucous membrane of the tonsil is supplied by the lesser palatine and glossopharyngeal nerves.

• The lingual nerve (A10) enters the mouth by passing beneath the lower border of the superior constrictor (A42), and immediately below this the nerve lies below and behind the third molar tooth (whose position is indicated by the asterisk in A), either in contact with the periosteum of the mandible or on the upper part of mylohyoid (as here, A38).

1 Sphenoidal sinus	30 Stylohyoid ligament	59 Masseter
2 Maxillary nerve	31 Middle constrictor of pharynx	60 Ramus of mandible
3 Sphenopalatine foramen and artery	32 Epiglottis	61 Palatal glands
4 Pterygopalatine ganglion	33 Vallecula	62 Hard palate
5 Greater palatine nerve	34 Lingual artery	63 Vestibule of mouth
6 Nerve of pterygoid canal	35 Hyoglossus	64 Base of styloid process
7 Tensor veli palatini	36 Vena comitans of hypoglossal nerve	65 Intra-articular disc of temporomandibular joint
8 Nerve to tensor veli palatini	37 Geniohyoid	66 Lateral pterygoid
9 Nerve to medial pterygoid	38 Mylohyoid	67 Inferior alveolar artery
10 Lingual nerve	39 Submandibular duct	68 Posterior part of submandibular gland
11 Otic ganglion	40 Submandibular ganglion	69 Superior thyroid artery
12 Mandibular nerve	41 Nerve to mylohyoid	70 Superior laryngeal artery
13 Greater petrosal nerve	42 Superior constrictor of pharynx	71 Inferior constrictor of pharynx
14 Trigeminal ganglion	43 Pterygomandibular raphe	72 Lamina of thyroid cartilage
15 Internal carotid artery	44 Buccinator	73 Piriform recess
16 Chorda tympani	45 Pterygoid hamulus	74 Aryepiglottic fold
17 Auriculotemporal nerve	46 Palatopharyngeus	75 Internal laryngeal nerve
18 Middle meningeal artery	47 Soft palate	76 Thyrohyoid
19 Maxillary artery	48 Dens of axis	77 Thyrohyoid membrane
20 Inferior alveolar nerve	49 Lateral mass of atlas	78 Greater horn of hyoid bone
21 Medial pterygoid	50 Nasal part of pharynx	79 Glossopharyngeal nerve
22 Occipital artery	51 Uvula	80 Palatine aponeurosis
23 Posterior belly of digastric	52 Tonsil (upper end)	81 Levator veli palatini
24 External carotid artery	53 Stylopharyngeus	82 Musculus uvulae
25 Facial artery	54 Vagus nerve	83 Cartilaginous part of auditory tube
26 Deep part of submandibular gland	55 Internal jugular vein	84 Longus capitis
27 Tendon of digastric	56 Stylohyoid	85 Posterior nasal aperture (choana)
28 Stylohyoid	57 Styloglossus	86 Nasal septum (vomer)
29 Hypoglossal nerve	58 Parotid gland	

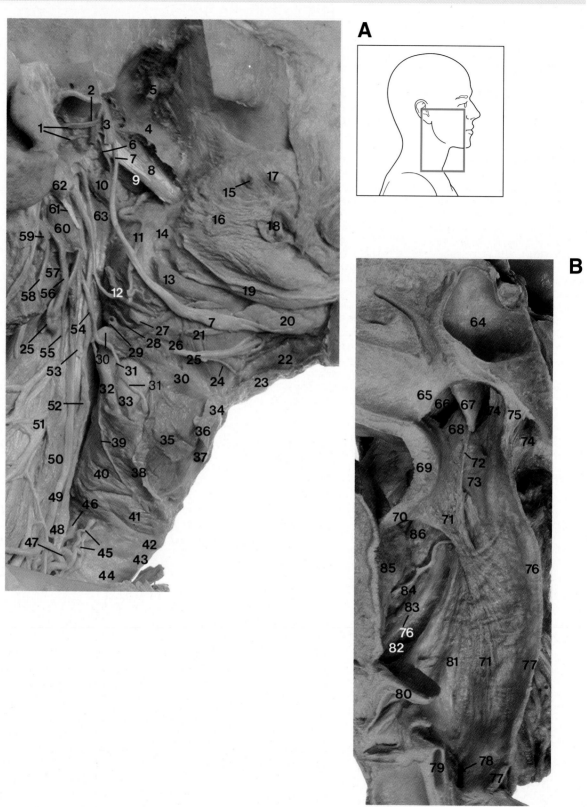

PHARYNX
The external and internal surfaces of the pharynx
A The external surface, from the right
B The right internal surface, from the left

In A the mandible, mastication muscles and great vessels have been removed. The superior constrictor (11) passes back from the pterygomandibular raphe (14), with the buccinator (16) running forwards from the raphe. The narrow origin of the middle constrictor (28) passes back from the angle between the stylohyoid ligament (27, whose upper end has been cut off) and the greater horn of the hyoid bone (30). The inferior constrictor (40) runs back from a broad origin from the thyroid cartilage behind the sternothyroid attachment (38) and from the side of the cricoid cartilage (42).

In B the muscular layer of the right side of the pharynx has been exposed from the inside by removing the mucous membrane. Palatopharyngeus (71) is the innermost muscle. The glossopharyngeal nerve (84) runs down in the 'tonsillar bed' between palatoglossus (86) in front and the upper anterior part of palatopharyngeus (71) behind.

- Palatopharyngeus (B71) (with salpingopharyngeus joining it, B72) passes downwards internal to the constrictor muscles.

- Stylopharyngeus (page 146, B11) passes downwards between the superior and middle constrictors (page 146, B32 and 30).

- Fibres from palatopharyngeus and stylopharyngeus reach the posterior border of the lamina of the thyroid cartilage (page 146, B38) and, together with the inferior constrictor, they act as elevators of the larynx during swallowing.

- All the muscles of the pharynx (page 137) are supplied by the pharyngeal plexus, except stylopharyngeus, which is supplied by the muscular branch of the glossopharyngeal nerve (A12). The lowest (cricopharyngeal) part of the inferior constrictor (A40) may receive an additional supply from the external laryngeal nerve (A39).

- Hyoglossus (A26) is a key landmark at the side of the tongue:
    passing superficial to it—lingual nerve (7), submandibular duct (21) and hypoglossal nerve (25).
    passing deep to its posterior border—glossopharyngeal nerve (12), stylohyoid ligament (27) and lingual artery (29).

1 Roots of auriculotemporal nerve	30 Greater horn of hyoid bone	60 Internal jugular vein
2 Middle meningeal artery	31 Internal laryngeal nerve	61 Stylohyoid
3 Mandibular nerve	32 Superior horn of thyroid cartilage	62 Styloid process
4 Lateral pterygoid plate	33 Thyrohyoid membrane	63 Longus capitis
5 Maxillary artery entering pterygomaxillary fissure	34 Body of hyoid bone	64 Sphenoidal sinus
6 Chorda tympani	35 Thyrohyoid	65 Vomer (posterior part of nasal septum)
7 Lingual nerve	36 Superior belly of omohyoid	66 Tensor veli palatini
8 Tensor veli palatini	37 Sternohyoid	67 Cartilaginous part of auditory tube
9 Levator veli palatini	38 Sternothyroid	68 Levator veli palatini
10 Pharyngobasilar fascia	39 External laryngeal nerve	69 Soft palate
11 Superior constrictor of pharynx and ascending palatine artery	40 Inferior constrictor of pharynx	70 Uvula
12 Stylopharyngeus and glossopharyngeal nerve	41 Cricothyroid	71 Palatopharyngeus
13 Styloglossus	42 Arch of cricoid cartilage	72 Salpingopharyngeus
14 Pterygomandibular raphe	43 Cricotracheal ligament	73 Superior constrictor
15 Parotid duct	44 Trachea	74 Longus capitis
16 Buccinator	45 Recurrent laryngeal nerve	75 Attachment of pharyngeal raphe to pharyngeal tubercle
17 Molar glands	46 Inferior laryngeal artery	76 Middle constrictor
18 Facial artery	47 Inferior thyroid artery	77 Inferior constrictor
19 Mucoperiosteum of mandible	48 Middle cervical sympathetic ganglion	78 Piriform recess
20 Sublingual gland	49 Vagus nerve	79 Lamina of cricoid cartilage
21 Submandibular duct	50 Scalenus anterior	80 Epiglottis
22 Geniohyoid	51 Ventral ramus of fourth cervical nerve	81 Pharyngeal wall overlying superior horn of thyroid cartilage
23 Mylohyoid	52 Sympathetic trunk	82 Greater horn of hyoid bone
24 Nerve to geniohyoid	53 Ascending pharyngeal artery	83 Stylohyoid ligament
25 Hypoglossal nerve	54 Superior laryngeal nerve	84 Glossopharyngeal nerve
26 Hyoglossus	55 Superior root of ansa cervicalis	85 Postsulcal part of dorsum of tongue
27 Stylohyoid ligament	56 Occipital artery	86 Palatoglossus
28 Middle constrictor of pharynx	57 Transverse process of atlas	
29 Lingual artery	58 Accessory nerve (spinal part)	
	59 Posterior auricular artery	

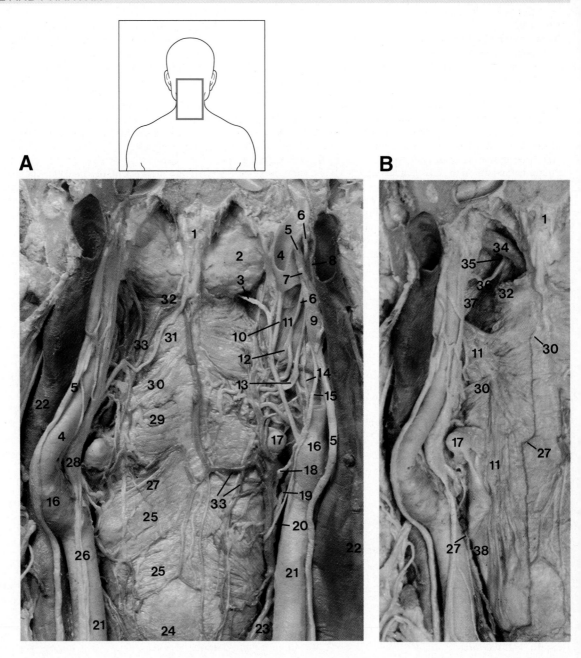

PHARYNX
The posterior surface of the pharynx
A The whole pharynx
B The left half

In A the skull has been sectioned coronally at the level of the pharyngeal tubercle (1). On the right, part of the internal carotid artery (4) has been removed to show the pharyngeal branches (12 and 13) of the glossopharyngeal and vagus nerves that make up the pharyngeal plexus. The pharyngeal venous plexus (33) is particularly prominent on the right.

In B removal of the pharyngobasilar fascia seen in A (2) reveals parts of the levator and tensor veli palatini (34 and 35), and with removal of parts of the middle and inferior constrictors (30 and 27), fibres of stylopharyngeus (11) can be traced down to the posterior border of the lamina of the thyroid cartilage (38).

---

1 Attachment of pharyngeal raphe to pharyngeal tubercle of base of skull
2 Pharyngobasilar fascia
3 Ascending pharyngeal artery
4 Internal carotid artery
5 Vagus nerve
6 Glossopharyngeal nerve
7 Accessory nerve
8 Hypoglossal nerve
9 Inferior ganglion of vagus nerve
10 Posterior meningeal artery
11 Stylopharyngeus
12 Pharyngeal branch of glossopharyngeal nerve
13 Pharyngeal branch of vagus nerve
14 Vagal branch to carotid body
15 Superior laryngeal branch of vagus nerve
16 Carotid sinus
17 Tip of greater horn of hyoid bone
18 Internal laryngeal nerve
19 Superior thyroid artery
20 External laryngeal nerve
21 Common carotid artery
22 Internal jugular vein
23 Lateral lobe of thyroid gland
24 Cricopharyngeal part ⎫ of inferior
25 Thyropharyngeal part ⎭ constrictor
26 Sympathetic trunk
27 Upper border of inferior constrictor
28 Superior cervical sympathetic ganglion
29 Middle constrictor
30 Upper border of middle constrictor
31 Superior constrictor
32 Upper border of superior constrictor
33 Pharyngeal veins
34 Levator veli palatini
35 Tensor veli palatini
36 Ascending palatine artery
37 Medial pterygoid
38 Posterior border of lamina of thyroid cartilage

• Fibres of all three constrictors converge in an upward direction on to the pharyngeal raphe (1); hence the importance of the inferior constrictor as an elevator of the larynx (see page 155).

• The pharyngobasilar fascia (A2) is the thickened submucosa of the pharynx that extends between the upper border of the superior constrictor and the base of the skull.

• The buccopharyngeal fascia (which is very much thinner than the pharyngobasilar fascia and must not be confused with it) lies on the external surface of the pharyngeal constrictors and is continuous anteriorly over the outer surface of the buccinator. It is really nothing more than the epimysium on the surface of the muscles.

• Some of the uppermost fibres of the superior constrictor and of the palatopharyngeus (page 145, C73 and 71) form a muscular band which, during swallowing, raises a transverse ridge (Passavant's ridge) on the posterior pharyngeal wall. With accompanying elevation of the soft palate, it closes off the nasal part of the pharynx from the oral part. It must be noted that the ridge only becomes evident during the act of swallowing; it is not seen in the living pharynx at rest or in the cadaver.

• The pharyngeal plexuses of nerves and veins are situated mainly on the posterior surface of the middle constrictor (A29).

• The pharyngeal plexus of nerves is formed by the pharyngeal branches of the glossopharyngeal and vagus nerves (A12 and 13). The glossopharyngeal component is afferent only; the vagal component is motor to the pharynx and palate as well as containing afferent fibres.

• Glossopharyngeal nerve paralysis:
    No detectable motor disability, as the nerve supplies only one small muscle, stylopharyngeus.
    Loss of taste from the posterior one-third of the tongue, with anaesthesia in the same area and in part of the pharyngeal mucous membrane.

• Vagus and cranial accessory nerve paralysis:
    Paralysis of the soft palate on the affected side (the palate is pulled towards the unaffected side on saying 'Ah').
    Dysphagia (difficulty in swallowing) due to paralysis of pharyngeal muscles.
    Hoarseness of voice due to paralysis of laryngeal muscles.

• Spinal accessory nerve paralysis:
    Paralysis of sternocleidomastoid and trapezius.

• Hypoglossal nerve paralysis:
    Paralysis of the tongue on the affected side (with deviation towards the affected side on protrusion, due to the unapposed action of the intact side).

EAR

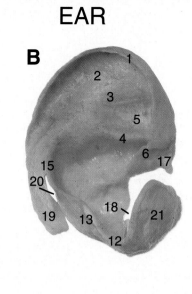

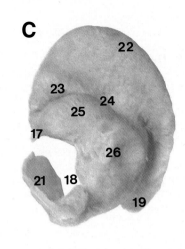

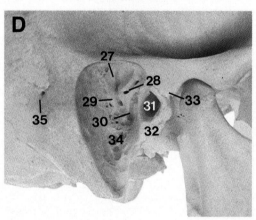

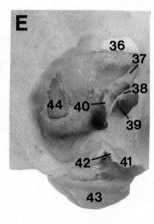

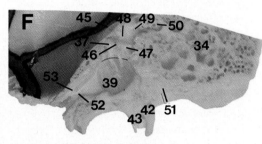

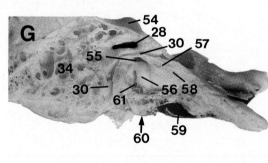

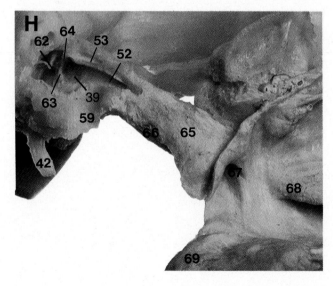

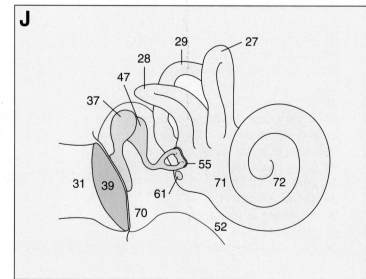

COMPONENTS OF THE EAR
The external, middle and internal ear
A Right auricle, from the right
B Right auricular cartilage, from the right
C Right auricular cartilage, from the left
D Dissection through the right mastoid process, from the right
E Similar to D but deeper, from the right and behind
F Section through the right middle ear, from the left
G Section through the right middle ear, from the right
H Left auditory tube, from the right (enlarged)
J Diagram of parts of the ear

A, B and C show the surface features and cartilaginous framework of the auricle (pinna).

In D part of the right mastoid process of a dried skull has been chipped away to open up the mastoid air cells (34) and the semicircular canals (27-29).

In E a deeper dissection of the area in D shows how near the sigmoid sinus (44) lies to the deepest mastoid air cells. The canal for the facial nerve (40) has been opened up where the chorda tympani branch (38) takes a recurrent course to pass through the mucous membrane of the tympanic membrane (39).

F and G are sections through the middle ear and adjacent parts of the temporal bone, showing the lateral (F) and medial (G) walls of the middle ear cavity. The narrow black bristle (unlabelled, below 46 and 47) indicates the course of the chorda tympani under the mucous membrane of the tympanic membrane (39).

In H the cartilaginous part of the auditory tube (65 and 66) has been dissected away from surrounding tissues but with the tubal opening (67) into the nasopharynx left intact.

The diagram (J) shows the parts of the right ear as seen from the front, with the external meatus and middle ear in coronal section.

• The lobule of the ear (A14), the part pierced for wearing earrings, is composed of dense fibrous tissue, not cartilage.

• The external ear consists of the auricle (pinna, A) and the external acoustic meatus (A10; D and J, 31), at the medial end of which lies the tympanic membrane (E, F and J, 39) separating the external ear from the middle ear.

• The middle ear (tympanic cavity, J70) is an irregular space in the temporal bone, lined with mucous membrane, containing the auditory ossicles (malleus, incus and stapes) and filled with air that communicates anteriorly with the nasopharynx through the auditory tube (Eustachian tube, H52, 65 and 66). For details of the walls of the middle ear cavity, see the notes on page 151.

• The epitympanic recess (F48) is the part of the tympanic cavity that projects upwards above the level of the tympanic membrane (F39) to accommodate the head of the malleus and the body of the incus (F37 and 47). It leads backwards through the aditus (F49) into the mastoid antrum (F50) which is an enlarged mastoid air cell (F34).

1 Helix	26 Ponticulus	51 Stylomastoid foramen
2 Scaphoid fossa	27 Anterior	52 Semicanal for auditory tube
3 Upper crus of antihelix	28 Lateral } semicircular canal	53 Semicanal for tensor tympani
4 Lower crus of antihelix	29 Posterior	54 Arcuate eminence (overlying anterior semicircular canal)
5 Triangular fossa	30 Canal for facial nerve	55 Oval window (fenestra vestibuli), with stapes in J
6 Crus of helix	31 External acoustic meatus	56 Promontory
7 Cymba conchae	32 Tympanic part of temporal bone	57 Trochleariform (cochleariform) process
8 Concha	33 Postglenoid tubercle	58 Position of opening of auditory tube
9 Cavum conchae	34 Mastoid air cells	59 Carotid canal
10 External acoustic meatus	35 Mastoid foramen	60 Jugular bulb
11 Tragus	36 Dura mater of middle cranial fossa	61 Round window (fenestra cochleae)
12 Intertragic notch	37 Head of malleus in epitympanic recess	62 Incudostapedial joint
13 Antitragus	38 Chorda tympani	63 Handle of malleus
14 Lobule	39 Tympanic membrane	64 Tendon of tensor tympani and 57
15 Antihelix	40 Facial nerve	65 Medial lamina } of cartilaginous
16 Position of auricular tubercle (if present)	41 Sheath of styloid process	66 Lateral lamina } part of auditory tube
17 Spine of helix	42 Styloid process	67 Opening of auditory tube
18 Terminal notch	43 Occipital condyle	68 Inferior nasal concha
19 Tail of helix	44 Dura mater of sigmoid sinus	69 Soft palate
20 Antitragohelicine meatus	45 Tegmen tympani	70 Middle ear (tympanic cavity)
21 Cartilage of external acoustic meatus	46 Incudomallear joint	71 Vestibule
22 Scaphoid eminence	47 Body of incus	72 Cochlea
23 Triangular eminence	48 Epitympanic recess	
24 Transverse antihelicine groove	49 Aditus to mastoid antrum	
25 Conchal eminence	50 Mastoid antrum	

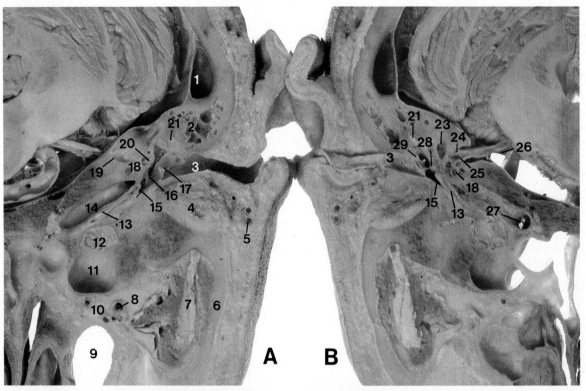

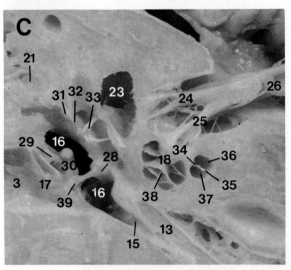

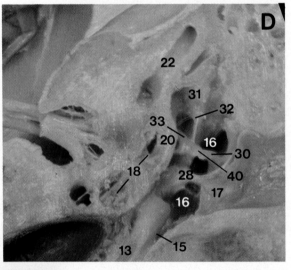

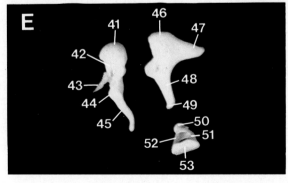

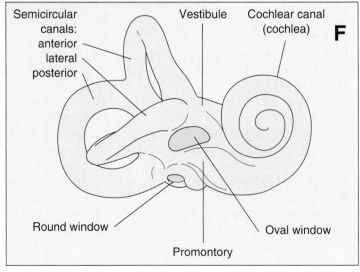

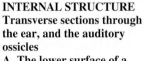

INTERNAL STRUCTURE
Transverse sections through the ear, and the auditory ossicles

A The lower surface of a section through the left ear from above

B The upper surface of the same section, from below

C The central area of B, enlarged

D The upper surface of a section through the right ear (enlarged), at a slightly lower level than the section in B

E The right auditory ossicles disarticulated and enlarged

F Diagram of the osseous labyrinth

G Diagram of the membranous labyrinth

The section in A is viewed looking down to the neck, and in B looking up to the top of the head; the sections were produced by the same saw cut and have been separated like opening a book, with the spine of the book in the centre at the auricle of the external ear. The section has passed through the external acoustic meatus (3), the middle ear cavity (16) and the horizontal part of the internal carotid artery within the carotid canal (14).

The enlargement of B in C shows the vestibular and cochlear parts of the vestibulo-cochlear nerve (24 and 25) in the internal acoustic meatus, coils of the cochlea (18), and the tendon of tensor tympani (28) bridging the tympanic cavity (16) to become attached to the handle of the malleus (39). The auditory tube (15) opens into the front of

F

Semicircular canals:
anterior
lateral
posterior

Vestibule

Cochlear canal (cochlea)

Round window

Promontory

Oval window

1	Sigmoid sinus	20	Promontory	35	Basilar membrane
2	Mastoid air cells	21	Facial nerve	36	Scala tympani
3	External acoustic meatus	22	Posterior semicircular canal	37	Scala vestibuli
4	Intra-articular disc of temporomandibular joint	23	Vestibular part of osseous labyrinth	38	Modiolus
5	Superficial temporal artery			39	Handle of malleus
6	Zygomatic arch	24	Vestibular part	40	Incudostapedial joint
7	Temporalis	25	Cochlear part	41	Head
8	Maxillary artery		of vestibulo-cochlear nerve in internal acoustic meatus	42	Neck
9	Maxillary sinus			43	Anterior process } of malleus
10	Pterygopalatine fossa	26	Labyrinthine artery	44	Lateral process
11	Sphenoidal sinus	27	Internal carotid artery in foramen lacerum	45	Handle
12	Cavernous sinus			46	Body
13	Semicanal with tensor tympani	28	Tendon of tensor tympani and trochleariform (cochleariform) process	47	Short limb } of incus
14	Internal carotid artery in carotid canal			48	Long limb
15	Opening of auditory tube	29	Chorda tympani	49	Lenticular process
16	Cavity of middle ear	30	Long limb of incus	50	Head
17	Tympanic membrane	31	Pyramid	51	Posterior limb } of stapes
18	Cochlea	32	Stapedius	52	Anterior limb
19	Floor of internal acoustic meatus	33	Stapes	53	Base (footplate)
		34	Osseous spiral lamina		

the cavity.

D is a similar section to C but at a slightly lower level, showing the stapedius muscle (32) emerging from the pyramid (31) to join the stapes (33). Much of the posterior semicircular canal (22) has been opened up.

E is an enlarged view of the three disarticulated auditory ossicles.

From the diagrams F and G it can be visualised that the semicircular ducts lie within the semicircular canals, the cochlear duct within the cochlear canal (cochlea), and the utricle and saccule within the vestibule.

• Features of the walls of the middle ear:
Lateral wall—tympanic membrane (page 148, F39); part of the petro-tympanic fissure (page 50, D42); anterior and posterior canaliculi for the chorda tympani (page 148, F, at either end of bristle).
Medial wall (from above downwards)—prominence due to lateral semicircular canal (page 148, G28); prominence due to canal for facial nerve (page 148, G30); promontory (A20 and page 148,

G56, due to first turn of cochlea), with oval window (fenestra vestibuli, page 148, G55) occupied by footplate of stapes above and behind promontory, and round window (fenestra cochleae, page 148, G61) below and behind promontory.
Roof—tegmen tympani (part of petrous part of temporal bone (page 148, F45 and page 50, C32).
Floor—above superior bulb of internal jugular vein in jugular fossa (page 50, D47) with canaliculus for tympanic branch of glossopharyngeal nerve (page 50, D45)
Anterior wall—carotid canal (page 148, G59) with (laterally) openings of semicanals for tensor tympani and auditory tube (page 50, E49 and 50).
Posterior wall—aditus to mastoid antrum (page 148, F49); pyramid (with stapedius emerging, C31 and 32) in front of vertical part of facial nerve (C21); fossa for incus (page 148, F47).

• The internal ear consists of the osseous (bony) labyrinth and the membranous labyrinth.

• The osseous labyrinth is a space within the temporal bone consisting of (from front to back) the cochlea (sometimes called the cochlear canal), the vestibule and the semicircular canals.

• The membranous labyrinth is inside the bony labyrinth and consists of the cochlear duct (within the cochlea), the utricle and saccule (within the vestibule), and the semicircular ducts (within the semicircular canals).

• The various parts of the membranous labyrinth are smaller than the osseous labyrinth and are separated from the walls of the osseous labyrinth by perilymph. The membranous labyrinth itself contains endolymph. These two fluids do not mix with one another, but the perilymph probably communicates with the cerebrospinal fluid in the subarachnoid space via the cochlear canaliculus.

• The cochlea is spiral-shaped, like a snail shell.

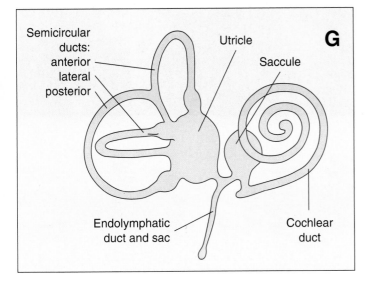

Semicircular ducts:
anterior
lateral
posterior

Utricle

Saccule

G

Endolymphatic duct and sac

Cochlear duct

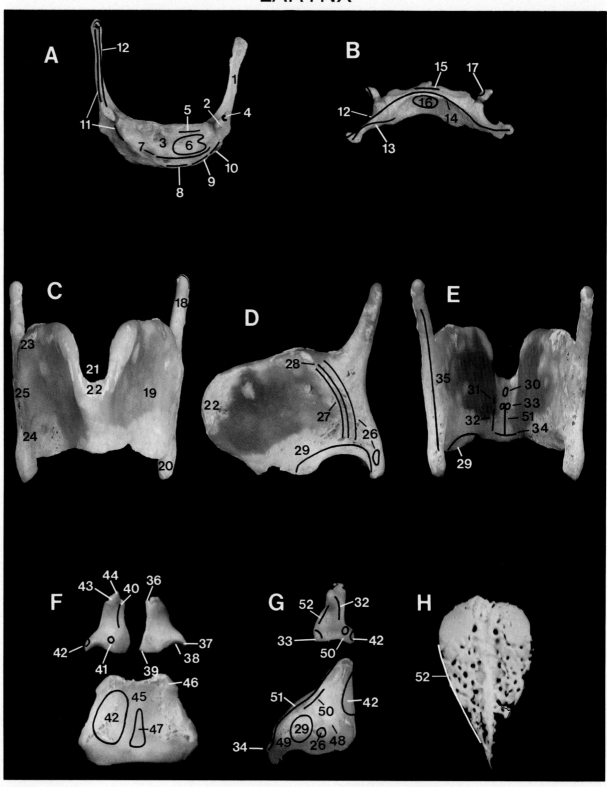

1 Greater horn ⎫
2 Lesser horn ⎬ of hyoid bone
3 Body ⎭
4 Stylohyoid ligament
5 Genioglossus
6 Geniohyoid
7 Mylohyoid
8 Sternohyoid
9 Omohyoid
10 Stylohyoid
11 Hyoglossus
12 Middle constrictor
13 Thyrohyoid
14 Thyrohyoid membrane
15 Hyoepiglottic ligament
16 Bursa
17 Chondroglossus
18 Superior horn ⎫
19 Lamina ⎬ of thyroid cartilage
20 Inferior horn ⎭
21 Thyroid notch
22 Laryngeal prominence (Adam's apple)
23 Superior ⎫
24 Inferior ⎬ tubercle of thyroid cartilage
25 Oblique line
26 Inferior constrictor
27 Sternothyroid
28 Thyrohyoid
29 Cricothyroid
30 Thyro-epiglottic ligament
31 Thyro-epiglottic muscle
32 Thyro-arytenoid
33 Vocal ligament
34 Conus elasticus
35 Stylopharyngeus and palatopharyngeus
36 Apex ⎫
37 Muscular process ⎬
38 Articular surface ⎬ of arytenoid cartilage
39 Vocal process ⎭
40 Transverse arytenoid
41 Oblique arytenoid
42 Posterior crico-arytenoid
43 Corniculate cartilage
44 Cuneiform cartilage
45 Lamina of cricoid cartilage
46 Articular surface for arytenoid cartilage
47 Tendon of oesophagus
48 Articular surface for inferior horn of thyroid cartilage
49 Arch of cricoid cartilage
50 Lateral crico-arytenoid
51 Cricothyroid ligament
52 Quadrangular membrane

HYOID BONE AND LARYNGEAL CARTILAGES
The hyoid bone and the cartilages of the larynx
A The hyoid bone, from above and in front, with attachments
B The hyoid bone, from behind, with attachments
C The thyroid cartilage, from the front
D The thyroid cartilage, from the left, with attachments
E The thyroid cartilage, from behind, with attachments
F The cricoid and arytenoid cartilages, from behind, with attachments
G The cricoid and arytenoid cartilages, from the left, with attachments
H The epiglottic cartilage, from behind

On the hyoid bone and laryngeal cartilages, attachments (unless central) have been shown for simplicity on one side only, though they are of course bilateral.

• The *hyoid bone*, not itself part of the larynx but attached to it by muscles and membranes, consists of a body (A3) with greater and lesser horns on each side (A1 and 2).

• The *thyroid cartilage* consists of two laminae (C19) united at the front and with superior and inferior horns at the back (C18 and 20). The gap above the united thyroid laminae is the thyroid notch (C21), which is bounded below by the laryngeal prominence (Adam's apple, C22). The angle between the laminae is more acute in males than in females, in whom the prominence is less obvious.

• The *cricoid cartilage* is shaped like a signet ring, with an arch at the front (G49) and a lamina at the back (F45).

• The paired *arytenoid cartilages* have the shape of a three-sided pyramid, with at the base an (anterior) vocal process (F39) to which the vocal ligament is attached (G33; page 156, C32), and a (lateral) muscular process (F37) to which the posterior and lateral crico-arytenoid muscles are attached (G42 and 50; page 156, B7 and 21).

• The thyroid, cricoid and almost all of the arytenoid cartilages are composed of hyaline cartilage and may undergo some degree of calcification with increasing age.

• The apex of the arytenoid cartilage (F36) is composed of elastic fibro-cartilage, like the epiglottic cartilage (which is leaf-shaped with numerous pits or perforations (H) and the corniculate and cuneiform cartilages (which are like small pips or rice grains, F43 and 44). The triticeal cartilages (not shown) are very small nodules that are often found in the posterior margin of the thyrohyoid membrane (page 156, D36).

LARYNX AND PHARYNX
The larynx with the pharynx, hyoid bone and trachea
A From the right, with the cervical vertebral column removed
B As in A, after removal of the thyroid gland and part of the inferior constrictor
C From the front and the right, after removal of muscles
D In a neck dissection, from the right

In the side view in A the lateral lobe of the thyroid gland (20) has been displaced backwards to show the part of the origin of the inferior constrictor (17) that arises from the tendinous band (18) over cricothyroid (19). The lingual artery (1) lies just above the tip of the greater horn of the hyoid bone (2) and then passes deep to the posterior border of hyoglossus (3). The internal

laryngeal nerve (30) runs just below the tip of the hyoid and pierces the thyrohyoid membrane (29) with the superior laryngeal branch (28) of the superior thyroid artery (27),

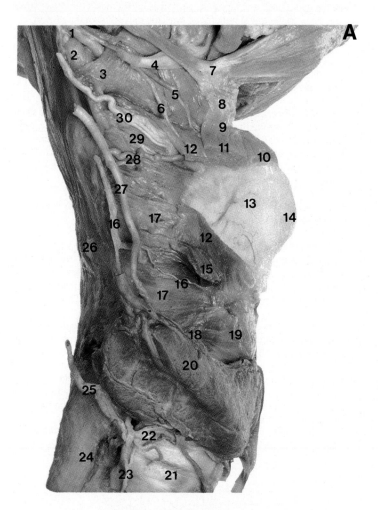

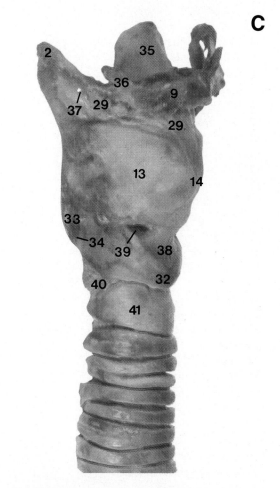

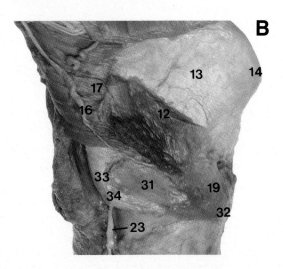

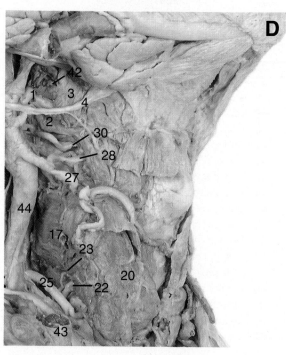

behind which runs the external laryngeal nerve (16). Much of thyrohyoid (12) has been removed to show part of the origin of the inferior constrictor (17) from the lamina of the thyroid cartilage (13).

In B with the thyroid gland taken away, the lowest (cricopharyngeus) part of the inferior constrictor has been removed to show the recurrent laryngeal nerve (23) passing up behind the cricothyroid joint (34).

In C all muscles, vessels and nerves have been removed to display the thyrohyoid membrane (29), the cricothyroid membrane (38 and 39), and the cricotracheal ligament (40) attached to the first tracheal ring (41, which is here unusually broad).

In D most of the internal jugular vein (43) has been removed and the common carotid artery (44) has been displaced backwards to show the inferior thyroid artery (25) and recurrent laryngeal nerve (23).

1 Lingual artery	17 Inferior constrictor	33 Inferior horn of thyroid cartilage
2 Tip of greater horn of hyoid bone	18 Tendinous band	34 Cricothyroid joint
3 Hyoglossus	19 Cricothyroid (straight part)	35 Epiglottis
4 Hypoglossal nerve	20 Lateral lobe of thyroid gland	36 Lesser horn of hyoid bone
5 Suprahyoid artery	21 Trachea	37 Aperture for internal laryngeal nerve and superior laryngeal artery
6 Nerve to thyrohyoid	22 Inferior laryngeal artery	
7 Tendon of digastric	23 Recurrent laryngeal nerve	38 Conus elasticus (central part of cricothyroid ligament)
8 Digastric sling	24 Oesophagus	
9 Body of hyoid bone	25 Inferior thyroid artery	39 Cricothyroid ligament (lateral part, cricovocal membrane)
10 Sternohyoid	26 Posterior pharyngeal wall	
11 Superior belly of omohyoid	27 Superior thyroid artery	40 Cricotracheal ligament
12 Thyrohyoid	28 Superior laryngeal artery	41 First tracheal ring (unusually large)
13 Lamina of thyroid cartilage	29 Thyrohyoid membrane	
14 Laryngeal prominence	30 Internal laryngeal nerve	42 Middle constrictor
15 Sternothyroid	31 Cricothyroid (oblique part)	43 Internal jugular vein
16 External laryngeal nerve	32 Arch of cricoid cartilage	44 Common carotid artery

• *Cartilages* of the larynx:
  Unpaired—thyroid, cricoid, epiglottic
  Paired—arytenoid, corniculate, cuneiform

• *Joints* of the larynx: cricothyroid (B and C, 34), crico-arytenoid (page 156, E42), arytenocorniculate (page 156, E44).

• *Membranes and ligaments* of the larynx:
  Extrinsic—thyrohyoid membrane (C29), hyo-epiglottic and thyro-epiglottic ligaments, cricotracheal ligament (C40).
  Intrinsic—quadrangular membrane (page 156, D37), whose upper margin forms the aryepiglottic fold (page 156, A3) and lower margin the vestibular (false vocal) fold (page 156, D28); cricothyroid ligament, whose upper margin (the vocal ligament, page 156, D32) forms the anterior part of the vocal fold (vocal cord). See notes on page 157.

• The *extrinsic muscles* of the larynx (those connecting it to surrounding structures) can be divided into elevators and depressors—those directly attached to the thyroid and cricoid cartilages and which raise the larynx, e.g during swallowing, and those that return it to the normal position:

Elevators: inferior constrictor (A17)
            stylopharyngeus (page 146, B11)
            palatopharyngeus (page 144, B71)   } attached to
            salpingopharyngeus (page 144, B72)   } the thyroid
            thyrohyoid (page 101, B9)   } cartilage

Depressors: sternothyroid (page 101, B48)—attached to thyroid
               cartilage
            upper oesophageal attachment (page 152, F47)—to
               cricoid cartilage
            elastic recoil of trachea

• The *intrinsic muscles* of the larynx move the vocal folds and alter the shape of the laryngeal inlet, and can be classified according to their main effects on the folds or the laryngeal inlet; i.e. they alter the shape of the rima of the glottis (the gap between the vocal folds of each side), or have a sphincteric action on the inlet:

Tensor: cricothyroid (B19 and 31)
Relaxor: thyro-arytenoid (page 156, B20)
Abductor: posterior crico-arytenoid (page 156, A7)
Adductor: lateral crico-arytenoid (page 156, B21)
           transverse arytenoid (page 156, A5)
           oblique arytenoid (page 156, A6)

• The vocalis part of the thyro-arytenoid may tighten segments of the vocal fold (as when singing a high note).

• The thyro-epiglottic, aryepiglottic and oblique arytenoid muscles constrict the inlet; their relaxation restores the normal shape.

• Cricothyroid (B19 and 31) is the only external intrinsic muscle of the larynx; it is easily seen on the outside of the larynx in dissections of the front of the neck (as on page 104, A9). The other intrinsic muscles are all inside the larynx and are only seen when the larynx itself is dissected (page 156).

• The intrinsic muscles of the larynx are all supplied by the recurrent laryngeal nerve (A and B, 23) except for cricothyroid, supplied by the external laryngeal nerve (A and B, 16).

• The mucous membrane of the larynx above the level of the vocal folds is supplied by the internal laryngeal nerve (A30), and below the vocal folds by the recurrent laryngeal nerve (A and B, 23).

• The internal laryngeal nerve (A30) first enters the *pharynx* by piercing the thyrohyoid membrane (A29), and from there fibres spread into the larynx.

• The recurrent laryngeal nerve (B23) lies immediately behind the cricothyroid joint (B34; page 156, B11) and enters the larynx by passing deep to the lower border of the inferior constrictor of the pharynx (A17).

155

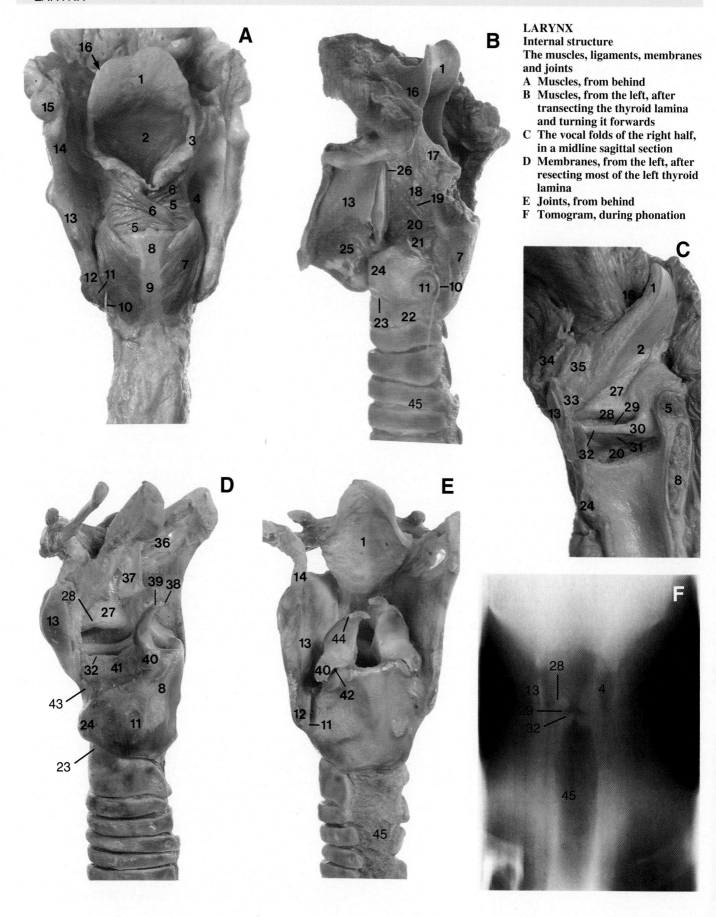

LARYNX
Internal structure
The muscles, ligaments, membranes and joints
A Muscles, from behind
B Muscles, from the left, after transecting the thyroid lamina and turning it forwards
C The vocal folds of the right half, in a midline sagittal section
D Membranes, from the left, after resecting most of the left thyroid lamina
E Joints, from behind
F Tomogram, during phonation

In A mucous membrane has been removed to show the most important of all laryngeal muscles, the posterior crico-arytenoid (7)—the only abductor of the vocal folds. The transverse arytenoid (5) is overlaid by the oblique arytenoids (6), whose fibres continue into the aryepiglottic fold (3) as the aryepiglottic muscles (B17).

In B most of the thyroid lamina (13) has been displaced forwards, revealing one above the other the lateral crico-arytenoid, thyro-arytenoid and thyro-epiglottic muscles (21, 20 and 18) (with some of the occasional overlying fibres that constitute the superior thyro-arytenoid, 19). The recurrent laryngeal nerve is seen passing up behind the (dislocated) cricothyroid joint (11).

In C removal of some mucous membrane below the vocal fold, formed by the vocal ligament (32) at the front and the vocal process of the arytenoid cartilage (30) at the back, shows the medial surface of the right thyro-arytenoid (20), whose upper fibres form the vocalis muscle (31). The vestibular fold (28) is at a higher level.

In D with all muscles and most of the left lamina of the thyroid cartilage removed, the left vocal ligament (32) is seen to be the upper margin of the cricovocal membrane (41). The vestibular fold (28) is the lower margin of the quadrangular membrane (37).

In E the capsules of the cricothyroid and crico-arytenoid joints (11 and 42) have been removed. This specimen is somewhat asymmetric.

The tomogram in F, produced by a radiographic method that allows a thin 'slice' of tissue to be visualised, illustrates the vestibular and vocal folds (28 and 32) in a living subject during phonation, with the vocal folds (32) approximated.

• The central (anterior) part of the cricothryoid ligament is often known as the conus elasticus (D43) (although some texts use this term for the whole ligament). The lateral part of the cricothyroid ligament is commonly known as the cricovocal membrane (D41).

• The upper (free) margin of the cricovocal membrane is thickened to form the vocal ligament (D32). It is attached at the front to the lamina of the thyroid cartilage adjacent to the midline, and at the back to the vocal process of the arytenoid cartilage. Covered by mucous membrane, the vocal ligament and vocal process together form the vocal fold or vocal cord (C30 and 32).

• The lower margin of the cricothyroid ligament is not free but attached to the upper border of the lamina and arch of the cricoid cartilage (D8 and 24).

• The surface marking of the vocal fold is at a level midway between the laryngeal prominence and lower border of the thyroid cartilage (page 90, 16).

• The quadrangular membrane, a very thin sheet of connective tissue that has been artificially thickened in D37 for emphasis, passes between the lateral side of the arytenoid cartilage (which is relatively short) to the lateral edge of the epiglottic cartilage (which is relatively long). The membrane is thus an irregular quadrilateral in shape and not rectangular.

• The upper (free) margin of the quadrangular membrane is covered by mucous membrane to form the aryepiglottic fold (A3).

• The lower (free) margin of the quadrangular membrane is covered by mucous membrane to form the vestibular fold (C28), also called the false vocal fold.

• The slitlike space between the vestibular and vocal folds is the ventricle (or sinus) of the larynx (C29), and is continuous with the saccule, a small pouch of mucous membrane that extends upwards for a few millimetres at the anterior part of the ventricle between the vestibular fold and the inner surface of the thyroid lamina. Mucous secretion from glands in the saccule trickles down to lubricate the vocal folds.

• The posterior crico-arytenoid (A7) is commonly accepted as the only muscle that can abduct the vocal folds, i.e. it opens the glottis.

• The lateral crico-arytenoid (B21) and the transverse and oblique arytenoids (A5 and 6) adduct the vocal folds (close the glottis).

• The cricothyroid (page 154, A19; page102, B67) lengthens (and may increase tension in) the vocal fold.

• In a *complete* recurrent laryngeal nerve lesion (e.g. complete transection during thyroidectomy), there is permanent hoarseness of the voice, and the affected vocal fold assumes a position midway between abduction and adduction.

• In an *incomplete* recurrent laryngeal nerve lesion (e.g. partial transection), the affected vocal fold takes up an adducted position (for reasons which have not yet been adequately explained). Bilateral incomplete lesions are thus liable to cause respiratory embarrassment because of the very narrow airway between the folds.

• In external laryngeal nerve lesions there may be no detectable abnormality. If there is any, there is some hoarseness of the voice due to loss of tension in the affected vocal fold from the paralysed cricothyroid; the fold may lie at a slightly lower level than that of the normal side. The hoarseness may disappear due to hypertrophy of the opposite cricothyroid, but with some residual loss of production of higher frequencies (as in the higher notes in singing).

1	Epiglottis	17	Aryepiglottic muscle	31	Vocalis part of thyro-arytenoid
2	Vestibule	18	Thyro-epiglottic muscle	32	Vocal ligament (anterior part of vocal fold)
3	Aryepiglottic fold	19	Superior thyro-arytenoid		
4	Piriform recess	20	Thyro-arytenoid	33	Thyro-epiglottic ligament
5	Transverse arytenoid	21	Lateral crico-arytenoid	34	Body of hyoid bone
6	Oblique arytenoid	22	First tracheal ring	35	Hyo-epiglottic ligament
7	Posterior crico-arytenoid	23	Cricotracheal ligament	36	Thyrohyoid membrane
8	Lamina of cricoid cartilage	24	Arch of cricoid cartilage	37	Quadrangular membrane
9	Site of attachment of oesophageal tendon	25	Cricothyroid	38	Cuneiform cartilage
		26	Internal laryngeal nerve	39	Corniculate cartilage
10	Recurrent laryngeal nerve	27	Mucous membrane overlying quadrangular membrane	40	Muscular process of arytenoid cartilage
11	Cricothyroid joint				
12	Inferior horn ⎫	28	Vestibular fold	41	Cricovocal membrane
13	Lamina ⎬ of thyroid cartilage	29	Ventricle of larynx	42	Crico-arytenoid joint
14	Superior horn ⎭	30	Vocal process of arytenoid cartilage (posterior part of vocal fold)	43	Conus elasticus
15	Greater horn of hyoid bone			44	Arytenocorniculate joint
16	Vallecula			45	Trachea

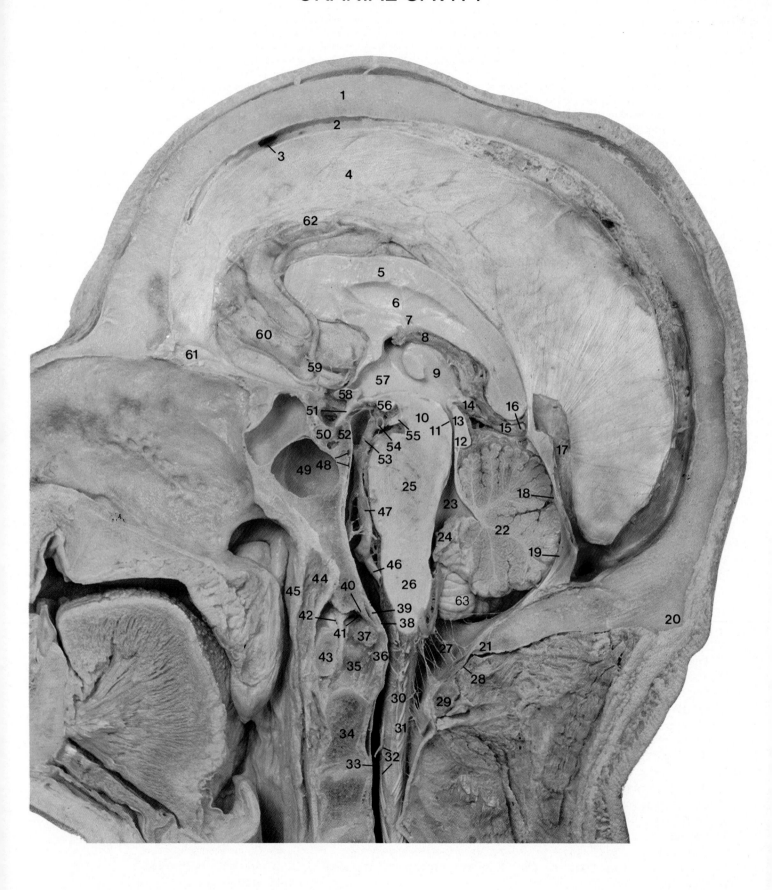

CRANIAL CAVITY AND BRAIN
The cranial cavity, brain and meninges, in a paramedian sagittal section

The section is slightly to the left of the midline so that the dens of the axis (35) and spinal cord (30) have escaped being cut. The vault of the skull (1) is thicker than usual. The superior sagittal and straight sinuses have been opened up (2 and 17). The corpus callosum (5) lies below the falx cerebri (4), and the cerebellum (22) is below and in front of the tentorium cerebelli (18). The tonsil of the cerebellum (63) is just above the foramen magnum (21), through which the medulla oblongata (26) passes, to become the spinal cord (30) at the level of the atlas (43 and 29). The basilar artery (47) passes up in front of the pons (25) with the posterior cerebral artery (54) arising at the upper end. The third ventricle (9) communicates with the fourth ventricle (23) via the aqueduct of the midbrain (11), and the pineal body (14) at the back of the third ventricle projects over the superior colliculus of the midbrain (13). (Details of the mouth and pharynx in this specimen are given on page 136.)

• The cranial cavity contains:
  the brain with its vessels and membranes
  the cranial nerves
  vessels on the outermost membrane

• The membranes of the brain, collectively called the meninges, consist of the dura mater, the arachnoid mater and the pia mater.

• The dura mater is sometimes called the pachymeninx; the arachnoid and pia mater together constitute the leptomeninges. For further details see page 161.

1	Vault of skull	33	Spinal subarachnoid space
2	Superior sagittal sinus	34	Body of axis
3	Aperture of a superior cerebral vein	35	Dens of axis (left side)
4	Falx cerebri	36	Transverse ligament of atlas
5	Corpus callosum	37	Alar ligament
6	Septum pellucidum	38	Dura mater
7	Body of fornix	39	Tectorial membrane
8	Choroid plexus of third ventricle	40	Superior longitudinal band of cruciform ligament
9	Thalamus and third ventricle	41	Apical ligament
10	Midbrain	42	Anterior atlanto-occipital membrane
11	Aqueduct of midbrain	43	Anterior arch of atlas
12	Inferior colliculus	44	Longus capitis
13	Superior colliculus	45	Posterior pharyngeal wall
14	Pineal body	46	Vertebral artery
15	Great cerebral vein	47	Basilar artery
16	Basal vein	48	Basilar sinus
17	Straight sinus	49	Sphenoidal sinus
18	Tentorium cerebelli	50	Pituitary gland
19	Falx cerebelli	51	Pituitary stalk
20	External occipital protuberance	52	Dorsum sellae
21	Posterior margin of foramen magnum	53	Superior cerebellar artery
22	Cerebellum	54	Posterior cerebral artery
23	Fourth ventricle	55	Oculomotor nerve
24	Choroid plexus of fourth ventricle	56	Mamillary body
25	Pons	57	Hypothalamus
26	Medulla oblongata	58	Optic chiasma
27	Filaments of arachnoid mater in cerebellomedullary cistern (cisterna magna)	59	Anterior cerebral artery
28	Posterior atlanto-occipital membrane and overlying dura mater	60	Arachnoid mater overlying medial surface of cerebral hemisphere
29	Posterior arch of atlas	61	Crista galli
30	Spinal cord (spinal medulla)	62	Lower border of falx cerebri and inferior sagittal sinus
31	Dorsal rootlets ⎫ of spinal nerves		
32	Ventral rootlets ⎭	63	Tonsil of cerebellum

BACK

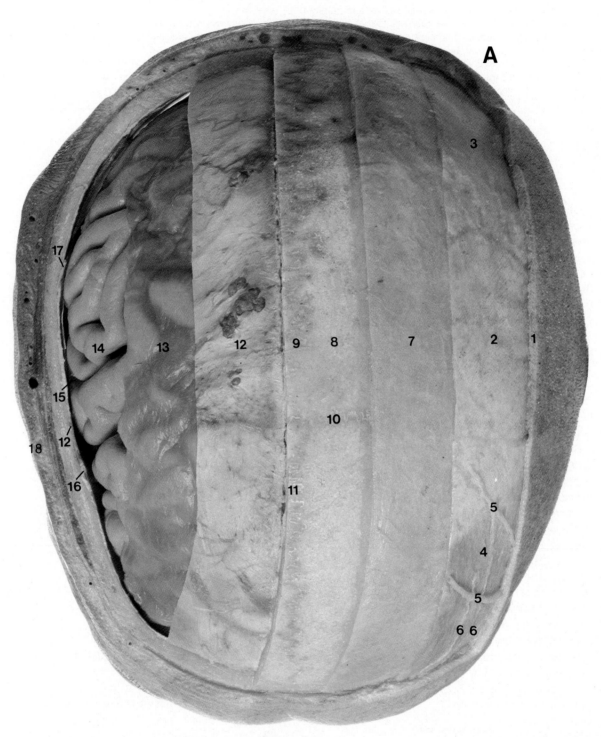

A

FRONT

CRANIAL VAULT, MENINGES AND BRAIN
Dissection of the scalp and cranial vault
A 'Stepped dissection', from above
B The dura mater and meningeal vessels on the right side

In A the bone of the cranial vault (8) has been removed on the right side of the head (left side of the picture) to show the dura mater (12), which itself has been partly removed to reveal the underlying arachnoid mater (13), in turn overlying the cerebral hemisphere (14). On the left side of the head are shown components of the scalp (1–7; see notes).

1 Skin and dense subcutaneous tissue
2 Epicranial aponeurosis (galea aponeurotica)
3 Occipital belly ⎫ of occipitofrontalis
4 Frontal belly ⎭
5 Branches of superficial temporal artery
6 Branches of supra-orbital nerve
7 Loose connective tissue and pericranium
8 Bone of cranial vault
9 Sagittal suture
10 Coronal suture
11 Frontal (metopic) suture
12 Dura mater
13 Arachnoid mater
14 Cerebral hemisphere covered by pia mater
15 Subarachnoid space
16 Frontal branch ⎫ of middle meningeal artery
17 Parietal branch ⎭
18 Scalp
19 Arachnoid granulation

In B the scalp (18) and cranial vault (8) of the right side have been removed to display branches of the middle meningeal artery (16 and 17). The dotted circle indicates the position of pterion, the region on the surface of the skull beneath which the main trunk of the artery lies (see the note on page 15).

• The *scalp* consists of five layers:
    skin (A1)
    dense connective tissue (A1)
    the epicranial aponeurosis and the occipitofrontalis muscle (A2, 3
        and 4)
    loose connective tissue (A7)
    the pericranium (periosteum of the cranial vault, A7)

• The *dura mater* (A12) is the outermost and thickest of the meninges. For further details see page 163.

• The *arachnoid mate*r (A13) lies inside the dura mater, separated from it by the subdural space which is merely a capillary interval: that is, the dura and arachnoid lie in contact like two pages of a closed book. Over parts of its inner surface within the cranium, the arachnoid has filamentous (spidery) projections attaching it to the pia mater (as on page 158, 27). The intervening space which is crossed by the filaments is the subarachnoid space (A15), filled with cerebrospinal fluid.

• The *pia mater* (A14) adheres intimately to the surface of the brain and spinal cord. It forms the denticulate ligament at the side of the spinal cord (page 200, B31, and the subarachnoid septum at the back of the cord (page 136, 12).

• The middle meningeal artery (B16 and 17) supplies the dura mater and bone but it does not supply the brain. It lies between the dura and cranial vault (B12 and 8).

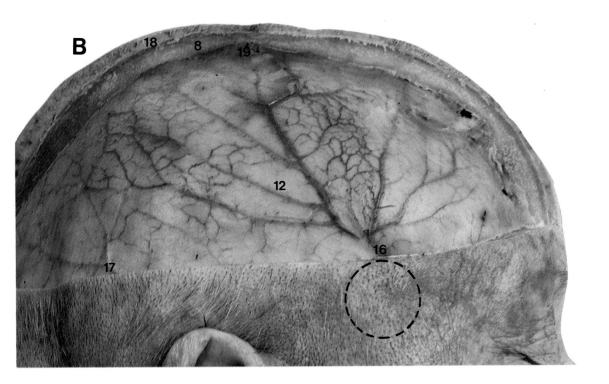

B

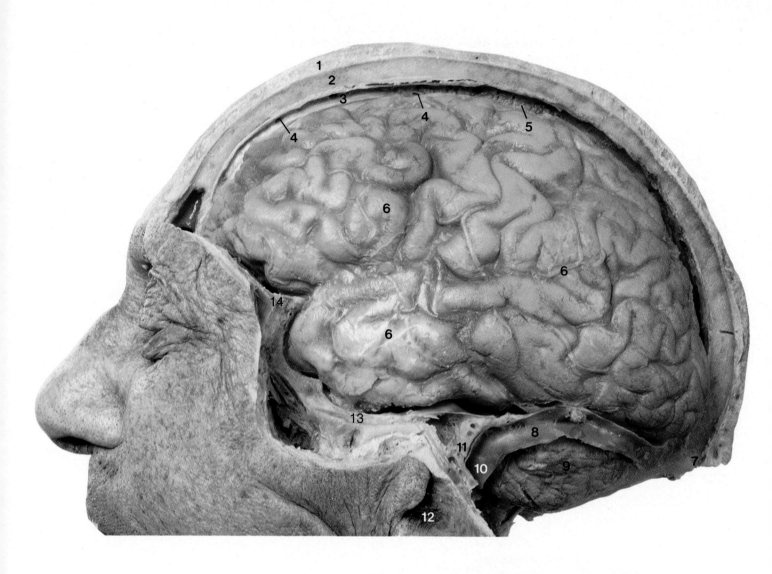

BRAIN AND MENINGES
The brain and arachnoid mater, from the left
The cranial vault and part of the base of the skull and dura mater have been dissected away, leaving the arachnoid mater covering the cerebral hemisphere, and the superior sagittal sinus (3), the left transverse sinus (8) and some of the mastoid air cells (11).

1	Scalp
2	Cranial vault
3	Superior sagittal sinus
4	Openings of superior cerebral veins
5	Arachnoid granulations
6	Vessels and arachnoid mater overlying cerebral hemisphere
7	External occipital protuberance
8	Transverse sinus
9	Cerebellar hemisphere
10	Sigmoid sinus
11	Mastoid air cells
12	External acoustic meatus
13	Floor of lateral part of middle cranial fossa
14	Floor of anterior cranial fossa

• The *dura mater* has cerebral and spinal parts.

• The cerebral part of the dura mater lines the inside of the cranium and consists of an outer endosteal layer (corresponding to periosteum), and an inner meningeal layer. The two layers blend with one another but in certain areas they become separated to form venous sinuses (see below).

• The meningeal layer forms sheaths for the cranial nerves as they pass out through skull foramina, and also forms four processes or partitions (see page 165):

falx cerebri (page 158, 4; page 164, 2)
tentorium cerebelli (page 164, 25)
falx cerebelli (page 158, 19)
diaphragma sellae (page 168, 31)

• The spinal part of the dura mater corresponds to the meningeal layer of the cerebral part and forms a sheath for the spinal cord within the vertebral canal (page 200, B35).

• The venous sinuses of the dura mater lie between the endosteal and meningeal layers. Some are situated in the midline and others are paired; they can be divided into two groups:

Posterosuperior	*Antero-inferior*
Superior sagittal	Cavernous (paired)
Inferior sagittal	Intercavernous
Straight	Sphenoparietal (paired)
Transverse (paired)	Superior petrosal (paired)
Sigmoid (paired)	Inferior petrosal (paired)
Petrosquamous (paired)	Basilar
Occipital	Middle meningeal veins (paired)

A

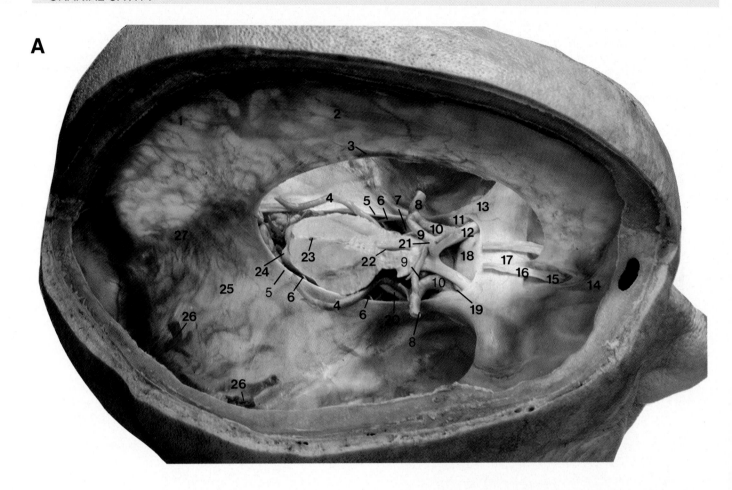

B

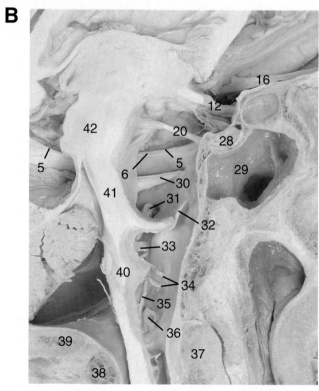

1 Superior sagittal sinus
2 Falx cerebri
3 Inferior sagittal sinus
4 Posterior cerebral artery
5 Free margin of tentorium cerebelli
6 Trochlear nerve
7 Attached margin of tentorium cerebelli and
  superior margin of petrous part of temporal
  bone with superior petrosal sinus
8 Middle cerebral artery
9 Anterior cerebral artery
10 Internal carotid artery
11 Anterior clinoid process
12 Optic nerve
13 Posterior margin of lesser wing of sphenoid
   bone and sphenoparietal sinus
14 Crista galli
15 Olfactory bulb
16 Olfactory tract
17 Jugum of sphenoid bone
18 Prechiasmatic groove
19 Ophthalmic artery
20 Oculomotor nerve
21 Anterior communicating artery
22 Third ventricle
23 Aqueduct of midbrain
24 Inferior colliculus
25 Tentorium cerebelli
26 Inferior cerebral veins
27 Straight sinus in junction of **2** and **25**
28 Pituitary gland
29 Left sphenoidal sinus
30 Trigeminal nerve
31 Facial and vestibulocochlear nerves and internal
   acoustic meatus
32 Abducent nerve
33 Roots of glossopharyngeal, vagus and cranial part of
   accessory nerves and jugular foramen
34 Roots of hypoglossal nerve and hypoglossal canal
35 Spinal root of accessory nerve
36 Vertebral artery
37 Dens of axis
38 Posterior arch of atlas
39 Margin of foramen magnum
40 Medulla oblongata
41 Pons
42 Midbrain

DURA MATER AND CRANIAL NERVES
A The falx cerebri and tentorium cerebelli, from the right and above
B The left half of the brainstem, with cranial nerves, in a midline sagittal section

In A the brain has been removed by cutting through the brainstem at the midbrain (23) and the lowest part of the third ventricle (22), level with the free margin of the tentorium cerebelli (5), leaving intact the optic chiasma (hidden by the anterior communicating and anterior cerebral arteries, 21 and 9) with the optic nerves (12) joining it. The olfactory tracts (16) and the anterior, middle and posterior cerebral arteries (9, 8 and 4) have been severed. The straight sinus (27) lies in the dura at the junction of the falx cerebri (2) and the tentorium cerebelli (25).

In B the anterior part of the brainstem has been dissected away, leaving the cranial nerves intact.

• The falx cerebri (A2) is the deep midline fold of dura mater, which hangs down from the cranial vault into the longitudinal fissure between the two cerebral hemispheres (page 158, 4). The superior sagittal sinus lies in its upper border (A1; page 158, 2; page 162, 3) and the inferior sagittal sinus in its lower (free) concave margin (A3; page 158, 62 and 5). Its narrow apex at the front is attached to the crista galli (page 158, 61), and its broad base at the back to the tentorium cerebelli with the straight sinus at the junction (A27; page 158, 18 and 17; page 166, A28).

• The tentorium cerebelli (A25) is the fold of dura mater forming the tent-like roof for much of the posterior cranial fossa (page 166, A27; page 168, 36). Its free margin (A5) forms the central gap over the anterior part of the fossa, which is occupied by the midbrain part of the brainstem (A23); at the front, the free margin runs forwards to form a ridge on the roof of the cavernous sinus (page 168, 33) and then becomes attached to the anterior clinoid process (A11; page 168, 32). Its attached margin adheres to the lips of the transverse and superior petrosal sinuses (page 168, 22 and 12), reaching the posterior clinoid process at the front (page 166, 8; page 168, 29). Note that the anterior end of the free margin crosses the anterior end of the attached margin before they reach their respective clinoid processes (best shown on page 168, 27 and 32, and 37 and 29).

• The falx cerebelli (page 158, 19) is a very small dural fold containing the occipital sinus, in the midline below the tentorium cerebelli.

• The diaphragma sellae (page 166, A17; page 168, 31) is a small circular fold of dura that forms a roof for the pituitary fossa. Part of the intercavernous sinus lies between its layers, and it is pierced by the pituitary stalk (page 166, A18; page 168, 30).

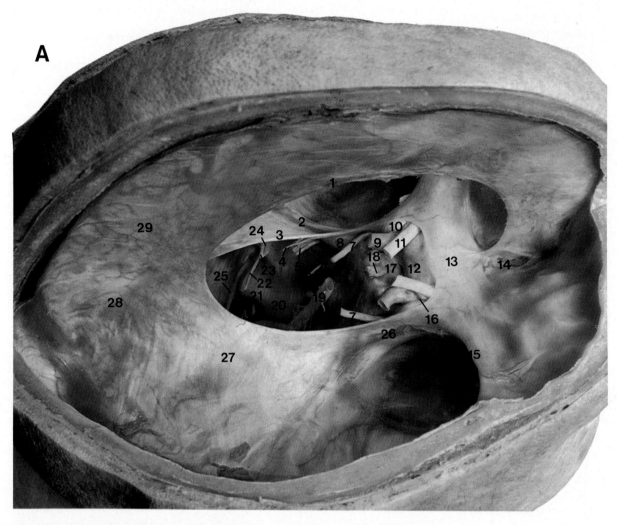

A

1
2
24 3
10
8 7 9 11
29
4
18
23 17 12 13 14
25 22
21 19 16
28 20
7
26
27 15

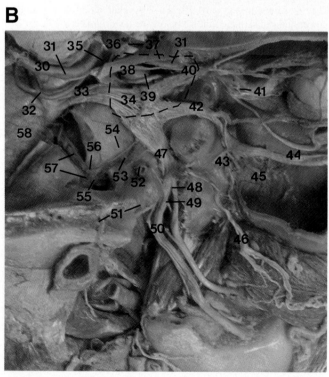

B

31 35 36 37 31
30 38 40
33 39 41
32 34
58 42
54 47 43 44
56 45
57 53 52
55 48
51 49
50 46

B and C

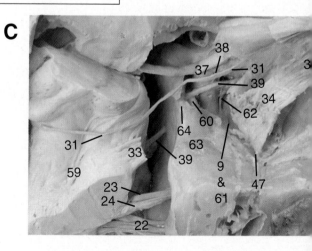

C

38
37 31
39
34
62
31 60
64 63 9
33 59 39 &
23 61 47
24
22

DURA MATER
The falx cerebri, tentorium cerebelli, cavernous sinus and the trigeminal nerve
A The falx and tentorium, from the right, above and behind
B The right cavernous sinus and trigeminal nerve, from the right
C The right cavernous sinus, from the right

In A the brainstem has been removed from the specimen shown on page 164 so that cranial nerves can be seen piercing the dura. The oculomotor nerve (7) enters the roof of the cavernous sinus (26); other nerves enter it from behind. The trochlear nerve (4) pierces the dura at the junction of the free and attached margins of the tentorium cerebelli (3 and 2), with the abducent nerve (6) lower down. The trigeminal nerve (5) runs forwards over the tip of the petrous part of the temporal bone, the facial and vestibulocochlear nerves (24 and 23) enter the internal acoustic meatus, and the roots of the glossopharyngeal, vagus and cranial part of the accessory nerves (22), with the spinal root of the accessory nerve (25), enter the jugular foramen. Compare with page 165, C.

In B much of the skull base of the right side has been dissected away and the superior orbital fissure (40), foramen rotundum (42) and foramen ovale (47) have been opened up, with removal of most of the dura but leaving part of the free margin of the tentorium (35) as a landmark. The dashed line indicates the extent of the cavernous sinus, whose contents (see notes) are seen from the lateral side. Bone of the petrous temporal has been removed to show the facial nerve (57) with its genicular ganglion (56) giving off the greater petrosal nerve (54) which runs forwards to the (hidden) foramen lacerum. The lesser petrosal nerve (53) emerges from the middle ear (55) to join the otic ganglion, hidden on the medial side of the mandibular nerve (47).

In C the lateral wall of the cavernous sinus has been opened up. The trigeminal nerve (33) has been transected and turned forwards, lifting the trigeminal ganglion (34) away from the trigeminal impression on the petrous bone (63) and giving a view of the oculomotor, trochlear and abducent nerves (37, 31 and 39) in the sinus.

• The cavernous sinus (A26; page 168, 33) contains the internal carotid artery with its sympathetic plexus (C38 and 62); the abducent nerve on the lateral side of the artery (B39); and the oculomotor, trochlear, ophthalmic and maxillary nerves in the lateral wall (B37, 31, 40 and 42).

• The trigeminal ganglion (B34) lies in the trigeminal cave of dura mater, in the trigeminal impression (C63; page 50, C37) at the apex of the petrous part of the temporal bone, below and behind the cavernous sinus.

• The facial nerve (B57) enters the internal acoustic meatus and runs laterally in the facial canal above the vestibule of the inner ear to the genicular ganglion (B56) in the medial wall of the epitympanic recess. The nerve then takes a right-angled turn backwards in the medial wall of the middle ear (B55) above the promontory, passes downwards in the medial wall of the aditus to the mastoid antrum, and finally emerges through the stylomastoid foramen.

• The greater petrosal nerve (B54, from the facial) is joined by the deep petrosal nerve (from the sympathetic plexus of the internal carotid artery, C62) within the foramen lacerum to form the nerve of the pterygoid canal (page 142, A6).

• After emerging from the brainstem between the pons and pyramid (page 188, A11), the abducent nerve runs forwards and slightly upwards and laterally through the cisterna pontis to pierce the dura mater on the clivus (C, lower 39). The nerve continues upwards beneath the dura to bend forwards over the tip of the petrous part of the temporal bone and beneath the petrosphenoidal ligament (C64) to enter the cavernous sinus. The nerve can be damaged in fractures of the skull that involve the petrous temporal or clivus, or by stretching if the brainstem is forced downwards. Displacement of the midbrain may also damage the oculomotor and trochlear nerves.

1	Inferior margin of falx cerebri and inferior sagittal sinus	**22**	Roots of glossopharyngeal, vagus and cranial part of accessory nerves	**43**	Posterior superior alveolar nerve
2	Attached margin of tentorium cerebelli and superior petrosal sinus	**23**	Vestibulocochlear nerve	**44**	Infra-orbital nerve
		24	Facial nerve	**45**	Maxillary sinus
3	Free margin of tentorium cerebelli	**25**	Spinal root of accessory nerve	**46**	Buccal nerve
4	Trochlear nerve	**26**	Cavernous sinus	**47**	Mandibular nerve in foramen ovale
5	Trigeminal nerve	**27**	Tentorium cerebelli	**48**	Lingual nerve
6	Abducent nerve	**28**	Straight sinus in junction between **27** and **29**	**49**	Chorda tympani
7	Oculomotor nerve			**50**	Inferior alveolar nerve
8	Posterior clinoid process	**29**	Falx cerebri	**51**	Auriculotemporal nerve
9	Internal carotid artery	**30**	Posterior cerebral artery	**52**	Middle meningeal artery in foramen spinosum
10	Anterior clinoid process	**31**	Trochlear nerve		
11	Optic nerve	**32**	Superior cerebellar artery	**53**	Lesser petrosal nerve
12	Prechiasmatic groove	**33**	Trigeminal nerve	**54**	Greater petrosal nerve
13	Jugum of sphenoid bone	**34**	Trigeminal ganglion	**55**	Middle ear (tympanic cavity)
14	Cribriform plate of ethmoid bone	**35**	Free margin of tentorium cerebelli	**56**	Genicular ganglion of facial nerve
15	Posterior margin of lesser wing of sphenoid bone and spheno-parietal sinus	**36**	Middle cerebral artery	**57**	Facial nerve
		37	Oculomotor nerve	**58**	Cerebellum
		38	Internal carotid artery	**59**	Pons
16	Ophthalmic artery	**39**	Abducent nerve	**60**	Apex of petrous part of temporal bone
17	Diaphragma sellae	**40**	Ophthalmic nerve entering superior orbital fissure		
18	Pituitary stalk			**61**	Upper margin of foramen lacerum
19	Basilar artery	**41**	Ciliary ganglion	**62**	Sympathetic plexus (internal carotid nerve)
20	Left vertebral artery	**42**	Maxillary nerve in foramen rotundum		
21	Hypoglossal nerve			**63**	Trigeminal impression
				64	Petrosphenoidal ligament

167

FRONT

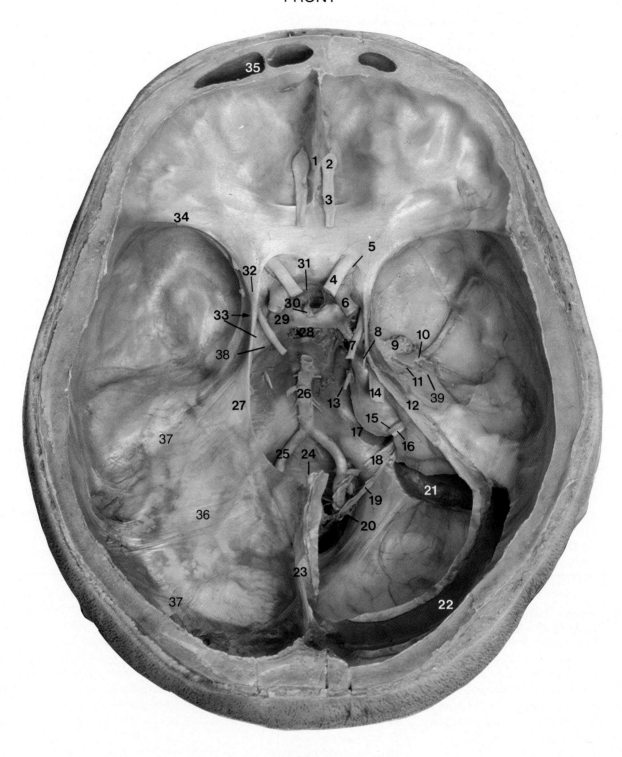

BACK

1 Falx cerebri attached to crista galli
2 Olfactory bulb
3 Olfactory tract
4 Optic nerve emerging from optic canal
5 Ophthalmic artery
6 Internal carotid artery
7 Oculomotor nerve
8 Trochlear nerve
9 Mandibular nerve and foramen ovale
10 Middle meningeal artery and foramen spinosum
11 Groove for greater petrosal nerve
12 Superior petrosal sinus and cut edges of attached margin of tentorium cerebelli
13 Abducent nerve
14 Trigeminal nerve
15 Facial nerve
16 Vestibulocochlear nerve
17 Inferior petrosal sinus
18 Roots of glossopharyngeal, vagus and cranial part of accessory nerves
19 Spinal root of accessory nerve
20 Hypoglossal nerve
21 Sigmoid sinus
22 Transverse sinus
23 Straight sinus at junction of falx cerebri and tentorium cerebelli
24 Great cerebral vein
25 Vertebral artery
26 Basilar artery
27 Free margin of tentorium cerebelli
28 Upper part of basilar plexus
29 Posterior clinoid process
30 Pituitary stalk
31 Diaphragma sellae
32 Anterior clinoid process
33 Cavernous sinus
34 Posterior margin of lesser wing of sphenoid bone and sphenoparietal sinus
35 Frontal sinus
36 Tentorium cerebelli
37 Attached margin of tentorium
38 Attached margin of tentorium passing to 29
39 Groove for lesser petrosal nerve

THE CRANIAL FOSSAE, FROM ABOVE

The right half of the tentorium cerebelli (36) has been removed. The right transverse, sigmoid and superior petrosal sinuses (22, 21 and 12) and the straight sinus (23) have been opened up, and part of the dura has been stripped off from the right lateral part of the middle cranial fossa to reveal the middle meningeal artery (10), the mandibular nerve (9) and the groove for the greater petrosal nerve (11). Compare this view of the various cranial nerves piercing the dura with that on page 166, A.

• The tentorium cerebelli (36) forms the roof of the posterior cranial fossa; the anterior and middle cranial fossae have no defined upper boundary.

• The *anterior cranial fossa* contains:
  the front parts of the frontal lobes of the cerebral hemispheres (page 163, 14)
  the olfactory nerves, olfactory bulbs and olfactory tracts (2 and 3)
  the anterior ethmoidal nerves and vessels (page 120, C32 and 35)

• The *middle cranial fossa* contains in its median part:
  the pituitary stalk and gland and the diaphragma sellae (30 and 31)
  the optic nerves (4) and optic chiasma (page188, A3 and 4)
  the intercavernous sinus (below the pituitary gland)
  and in its lateral parts:
  the cavernous sinus (33) containing the internal carotid artery and sympathetic plexus, the oculomotor, trochlear and abducent nerves, and the ophthalmic and maxillary branches of the trigeminal nerve (see pages 166 and 167)
  the trigeminal ganglion and the mandibular branch of the trigeminal nerve (see pages 166 and 167)
  the greater and lesser petrosal nerves (11 and 39)
  the middle meningeal (10) and accessory meningeal vessels, and meningeal branches of the ascending pharyngeal, ophthalmic and lacrimal arteries
  the temporal lobes of the cerebral hemispheres (page 163, 13)

• The *posterior cranial fossa* contains:
  the lowest part of the midbrain, and the pons, medulla oblongata and cerebellum (page 158, 10, 25, 26 and 22)
  the vertebral and basilar arteries and their branches (25 and 26), and meningeal branches of the ascending pharyngeal and occipital arteries
  the sigmoid (21), inferior petrosal (17), basilar and occipital sinuses, with the straight, transverse and superior petrosal sinuses in the tentorium cerebelli that forms the roof (23, 22 and 12)
  the trigeminal (14), abducent (13), facial (15), vestibulocochlear (16), glossopharyngeal, vagus and accessory (18 and 19) and hyoglossal nerves (i.e. the fifth to twelfth cranial nerves), and meningeal branches of upper cervical nerves
  the falx cerebelli (page 158, 19).

• The posterior (lower) end of the superior sagittal sinus is known as the confluence of the sinuses, where there is communication with the straight and occipital sinuses and the transverse sinuses of both sides.

BRAIN

FRONT

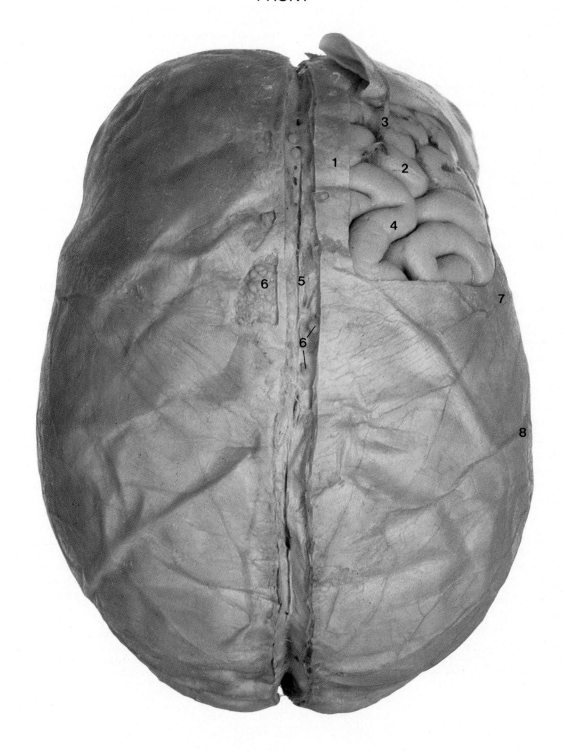

BACK

BRAIN AND MENINGES
The brain within the meninges, from above

Here the whole of the dura mater has been stripped off from the inside of the cranial vault and removed intact with the brain; this is an unusual dissection—the dura is normally left within the cranium (as on page 161, B) and the brain removed with the arachnoid surrounding it (as on pages 172 and 174). A window has been cut in the dura over the front of the right cerebral hemisphere, and the flap of dura turned forwards to show the underlying filmy and transparent arachnoid mater; some arachnoid has been removed, and it is labelled (2) at the cut edge. The dura forming the roof of the superior sagittal sinus (5) has also been removed, to show the arachnoid granulations (6) projecting into the sinus (cerebrospinal fluid drains into the venous blood through the walls of these projections).

```
1  Dura mater
2  Arachnoid mater (cut edge)
3  A superior cerebral vein
4  Cerebral hemisphere (and pia mater)
5  Superior sagittal sinus
6  Arachnoid granulations
7  Frontal branch  ⎫
                    ⎬ of middle meningeal artery
8  Parietal branch ⎭
```

• For notes on the meninges see page 159

• The central nervous system consists of the brain and spinal cord (properly known as the spinal medulla).

• The brain consists of:
   the hindbrain (rhombencephalon), comprising the medulla oblongata (myelencephalon), pons (metencephalon) and the cerebellum
   the midbrain (mesencephalon)
   the forebrain (prosencephalon), comprising the diencephalon (structures surrounding the third ventricle) and the cerebral hemispheres (telencephalon)

• The cavity of the hindbrain is the fourth ventricle.

• The cavity of the midbrain is the aqueduct.

• The cavities of the forebrain are the third ventricle (centrally) and the lateral ventricles (one in each cerebral hemisphere).

• For notes on the ventricles see page 191.

• The brainstem (see page 181) consists of:
   the midbrain
   the pons
   the medulla oblongata

• The peripheral nervous system consists of:
   the cranial nerves (12 pairs)
   the spinal nerves (31 pairs)
   the autonomic system of nerves and their associated ganglia

BACK

A

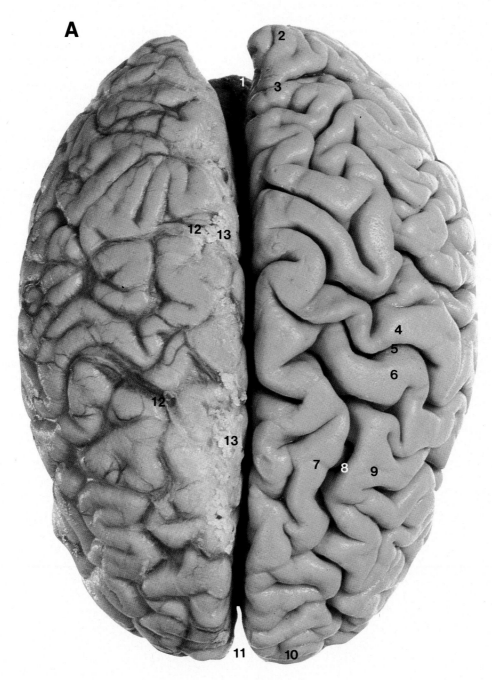

FRONT

1 Cerebellum
2 Occipital pole
3 Parieto-occipital sulcus
4 Postcentral gyrus
5 Central sulcus
6 Precentral gyrus
7 Superior frontal gyrus
8 Superior frontal sulcus
9 Middle frontal gyrus
10 Frontal pole
11 Longitudinal fissure
12 Superior cerebral veins
13 Arachnoid granulations
14 Cerebellar hemisphere
15 Arachnoid mater of cerebellomedullary cistern (cisterna magna)

CEREBRAL HEMISPHERES AND CEREBELLUM
The cerebral and cerebellar hemispheres
A The cerebral hemispheres, from above
B The lower part of the brain, from behind, showing the cerebellum

The arachnoid, with the underlying blood vessels, remains intact over the right cerebral hemisphere in A and B, and over the cerebellum in B, but it has been removed from the left hemisphere. In life, cerebrospinal fluid would raise the arachnoid from the brain surface. The larger gaps beneath the arachnoid form various cisterns (cisternae), such as the cerebellomedullary cistern (cisterna magna, 15)

• The cerebral cortex is thrown into broad convoluted folds known as gyri (singular—gyrus). The spaces between the gyri are the sulci (singular—sulcus).

No two brains have identical gyri and sulci, but the general pattern is sufficiently constant to allow the gyri and sulci to be named. Only those of major clinical importance are identified here and on pages 176 and 182

• The cerebellar cortex is thrown into narrow closely-packed folds known as folia. Unlike the gyri of the cerebral cortex, the cerebellar folia are not individually identified, but names are given to particular areas.

B

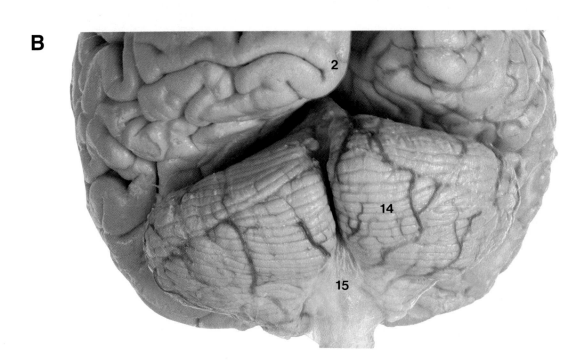

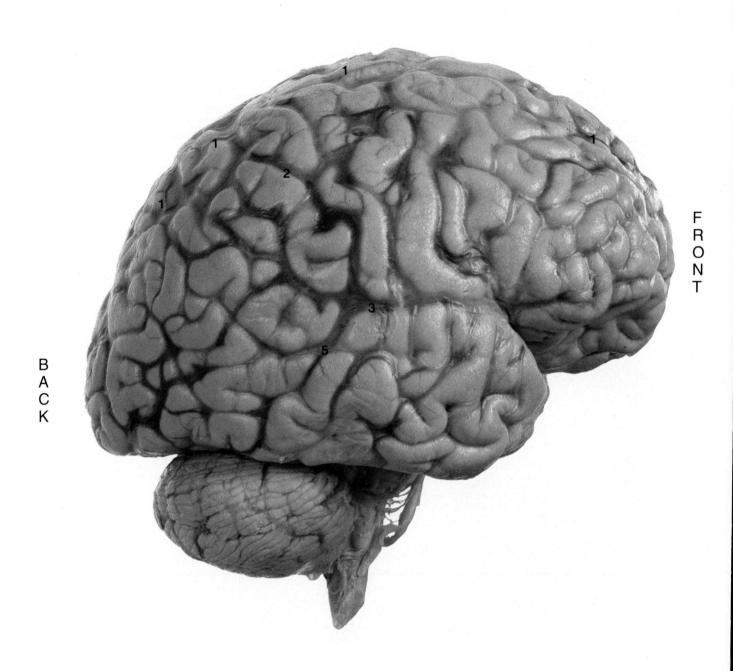

BACK

FRONT

CEREBRAL VEINS
The external cerebral veins, from the right
The arachnoid mater has been left intact over the cerebral hemispheres, leaving vessels visible underneath the the arachnoid. The larger ones are veins and the more important are identified. (For arteries see page 178.)

1 Superior cerebral veins
2 Superior anastomotic vein
3 Superficial middle cerebral vein overlying posterior ramus of lateral sulcus
4 Inferior cerebral veins
5 Inferior anastomotic vein

• Most cerebral veins do not accompany arteries and are named differently. The main exceptions are the anterior cerebral veins.

• Veins of the brain can be divided into internal and external groups.

• The two internal cerebral veins (right and left) receive blood from the inner parts of the brain, and unite to form the great cerebral vein (page 180, 14; page 158, 15).

• Various external veins drain the surfaces: superior and inferior cerebral veins, superficial and deep middle cerebral veins, superior and inferior anastomotic veins, and the basal vein. Most of them enter the nearest convenient venous sinus.
　The superior cerebral veins (as at 1), 8–12 in number, drain into the superior sagittal sinus (page 170, 5; page 158, 2 and 3), the more posterior veins entering obliquely in a forward direction (against the normal current in the sinus, which is from front to back).
　The superficial middle cerebral vein (3) runs forwards along the surface of the main part of the lateral sulcus and drains into the cavernous sinus (page 168, 33).
　The inferior cerebral veins (4) are small. Those under the frontal lobe join superior cererbal veins and drain into the superior sagittal sinus. From the temporal lobe they drain into the cavernous, superior petrosal and transverse sinuses (page 168, 33, 12 and 22).
　The superior anastomotic vein (2) runs upwards and backwards from the superficial middle cerebral vein (3) to the superior sagittal sinus, and the inferior anastomotic vein (5) passes downwards and backwards to the transverse sinus (page 168, 22).

• The internal cerebral vein (page 191, B31) is formed by the union of the thalamostriate and choroidal veins (with some smaller adjacent veins from the choroid plexus, page 191, B8) and runs backwards in the tela choroidea of the roof of the third ventricle (see the note on page 191), to unite with its fellow of the opposite side beneath the splenium of the corpus callosum to form the great cerebral vein (page 191, B32; page 180, 14; page 158, 15).

• The basal vein (page 159, 16) is formed by the union of the anterior cerebral vein (which accompanies the artery of the same name, page 158, 59), the deep middle cerebral vein (from the insula, page 177, B), and the striate veins (from the anterior perforated substance, page 188, B32). It passes backwards round the lateral side of the cerebral peduncle to join the great cerebral vein (page 158, 15).

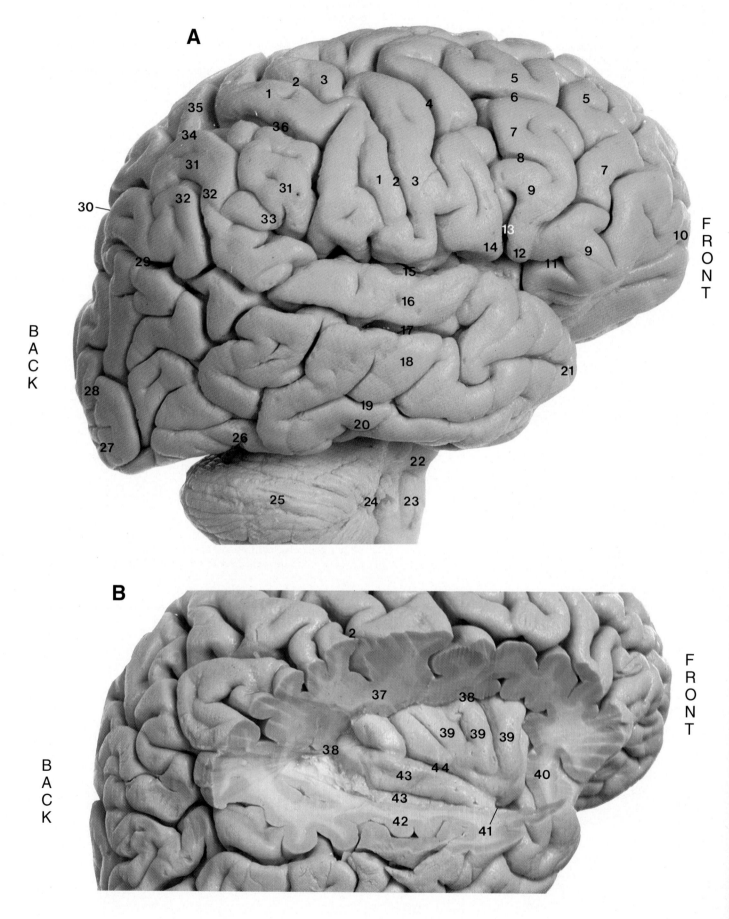

CEREBRAL HEMISPHERES
The right cerebral hemisphere
A The superolateral surface, from the right
B The insula, from the right
C Diagram of principal cortical areas, superolateral surface
D Diagram of principal cortical areas, medial surface
In A the major sulci and gyri are identified.

In B the cortex bounding the lateral sulcus (A15) has been removed to show the insula—the cortex buried in the depths of the lateral sulcus and only seen when the overlapping margins of the sulcus (the opercula or lids) are displaced or removed. On the diagrams in C and D the principal functional areas of the cortex are indicated.

1	Postcentral gyrus
2	Central sulcus
3	Precentral gyrus
4	Precentral sulcus
5	Superior frontal gyrus
6	Superior frontal sulcus
7	Middle frontal gyrus
8	Inferior frontal sulcus
9	Inferior frontal gyrus
10	Frontal pole
11	Anterior ramus of lateral sulcus
12	Pars triangularis of inferior frontal gyrus
13	Ascending ramus of lateral sulcus
14	Pars opercularis of inferior frontal gyrus
15	Lateral sulcus (posterior ramus)
16	Superior temporal gyrus
17	Superior temporal sulcus
18	Middle temporal sulcus
19	Inferior temporal sulcus
20	Inferior temporal gyrus
21	Temporal pole
22	Pons
23	Medulla oblongata
24	Flocculus
25	Cerebellar hemisphere
26	Pre-occipital notch
27	Occipital pole
28	Lunate sulcus
29	Transverse occipital sulcus
30	Parieto-occipital sulcus
31	Inferior parietal lobule
32	Angular gyrus
33	Supramarginal gyrus
34	Intraparietal sulcus
35	Superior parietal lobule
36	Postcentral sulcus
37	Frontoparietal operculum
38	Circular sulcus of insula
39	Short gyri of insula
40	Frontal operculum
41	Limen of insula
42	Temporal operculum
43	Long gyri of insula
44	Central sulcus of insula

• The cerebral hemisphere has frontal, parietal, occipital and temporal lobes.

The frontal lobe is the part lying in front of the central sulcus (2).

The parietal lobe is bounded in front by the central sulcus (2) and behind by the upper part of a line drawn from the parieto-occipital sulcus (30) to the pre-occipital notch (26). The lower limit is the posterior ramus of the lateral sulcus (15) (and an arbitrary line continued backwards in the main line of this ramus to the posterior boundary).

The occipital lobe lies behind the line joining the parieto-occipital sulcus (30) to the pre-occipital notch (26).

The temporal lobe lies below the lateral sulcus (15), and is bounded behind by the lower part of the line drawn from the parieto-occipital sulcus (30) to the pre-occipital notch (26).

• The lateral sulcus consists of short anterior and ascending rami (A11 and 13) and a longer posterior ramus (15), which itself is commonly known as the lateral sulcus.

• The areas around the anterior and ascending rami of the lateral sulcus (A11 and 13) of the *left* cerebral hemisphere constitute the motor speech area (of Broca).

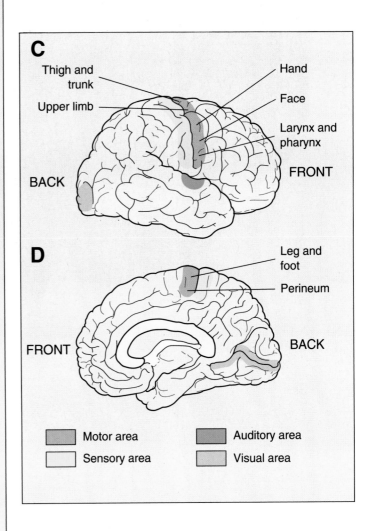

C

Thigh and trunk
Hand
Upper limb
Face
Larynx and pharynx
BACK
FRONT

D

Leg and foot
Perineum
FRONT
BACK

Motor area	Auditory area
Sensory area	Visual area

A

FRONT

BACK

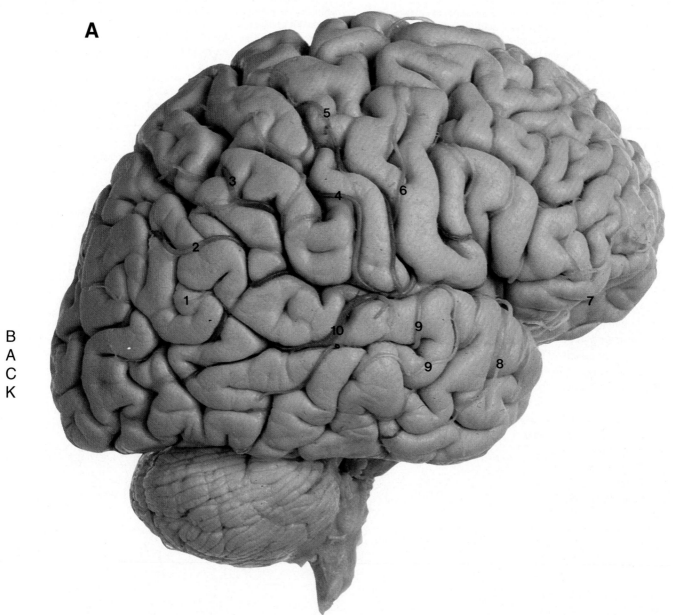

CEREBRAL HEMISPHERES
Blood supply of the cerebral cortex
A The right middle cerebral artery, from the right
B Diagram of cortical blood supplies, superolateral surface
C Diagram of cortical blood supplies, medial surface

In A the arachnoid mater and all veins have been removed. Branches of the middle cerebral artery emerge from the lateral sulcus to spread out over much of the superolateral surface of the cortex.

The diagrams in B and C indicate the areas of cortex supplied by the three cerebral arteries.

• The middle cerebral artery supplies a large part of the superolateral aspect of the cerebral cortex, except for a strip about 1 cm wide along the upper border (B, anterior cerebral, extending over from the medial surface, C, and page 183), and the lower border (B and C, posterior cerebral, and page 183).

• The cortex supplied by the middle cerebral artery includes much of the motor area of the precentral gyrus (but excluding the perineal and leg areas, page 177, D), and the insula in the depths of the lateral sulcus (page 176, B).

• Some small middle cerebral branches extend as far back as the most lateral part of the visual area (page 183).

• For branches of the anterior and posterior cerebral arteries see page182, B.

B BACK   FRONT

C FRONT   BACK

Anterior cerebral artery
Posterior cerebral artery
Middle cerebral artery

1 Artery of angular gyrus ⎫
2 Posterior parietal artery ⎪
3 Anterior parietal artery ⎬ branches of terminal (cortical) part
4 Artery of postcentral sulcus ⎪
5 Artery of central sulcus ⎪
6 Artery of precentral sulcus ⎭
7 Lateral frontobasal artery ⎫
8 Anterior temporal artery ⎬ branches of insular part
9 Intermediate temporal artery ⎪
10 Posterior temporal artery ⎭

179

BRAIN AND BRAINSTEM
The right half of the brain and brainstem
A In a midline sagittal section, from the left
B Magnetic resonance (MR) image

In A the brain has been cut in half longitudinally, exactly in the
midline, and the right half is seen from the left. The corpus callosum
(3–6), which connects the two cerebral hemispheres together, forms an
obvious central feature. The aqueduct of the midbrain (22) connects the
third ventricle (11) with the fourth ventricle (19). The optic chiasma
(31) is at the front lower corner of the third ventricle, with the stalk of
the pituitary gland (30) just behind the chiasma. Compare this section
with the MR image in B and with the similar section within the cranial
cavity (page 158).

• The brainstem consists of the midbrain (21), pons (20) and medulla
oblongata (17).

• The midbrain consists of the two cerebral peduncles (page 188, A26;
page 188, B39).

• Each cerebral peduncle consists of a ventral part, the crus of the
peduncle (basis pedunculi), and a dorsal part, the tegmentum. Between
the crus and tegmentum is a layer of pigmented grey matter, the
substantia nigra.

The tegmentum contains the aqueduct of the midbrain (22), and the
part of the tegmentum dorsal to the aqueduct is the tectum, which
includes the superior and inferior colliculi (24 and 23).

• When removing the brain from the cranial cavity, the pituitary stalk
(30) is torn, leaving the gland in the pituitary fossa (page 158, 50).

• The pituitary gland (hypophysis cerebri) consists of two
developmentally and functionally different parts, the adenohypophysis
and neurohypophysis.

The adenohypophysis (the more anterior part of the gland) is
developed from an outgrowth of ectoderm (Rathke's pouch) from the
primitive mouth, and consists histologically of the pars distalis (pars
anterior), pars tuberalis and pars intermedia.

The neurohypophysis (the more posterior part of the gland) is
developed from an outgrowth of neuro-ectoderm from the primitive
forebrain, and consists of the pars nervosa, the infundibulum and the
median eminence.

• The term 'anterior pituitary' or 'anterior lobe of the pituitary' is
commonly understood to mean the pars distalis of the adenohypophysis,
and 'posterior pituitary' or 'posterior lobe of the pituitary' to mean the
pars nervosa.

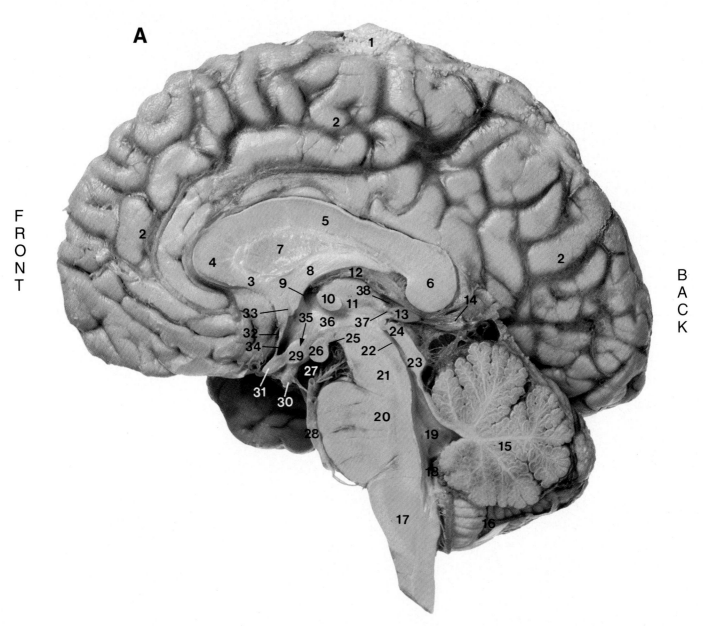

• The infundibulum is the upper hollow part of the pituitary stalk (30) and contains the infundibular recess of the third ventricle (35).

• The tuber cinereum, the part of the floor of the third ventricle between the mamillary bodies (26) and the optic chiasma (31), includes an area at the base of the infundibulum known as the median eminence. This is the site of the neurosecretory cells whose products (regulatory factors) enter the hypophysial portal system of blood vessels to control the release of hormones from the cells of the anterior pituitary.

• The main hormones of the anterior pituitary are growth hormone, prolactin, TSH, ACTH, LH and FSH.

• The hormones of the posterior pituitary are produced in neurosecretory cells of the paraventricular and supra-optic nuclei in the lateral wall of the third ventricle. The axons of these cells run down in the pituitary stalk to the posterior pituitary, and the secretory products are stored within the nerve fibres.

• The main hormones of the posterior pituitary are oxytocin and vasopressin (ADH).

1 Arachnoid granulations	13 Pineal body	26 Mamillary body
2 Arachnoid mater and vessels overlying medial surface of cerebral hemisphere	14 Great cerebral vein	27 Interpeduncular cistern
	15 Cerebellum	28 Basilar artery
	16 Cerebellomedullary cistern (cisterna magna)	29 Tuber cinereum
3 Rostrum	17 Medulla oblongata	30 Pituitary stalk (infundibulum)
4 Genu } of corpus callosum	18 Choroid plexus of fourth ventricle	31 Optic chiasma
5 Body	19 Fourth ventricle	32 Lamina terminalis
6 Splenium	20 Pons	33 Anterior commissure
7 Septum pellucidum	21 Midbrain	34 Optic recess
8 Body of fornix	22 Aqueduct of midbrain	35 Infundibular recess
9 Interventricular foramen	23 Inferior colliculus	36 Hypothalamus
10 Interthalamic adhesion	24 Superior colliculus	37 Pineal recess
11 Third ventricle	25 Posterior perforated substance	38 Suprapineal recess
12 Choroid plexus of third ventricle		39 Pituitary gland

B

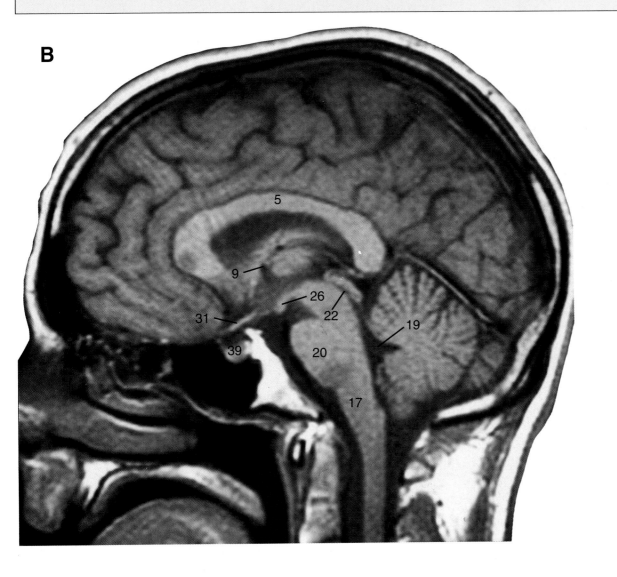

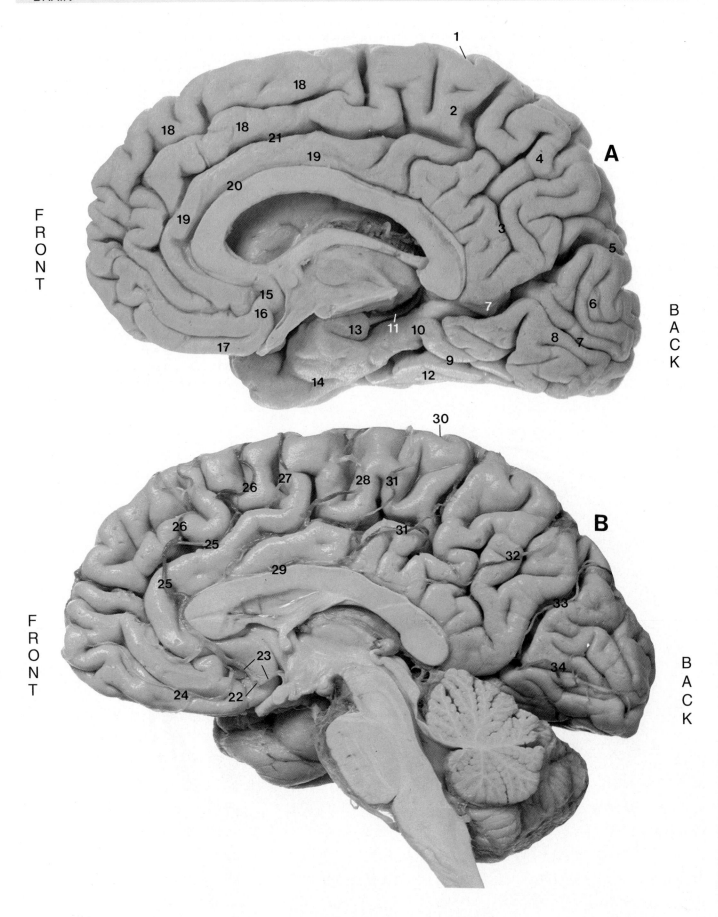

1 Central sulcus
2 Paracentral lobule
3 Subparietal sulcus
4 Precuneus
5 Parieto-occipital sulcus
6 Cuneus
7 Calcarine sulcus
8 Lingual gyrus
9 Collateral sulcus
10 Parahippocampal gyrus
11 Dentate gyrus
12 Medial occipitotemporal gyrus
13 Uncus
14 Rhinal sulcus
15 Paraterminal gyrus
16 Subcallosal area
17 Gyrus rectus
18 Medial frontal gyrus
19 Cingulate gyrus
20 Corpus callosal sulcus
21 Cingulate sulcus
22 Anterior communicating artery
23 Anterior cerebral artery
24 Medial frontobasal artery
25 Callosomarginal artery
26 Anteromedial frontal artery
27 Intermediomedial frontal artery
28 Posteromedial frontal artery   } from the anterior
29 Pericallosal artery   cerebral artery
30 Central sulcus
31 Paracentral artery
32 Precuneal artery
33 Parieto-occipital branch } of posterior cerebral artery
34 Calcarine branch

CEREBRAL HEMISPHERES AND BRAINSTEM
The medial surface of the hemispheres and cerebral arteries
A **The medial surface of the right cerebral hemisphere, in a midline sagittal section with the brainstem removed, from the left**
B **The right half of a midline sagittal section of the brain and brainstem, with branches of the anterior and posterior cerebral arteries, from the left**

In A removal of the brainstem allows more of the medial surface of the temporal lobe to be seen, e.g. the parahippocampal gyrus (10), the collateral sulcus (9) and the anterior part of the calcarine sulcus (7).

In B various cortical branches of the anterior and posterior cerebral arteries are shown; the most important are the posterior cerebral branches to the visual cortex. (For branches of the middle cerebral artery, see 178.)

• On the surface of the cerebral hemisphere the anterior cerebral artery (B23) supplies the cortex on the medial aspect as far back as the parieto-occipital sulcus (A5), and a strip on the upper part of the superolateral surface adjacent to the midline (page 179, B). The cortex supplied includes the perineal and leg areas on the medial surface (page 177, D).

• The posterior cerebral artery (page 186, A and B, 9) supplies the cortex of the occipital lobe and an area continuing forwards on the medial and inferior surfaces of the temporal lobe as far as and including the uncus (A13), but not including the temporal pole which has a middle cerebral supply. The cortex supplied includes the visual area (striate cortex, page 177, D; page 192, B39).

FRONT

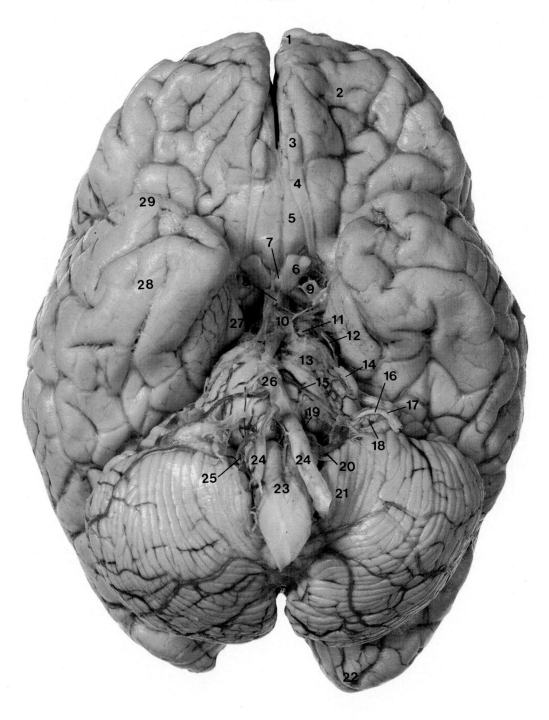

BACK

1 Frontal pole
2 Inferior surface of frontal lobe
3 Olfactory bulb
4 Olfactory tract
5 Gyrus rectus
6 Optic nerve
7 Optic chiasma
8 Pituitary stalk
9 Internal carotid artery
10 Arachnoid mater overlying mamillary bodies
11 Oculomotor nerve
12 Trochlear nerve
13 Pons
14 Trigeminal nerve
15 Labyrinthine artery
16 Facial nerve
17 Vestibulocochlear nerve
18 Flocculus
19 Abducent nerve
20 Rootlets of glossopharyngeal, vagus and cranial part
   of accessory nerves
21 Tonsil of cerebellum
22 Occipital pole
23 Medulla oblongata
24 Vertebral artery
25 Posterior inferior cerebellar artery
26 Basilar artery
27 Uncus
28 Inferior surface of temporal lobe
29 Temporal pole

BASE OF THE BRAIN
The brain with the brainstem, from below
This is the view of the base of the brain as typically seen after removal from the cranial cavity; some arachnoid mater is still adherent. The medulla oblongata (23), and the two vertebral arteries (24), internal carotid arteries (9) and optic nerves (6) are the largest structures which have to be cut through in order to remove the brain. The remaining cranial nerves must also be cut, although the filaments of the olfactory nerve are invariably avulsed from the olfactory bulb (3) if the bulb itself is removed with the brain. The pituitary stalk (8) is severed, leaving the gland in its fossa in the base of the skull (page 158, 50). Details of the blood vessels and nerves are given on pages 186–189.

• The inferior surface of the frontal lobe (2) shows a slight concavity due to the convexity of the orbital part of the frontal bone in the anterior cranial fossa (page 28, A10).

• The inferior surface of the temporal lobe (28) lies in the lateral part of the middle cranial fossa (page 28, A21).

• The pons (13) and the overlying basilar artery (26) lie behind the clivus (page 28, A42).

• The medulla oblongata (23) has been transected at the level where it passes through the foramen magnum (page 28, A40) to become continuous with the spinal cord (page 158, 30).

• The tonsils of the cerebellum (21) lie just above the lateral margins of the foramen magnum (page 158, 63); increased intracranial pressure may force them into the top of the foramen and so impede the circulation of cerebrospinal fluid into the spinal subarachnoid space.

BASE OF THE BRAIN
The arteries of the base of the brain and brainstem
A The brain, from below, with arteries in place
B The arterial circle and associated vessels
The arteries taking part in the arterial circle (see note) are displayed: anterior communicating (38, in the midline), and on each side the anterior cerebral (3), internal carotid (6), posterior communicating (8) and posterior cerebral (9, from the basilar, 15).

In A removal of the front part of the right temporal lobe has opened up the lateral sulcus to show how the middle cerebral artery courses laterally through it, giving off the cortical branches (as at 34 and 35), which emerge on to the lateral surface of the cerebral hemisphere (page 178). Also revealed is the optic tract (32), passing back from the optic chiasma (4) round the side of the cerebral peduncle (31) to the lateral geniculate body (29). Superficial to the optic tract lies the anterior choroidal artery (33), running into the choroid plexus of the inferior horn of the lateral ventricle (30) and so forming the main supply of the choroid plexus of the lateral and third ventricles.

In B the various arteries have been removed en bloc and spread out to indicate their anastomotic connexions.

FRONT

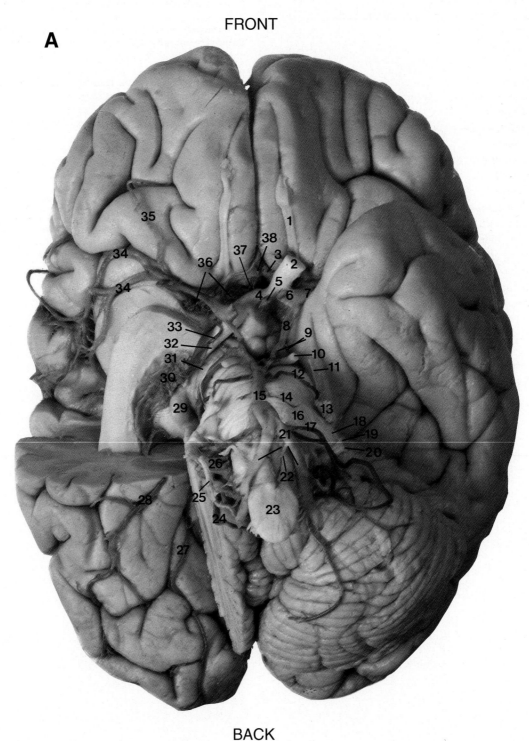

BACK

1 Olfactory tract
2 Optic nerve
3 Anterior cerebral artery
4 Optic chiasma
5 Pituitary stalk
6 Internal carotid artery
7 Middle cerebral artery
8 Posterior communicating artery
9 Posterior cerebral artery
10 Oculomotor nerve
11 Trochlear nerve
12 Superior cerebellar artery
13 Trigeminal nerve
14 Labyrinthine artery
15 Basilar artery
16 Pons
17 Anterior inferior cerebellar artery
18 Middle cerebellar peduncle
19 Facial nerve
20 Vestibulocochlear nerve
21 Vertebral artery
22 Anterior spinal artery
23 Medulla oblongata
24 Posterior inferior cerebellar artery
25 Spinal root of accessory nerve
26 Rootlets of glossopharyngeal, vagus and cranial part of accessory nerves
27 Posterior temporal ⎫ branch of posterior
28 Middle temporal ⎭ cerebral artery
29 Lateral geniculate body
30 Choroid plexus of inferior horn of lateral ventricle
31 Cerebral peduncle
32 Optic tract
33 Anterior choroidal artery
34 Cortical branches of middle cerebral artery
35 Lateral frontobasal artery
36 Striate branches of middle and anterior cerebral arteries
37 Long central (recurrent) branch of anterior cerebral artery
38 Anterior communicating artery

• The arterial circle (of Willis) is an anastomosis between the internal carotid and vertebral systems of vessels. It is hexagonal rather than circular in shape. The anterior cerebral branches (3) of each internal carotid artery (6) are joined by the (single) anterior communicating artery (38). On each side a posterior communicating artery (8) joins the internal carotid (6) to the posterior cerebral artery (9), the two posterior cerebrals being the terminal branches of the (single midline) basilar artery (15) which itself has been formed by the union of the two vertebral arteries (21). At the point where the anterior and posterior communicating vessels come off the internal carotid (passing forwards and backwards, respectively), the middle cerebral artery (7) runs laterally.

• The various striate branches of the middle and anterior cerebral arteries (36) which enter the anterior perforated substance (page 188, B32) supply (among other structures) the internal capsule (page 193). One such branch of the middle cerebral artery has become known as the 'artery of cerebral haemorrhage', since it is particularly liable to rupture and damage the corticonuclear and corticospinal fibres that course through the capsule. This type of cerebral damage causes varying degrees of paralysis, especially of the limbs, and is commonly called a 'stroke'.

• The third (oculomotor) and fourth (trochlear) nerves (10 and 11) pass between the posterior cerebral and superior cerebellar arteries (9 and 12).

FRONT

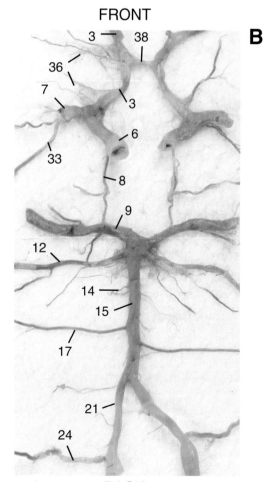

B

BACK

187

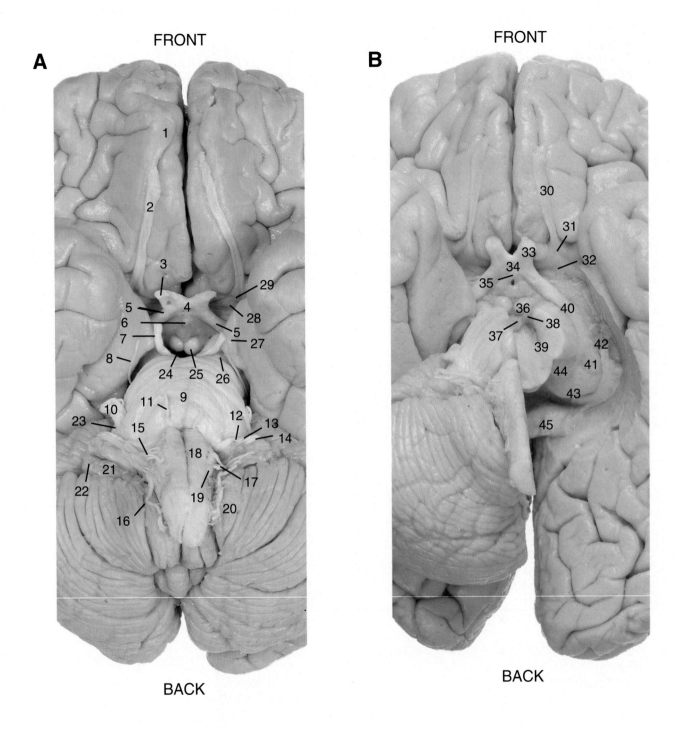

FRONT

A

1
2
3
29
5   4
6   28
7   5
8   27
24 25 26
9
10   11
23   12 13
15   14
21   18
22   17
19   20
16

BACK

FRONT

B

30
31
33
34   32
35
36   40
38
37   39   42
44   41
43
45

BACK

BASE OF THE BRAIN
The brainstem, cranial nerves and geniculate bodies
A Brain with the brainstem, from below
B With most of the left half of the brainstem removed
In A all vessels have been removed to give a clear view of the cranial nerves and their relationship to the brainstem (see notes).

In B the left half of the brainstem has been removed at midbrain level to show the optic tract (40) winding backwards round the side of the cerebral peduncle (39) and leading to the lateral geniculate body (41), with the medial geniculate body adjacent (44).

1 Olfactory bulb
2 Olfactory tract
3 Optic nerve
4 Optic chiasma
5 Optic tract
6 Pituitary stalk
7 Oculomotor nerve
8 Trochlear nerve
9 Pons
10 Trigeminal nerve
11 Abducent nerve
12 Motor root ⎫
13 Sensory root ⎭ of facial nerve
14 Vestibulocochlear nerve
15 Roots of glossopharyngeal, vagus and cranial part of accessory nerves
16 Spinal part of accessory nerve
17 Rootlets of hypoglossal nerve
18 Pyramid of medulla oblongata
19 Olive
20 Tonsil of cerebellum
21 Choroid plexus of fourth ventricle
22 Flocculus
23 Middle cerebellar peduncle
24 Posterior perforated substance
25 Mamillary body
26 Cerebral peduncle
27 Uncus
28 Anterior perforated substance
29 Olfactory trigone
30 Olfactory tract
31 Olfactory trigone
32 Anterior perforated substance
33 Optic nerve
34 Optic chiasma
35 Pituitary stalk
36 Mamillary body
37 Posterior perforated substance
38 Oculomotor nerve
39 Cerebral peduncle
40 Optic tract
41 Lateral geniculate body
42 Choroid plexus of inferior horn of lateral ventricle
43 Pulvinar
44 Medial geniculate body
45 Splenium of corpus callosum

• The cranial nerves are numbered (by long tradition with Roman numerals) as well as named:

I	First	Olfactory
II	Second	Optic
III	Third	Oculomotor
IV	Fourth	Trochlear
V	Fifth	Trigeminal
VI	Sixth	Abducent
VII	Seventh	Facial
VIII	Eighth	Vestibulocochlear
IX	Ninth	Glossopharyngeal
X	Tenth	Vagus
XI	Eleventh	Accessory
XII	Twelfth	Hypoglossal

• The olfactory nerve (I) consists of about 20 filaments that pass through the cribriform plate of the ethmoid bone to enter the olfactory bulb (A1) at the front end of the olfactory tract (A2), on the undersurface of the frontal lobe.

• The optic nerve (II) (A3) passes backwards from the eye through the optic canal (page 168, 4) to the optic chiasma (A4).

• The oculomotor nerve (III) (A7; B38) emerges on the medial side of the cerebral peduncle (A26).

• The trochlear nerve (IV) (A8) is the only cranial nerve to emerge from the dorsal surface of the brainstem (from the midbrain, behind the inferior colliculus, page 198, C and D, 38). It winds round the lateral side of the cerebral peduncle.

• The trigeminal nerve (V) (A10) emerges from the lateral side of the pons (A9), where the pons continues into the middle cerebellar peduncle (A23).

• The abducent nerve (VI) (A11) emerges near the midline at the junction of the pons (A9) and the pyramid of the medulla (A18).

• The facial nerve (VII) (A12 and 13) and the vestibulocochlear nerve (VIII) (A14) emerge from the lateral pontomedullary angle.

• The glossopharyngeal (IX) and vagus (X) nerves and the cranial part of the accessory nerve (XI) (A15) emerge from the medulla lateral to the olive (A19).

• The spinal part of the accessory nerve (A16) emerges as a series of roots from the lateral side of the upper five or six cervical segments of the spinal cord, dorsal to the denticulate ligament (page 198, F47), and runs up at the side of the medulla to join the cranial part.

• The hypoglossal nerve (XII) (A17) emerges from the medulla between the pyramid and the olive (A18 and 19).

FRONT

A

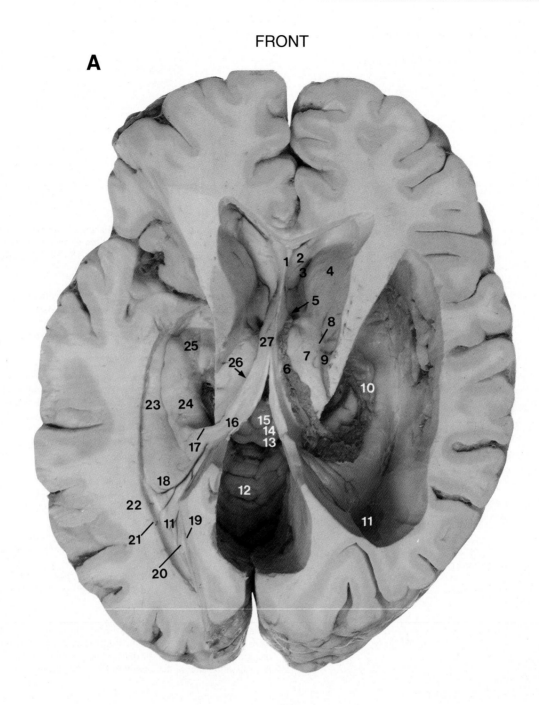

1
2
3
4
5
8
25
27
7
9
26
6
10
23
24
16
15
14
13
17
18
12
22
11
19
21
20
11

BACK

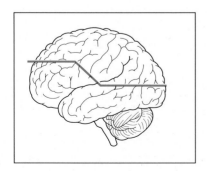

INTERIOR OF THE CEREBRAL HEMISPHERES
Ventricles of the brain
The lateral ventricles and their horns, from above
The lateral ventricles and the roof of the third ventricle, from above

In A the cerebral hemispheres have been dissected away from above, to open up the lateral ventricles. On the right side, the body of the lateral ventricle (the region containing in its floor the key numbers 6-9) becomes the anterior horn (3) in front of the interventricular foramen (5). At the back the ventricle curves downwards and forwards as the inferior horn (10) and backwards as the posterior horn (11). On the left side, there has been further dissection of the inferior and posterior horns. In the floor of the inferior horn are seen the hippocampus (24 and 25) and the collateral eminence (23, the bulge produced by the collateral sulcus seen on page 182, A9). The collateral trigone (18) is at the junction of the inferior and posterior horns. The bulb (19, caused by fibres of the corpus callosum) and the calcar (20, caused by the bulge of the calcarine sulcus seen on page 182, A7) are in the medial wall of the posterior horn. The optic radiation (22) is immediately lateral to the posterior horn.

In B the front part of the bluish diamond-shaped area with the key numbers 30 and 31 is the roof of the third ventricle (B30).

The ventricles of the brain:
- the third ventricle (page 180, 11), with on each side an interventricular foramen (5; page 180, 9) leading into
- the lateral ventricle, consisting of a body (6) with anterior, inferior and posterior horns (3, 10 and 11);
- the aqueduct of the midbrain (page 180, 22) connecting the third ventricle (page 180, 11) with
- the fourth ventricle, behind the lower part of the pons and upper part of the medulla oblongata (page 180, 17), with a median aperture in the roof (page 198, E40) and a lateral aperture in each lateral recess (page 198, C31) through which cerebrospinal fluid escapes into the subarachnoid space.

Tela choroidea is the name given to a double layer of pia mater (as at 29). When it contains a mass of capillary blood vessels and is covered by ependyma (the epithelium lining the ventricles) it becomes the choroid plexus (as at A and B, 6).

Cerebrospinal fluid is produced by the choroid plexuses. One mass of choroid plexus is in the roof of the third ventricle (B30) and extends on each side through the interventricular foramen (A and B, 5) into the body of the lateral ventricle (A and B, 6) and then into its inferior horn (A10) (but not into its anterior or posterior horns, 3 and 11).

• A separate choroid plexus, not connected with the above, lies in the roof of the fourth ventricle (page 180, 18; page 198, D,39) and extends out through the lateral recesses to become visible on the undersurface of the brain near the pontomedullary angle (page 188, A21).

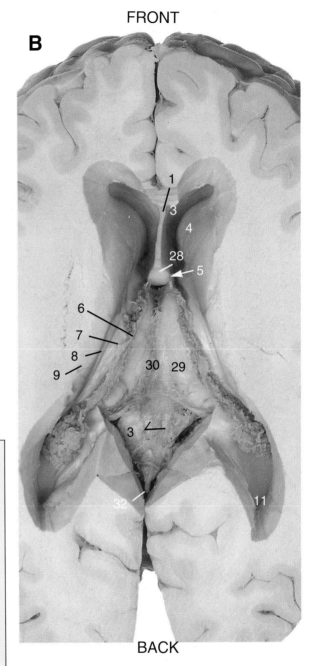

FRONT

B

BACK

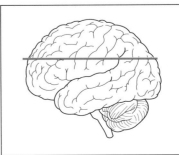

1 Septum pellucidum	16 Crus of fornix
2 Rostrum of corpus callosum (posterior surface)	17 Fimbria
	18 Collateral trigone
3 Anterior horn of lateral ventricle	19 Bulb
	20 Calcar
4 Head of caudate nucleus	21 Tapetum of corpus callosum
5 Interventricular foramen	22 Optic radiation
6 Choroid plexus of body of lateral ventricle	23 Collateral eminence
	24 Hippocampus
7 Thalamus	25 Pes hippocampi
8 Thalamostriate vein	26 Choroid fissure
9 Body of caudate nucleus	27 Body of fornix
10 Choroid plexus of inferior horn of lateral ventricle	28 Anterior column of fornix
	29 Tela choroidea of third ventricle
11 Posterior horn of lateral ventricle	30 Choroid plexus in third ventricle (visible below 29)
12 Vermis of cerebellum	31 Internal cerebral vein
13 Inferior colliculus	32 Great cerebral vein
14 Superior colliculus	
15 Pineal body	

INTERIOR OF THE CEREBRAL HEMISPHERES
The internal capsule and basal nuclei
A Transverse sections of the cerebral hemispheres, from above
B Transverse section of the left cerebral hemisphere, from below
C MR image at a similar level to the sections in A

In A the left hemisphere has been sectioned at the level of the interventricular foramen (6), and the right hemisphere about 1 cm higher. On the left side the internal capsule (27-29) is seen between the caudate nucleus (7) and thalamus (26) medially and the lentiform nucleus (30 and 31) laterally. In the higher section on the right, the nerve fibres that form the internal capsule occupy the corona radiata (13). The view on the right looks down into the body of the lateral ventricle with the choroid plexus (11) and the upper surface of the thalamus (10) in the floor of the ventricle. At the lower level on the left the thalamus is seen in section (26). The anterior horn of the lateral ventricle (4) extends forwards into the frontal lobe, and the posterior horn (18) backwards into the occipital lobe. The optic radiation (20) runs lateral to the posterior horn, separated from it by the tapetum (19), which is a thin sheet of fibres derived from the corpus callosum (14) whose main bulk lies medial to the horn as the forceps major (15).

In B, looking upwards at a similar level to that on the left side of A, the third ventricle (24)

is in the midline, communicating at the front with the anterior horn of the lateral ventricle (4) through the interventricular foramen (6), which is bounded medially by the anterior column of the fornix (36) and laterally by the thalamus (26). Compare with major features in the MR image (C).

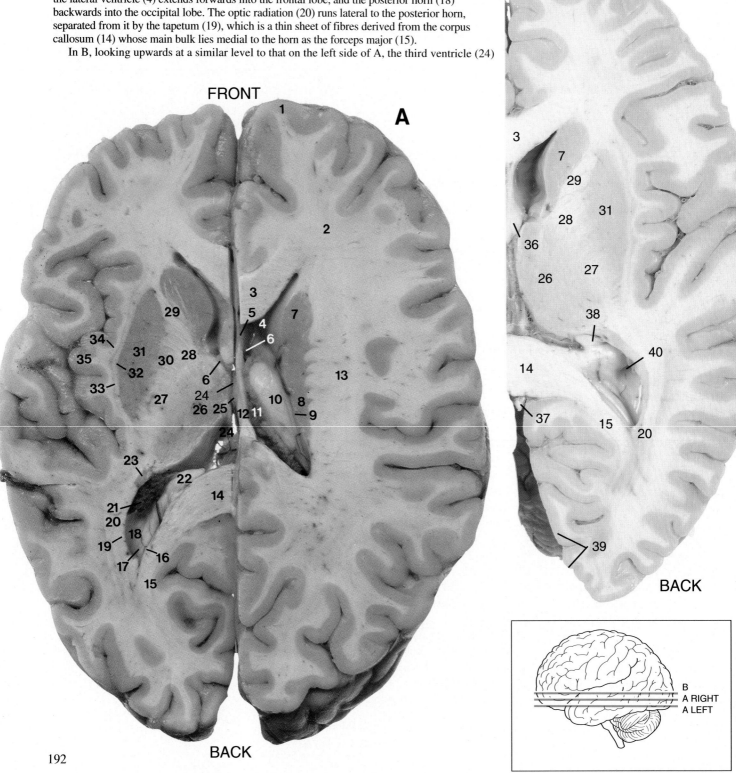

FRONT

A

FRONT

BACK

BACK

B
A RIGHT
A LEFT

1 Frontal pole	16 Bulb	30 Globus pallidus ⎫
2 Forceps minor	17 Calcar	31 Putamen ⎭ lentiform nucleus
3 Genu of corpus callosum	18 Posterior horn of lateral ventricle	32 External capsule
4 Anterior horn of lateral ventricle	19 Tapetum of corpus callosum	33 Claustrum
5 Septum pellucidum	20 Optic radiation	34 Extreme capsule
6 Interventricular foramen	21 Choroid plexus passing forwards into inferior horn of lateral ventricle	35 Insula
7 Head ⎫ of caudate nucleus		36 Anterior column of fornix
8 Body ⎭		37 Pineal body
9 Thalomostriate vein	22 Crus of fornix	38 Fimbria
10 Thalamus	23 Tail of caudate nucleus	39 Visual (striate) area of cerebral cortex
11 Choroid plexus of body of lateral ventricle	24 Third ventricle	
	25 Interthalamic adhesion	40 Junction of posterior and inferior horns of lateral ventricle
12 Body of fornix	26 Thalamus	
13 Corona radiata	27 Posterior limb ⎫	
14 Splenium of corpus callosum	28 Genu ⎬ of internal capsule	
15 Forceps major	29 Anterior limb ⎭	

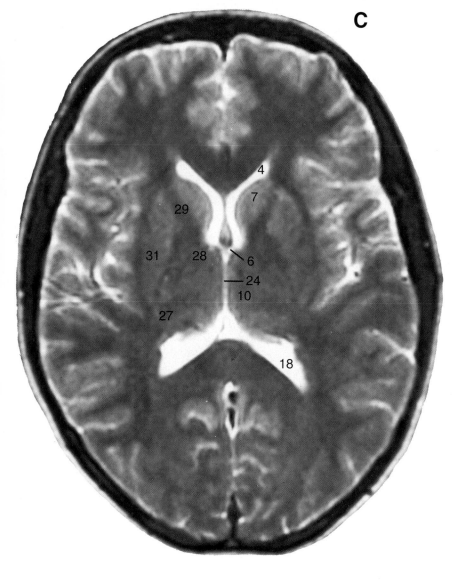

C

• The *internal capsule* consists of:
  the anterior limb
  the genu
  the posterior limb
  the sublentiform part
  the retrolentiform part

• The anterior limb (29) lies between the head of the caudate nucleus (7) and the lentiform nucleus (30 and 31). Its main fibre constituents are those passing between the various parts of the frontal cortex and thalamus (in both directions) and to pontine nuclei.

• The genu (28) is between the anterior and posterior limbs (29 and 27). Its most important fibres are the corticonuclear fibres (formerly called corticobulbar), passing from the head and neck area of the motor cortex (precentral gyrus) to the motor nuclei of cranial nerves.

• The posterior limb (27) lies between the thalamus (26) and the lentiform nucleus (30 and 31). Apart from fibres to pontine nuclei, it also contains those fibres of the sensory pathway that run from the thalamus to the postcentral gyrus (thalamocortical fibres), and the corticospinal fibres from the motor cortex to the anterior horn cells of the spinal cord. These motor fibres mainly occupy the anterior two-thirds of the posterior limb.

• The sublentiform part consists of fibres passing below the posterior end of the lentiform nucleus. Among its most important fibres are those of the auditory radiation, running from the medial geniculate body to the auditory area of the cortex.

• The retrolentiform part consists of fibres at the posterior end of the posterior limb, passing from the lateral geniculate body to the visual area of the cortex and constituting the optic radiation (20).

• Clinically the most important parts of the internal capsule are the genu and anterior two-thirds of the posterior limb, because this is where the motor fibres from the cortex to cranial nerve nuclei and anterior horn cells are situated. It is damage to these 'upper motor neurons' by haemorrhage or thrombosis that causes the characteristic paralysis of a stroke (page 187).

1 Corpus callosum
2 Septum pellucidum
3 Body of fornix
4 Choroid plexus
5 Body of lateral ventricle
6 Thalamus
7 Thalamostriate vein
8 Body of caudate nucleus
9 Corona radiata
10 Internal capsule
11 External capsule
12 Extreme capsule
13 Insula
14 Tail of caudate nucleus
15 Inferior horn of lateral ventricle
16 Collateral sulcus
17 Parahippocampal gyrus
18 Hippocampus
19 Choroid plexus of inferior horn of lateral ventricle
20 Choroid fissure
21 Optic tract
22 Corticospinal and corticonuclear fibres in cerebral peduncle
23 Corticospinal and corticonuclear fibres in pons
24 Corticospinal fibres in pyramid of medulla oblongata
25 Substantia nigra
26 Red nucleus
27 Subthalamic nucleus
28 Third ventricle
29 Globus pallidus ⎫ lentiform nucleus
30 Putamen ⎭
31 Claustrum
32 Basilar artery

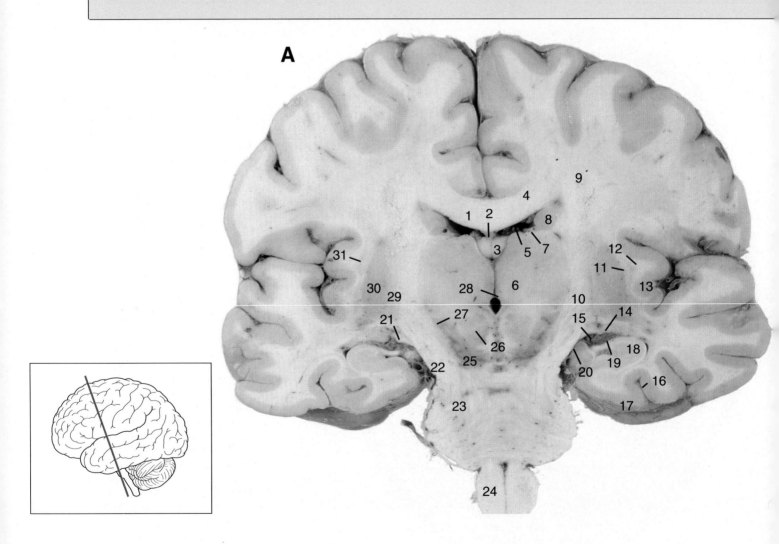

A

INTERIOR OF THE CEREBRAL HEMISPHERES
The hemispheres and brainstem in coronal section
A Oblique coronal section, from the front
B MR image, coronal

The section in A, looking from front to back, has been cut slightly obliquely in order to show how the motor fibres of the internal capsule (10) pass from the hemispheres and down through the midbrain (cerebral peduncle, 22), pons (23) and medulla (24). The sloping floor of the body of the lateral ventricle (5) is formed by the thalamus (6) and caudate nucleus (8) with the thalamostriate vein (7) in between. The roof is the corpus callosum (1), with the septum pellucidum (2) separating the two ventricles in the midline. The hippocampus (18) is in the floor of the inferior horn (15), with the tail of the caudate nucleus (14) in its roof.

The MR image in B is at a more anterior and vertical level than A, and shows the basilar artery (32) at the front of the pons (seen in a lateral view on page 180, A28).

• The **basal nuclei** (still often known clinically by their old name, basal ganglia) include certain subcortical cell groups in the white matter of the cerebral hemispheres, in particular the caudate and lentiform nuclei (A8, 29 and 30). On functional grounds it is now usual to include the substantia nigra (A25) and the subthalamic nucleus (A27) (both in the midbrain, not in the cerebrum), and to exclude the amygdaloid nucleus (at the front end of the tail of the caudate nucleus) because it is functionally associated with the limbic system.

• The basal nuclei are functionally part of the extrapyramidal system. Extrapyramidal diseases do not cause paralysis but lead to abnormal involuntary movements and disturbances of reflexes and muscle tone: for example, Parkinsonism, where there is loss of the neurotransmitter dopamine in the substantia nigra.

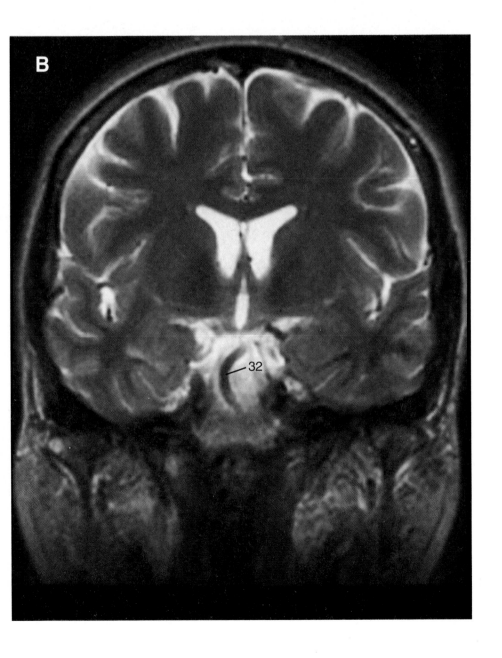

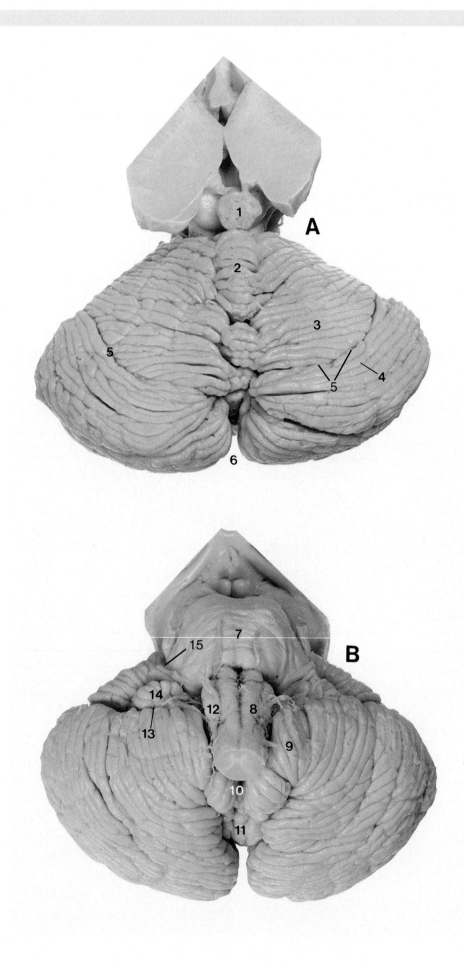

CEREBELLUM
The cerebellum and the brainstem
A From above
B From below

The view in A, looking down from above, shows the central vermis of the cerebellum (2) with the hemispheres on each side (3). The pineal body (1) projects backwards from the (unlabelled) third ventricle to overlie the midbrain (compare with the side view on page 180, 13).

In B the anterior or ventral view shows the pons (7) passing laterally to become the middle cerebellar peduncle, which disappears into the cerebellar hemisphere (as on page 188, A23). The flocculus (14) lies behind the peduncle, and the tonsil (9) is the part of the hemisphere that overlies the margin of the foramen magnum (as on page 158, 63)

• The cerebellum occupies much of the posterior cranial fossa (page 158, 22) and is covered by the tentorium cerebelli (page 168, 36).

• The cerebellum consists of a central longitudinal region, the vermis (A2), with a cerebellar hemisphere on each side (A3).

• Like the cerebrum, the cerebellum has a cortex of grey matter on the surface, with underlying white matter.

• In each hemisphere the white matter contains four subcortical cell groups—the dentate, globose, emboliform and fastigial nuclei. The nuclei give rise to most of the fibres that leave the cerebellum; the most important is the dentate nucleus (page 198, B23).

1	Pineal body
2	Vermis of cerebellum
3	Cerebellar hemisphere
4	A cerebellar folium
5	Primary fissure
6	Cerebellar notch
7	Pons
8	Pyramid of medulla oblongata
9	Tonsil of cerebellum
10	Uvula of vermis
11	Pyramid of vermis
12	Olive
13	Dorsolateral (posterolateral) fissure
14	Flocculus
15	Middle cerebellar peduncle

• The cerebellum is connected to the brainstem by three pairs of peduncles, one pair to each part of the brainstem:
 by the superior cerebellar peduncles to the midbrain (page 198, C24)
 by the middle cerebellar peduncles to the pons (B15; page 198, C25)
 by the inferior cerebellar peduncles to the medulla oblongata (page 198, C26)

• The following notes, correlating cerebellar form and function, are a simplified synopsis of a complicated organ, but are sufficient to give a general understanding of its significance.

• Functionally, the cerebellum is concerned with the co-ordination of muscular movement; it has nothing to do with conscious sensation. Each cerebellar hemisphere affects its own side of the body (the ipsilateral side): for example, the left cerebellar hemisphere helps to control the left arm and leg, in contrast to the left cerebral hemisphere, which exerts its influence on the right arm and leg (the contralateral side), due to the decussation of corticospinal fibres in the medulla oblongata.

• The various named parts are best appreciated in a midline sagittal section (as on page 198, A), and can conveniently be grouped according to their phylogenetic (evolutionary) significance.

• The lingula at the front (page 198, A21), and the nodule at the back (page 198, A10), which is continuous at each side with the flocculus (A 14, forming the flocculonodular lobe), constitute the oldest or vestibular part of the cerebellum (archaeocerebellum) and are mainly concerned with vestibular functions (balance).

• The central lobule and culmen of the front part of the vermis (page 198, A20 and 19), the uvula and pyramid of the back part of the vermis (page 198, A11 and 13) and the hemisphere in front of the primary fissure (A5; page 198, A18) forming the anterior lobe, constituting the palaeocerebellum or spinal part, receiving fibres from the spinal cord and being largely concerned with posture and muscle tone.

• The remainder of the vermis (page 198, A15–17) and the hemisphere behind the primary fissure (page 198, A11–18) constitute the middle lobe (sometimes also known confusingly as the posterior lobe). This is the largest and most recently evolved part of the cerebellum, the neocerebellum, and receives input from the cerebral cortex via the pontine nuclei. It is mainly concerned with the control of muscle tone and fine movements.

• It follows from the above that disturbances of cerebellar function, e.g. by the pressure of tumours, result in disorders of balance and inco-ordinated movements of the arms and legs (ataxia), with loss of muscle tone (hypotonia) and nystagmus (oscillating eye movements) but no paralysis.

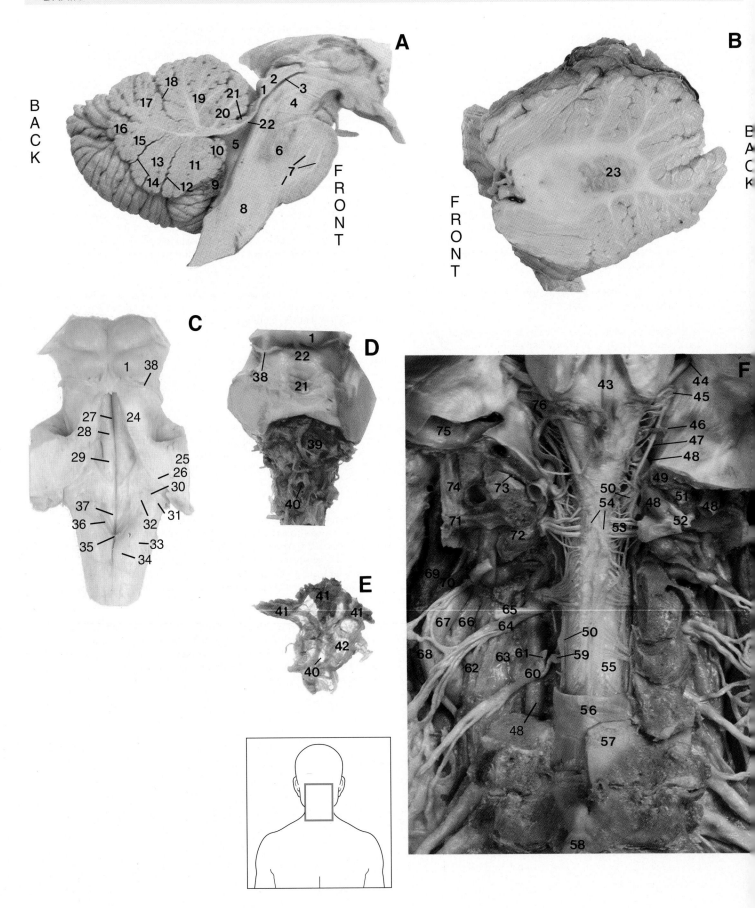

CEREBELLUM, BRAINSTEM AND SPINAL CORD
Sections of the cerebellum and brainstem, and the cervical cord
A **The left half of the brainstem and cerebellum, in a midline sagittal section, from the right**
B **The right cerebellar hemisphere in an oblique sagittal section, from the left**
C **The floor of the fourth ventricle, from behind**
D **The roof of the fourth ventricle, from behind**
E **The isolated choroid plexus of the fourth ventricle, from behind**
F **The lower brainstem and cervical part of the spinal cord, from behind**

In the sagittal section in A, various parts of the cerebellum are labelled (9-21). In the pons (6) corticospinal and corticonuclear fibres (7) are seen coursing down through the ventral part to reach the medulla (8).

The section of a hemisphere in B shows the dentate nucleus (23), the largest of the subcortical cerebellar nuclei.

At the side of the floor of the fourth ventricle in C are seen the cut edges of the three cerebellar peduncles (24–26) which connect the cerebellum to the midbrain, pons and medulla.

In D the tela choroidea and choroid plexus (39) of the posterior part of the roof of the fourth ventricle are shown *in situ*.

In E they have been dissected free to emphasise the T-shaped plexus (41) and the median aperture (40) in the tela (42).

In F the posterior parts of the skull and upper vertebrae have been removed to show the continuity of the brainstem with the spinal cord, from which dorsal nerve rootlets are seen to emerge (as at 53). The spinal part of the accessory nerve (47) runs up through the foramen magnum (49) to join the cranial part in the jugular foramen (45). Ventral nerve rootlets (as at 59), ventral to the denticulate ligament (50), unite to form a ventral nerve root which joins with a dorsal nerve root (61, whose formative rootlets dorsal to the ligamentum have been cut off from the cord in order to make the ventral rootlets visible) to form a spinal nerve immediately beyond the dorsal root ganglion (60). The nerve immediately divides into ventral and dorsal rami (as at 64 and 65).

1	Inferior colliculus	41	Choroid plexus
2	Tectum	42	Tela coroidea
3	Aqueduct } of midbrain	43	Floor of the fourth ventricle
4	Tegmentum	44	Internal acoustic meatus with facial and vestibulo-cochlear nerves and labyrinthine artery
5	Fourth ventricle	45	Roots of glossopharyngeal, vagus and cranial part of accessory nerves and jugular foramen
6	Pons	46	Posterior inferior cerebellar artery
7	Corticonuclear and corticospinal fibres	47	Spinal part of accessory nerve
8	Medulla oblongata	48	Vertebral artery
9	Choroid plexus of fourth ventricle	49	Margin of foramen magnum
10	Nodule	50	Denticulate ligament
11	Uvula of vermis	51	Lateral mass of atlas
12	Secondary (postpyramidal) fissure	52	First cervical nerve and posterior arch of atlas
13	Pyramid of vermis	53	Dorsal rootlets of second cervical nerve
14	Prepyramidal fissure	54	Posterior spinal arteries
15	Tuber of vermis	55	Arachnoid mater
16	Folium of vermis	56	Dura mater
17	Declive	57	Lamina of sixth cervical vertebra
18	Primary fissure	58	Spinous process of seventh cervical vertebra
19	Culmen	59	Ventral rootlets
20	Central lobule	60	Dorsal root ganglion } of fourth cervical nerve
21	Lingula	61	Dorsal root
22	Superior medullary velum	62	Scalenus anterior
23	Dentate nucleus	63	Longus capitis
24	Superior	64	Ventral ramus } of third cervical nerve
25	Middle } cerebellar peduncle	65	Dorsal ramus
26	Inferior	66	External carotid artery
27	Median groove	67	Internal carotid artery
28	Medial eminence	68	Vagus nerve
29	Facial colliculus	69	Internal jugular vein
30	Medullary striae	70	A vein from vertebral venous plexuses
31	Lateral recess	71	Transverse process of atlas
32	Vestibular area	72	Capsule of lateral atlanto-axial joint
33	Cuneate tubercle	73	Atlanto-occipital joint
34	Gracile tubercle	74	Rectus capitis lateralis
35	Obex	75	Sigmoid sinus
36	Vagal triangle	76	Choroid plexus emerging from lateral recess of fourth ventricle
37	Hypoglossal triangle		
38	Trochlear nerve		
39	Tela choroidea and choroid plexus		
40	Median aperture		

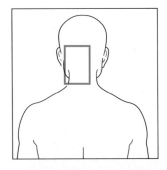

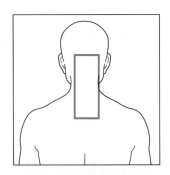

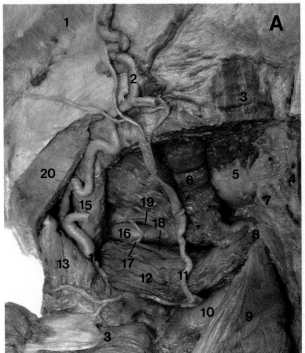

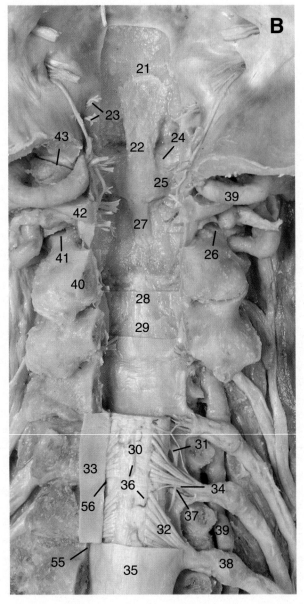

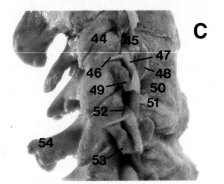

CERVICAL VERTEBRAL COLUMN
Posterior neck and vertebral joints
The suboccipital region, vertebral column and spinal nerves
A The left suboccipital triangle
B The vertebral column and spinal cord, from behind
C Intervertebral foramina and spinal nerves, from the right

In A the suboccipital region has been exposed by removing trapezius and parts of splenius (20) and semispinalis (3). The principal structure in the suboccipital triangle (see the note below) is the vertebral artery (16).

In B the vertebral arches and much of the skull have been removed, together with parts of the meninges and spinal cord. The tectorial membrane (28) is the upward continuation of the posterior longitudinal ligament (29). The transverse ligament of the atlas (25) forms the transverse part of the cruciform ligament (22 and 27); all are displayed by removing the tectorial membrane.

The side view of the cervical vertebral column in C shows a typical dorsal root ganglion (as at 52) in an intervertebral foramen (see page 183), and spinal nerves dividing into a small dorsal ramus (as at 46) and a large ventral ramus (47).

• The suboccipital triangle:
Boundaries—rectus capitis posterior major (A6), obliquus capitis superior (15) and obliquus capitis inferior (12).
Floor—posterior atlanto-occipital membrane (19) and posterior arch of atlas (18).
Contents—vertebral artery (16); dorsal ramus of C1 nerve (17).

• Do not confuse the three spaces associated with the meninges: the *extradural space* (sometimes called the epidural space), outside the dura in the vertebral canal; the *subdural space*, inside the dura (between the dura and arachnoid); and the *subarachnoid space*, inside the arachnoid (between the arachnoid and the pia mater on the surface of the brain and spinal cord) and filled with cerebrospinal fluid.

1	Occipital belly of occipitofrontalis	29	Posterior longitudinal ligament
2	Occipital artery	30	Spinal cord
3	Semispinalis capitis	31	Denticulate ligament
4	Ligamentum nuchae	32	Dorsal rootlets of spinal nerve
5	Rectus capitis posterior minor	33	Arachnoid and dura mater (reflected)
6	Rectus capitis posterior major	34	Radicular artery
7	Posterior tubercle of atlas	35	Dura mater
8	Spinous process of axis	36	Posterior spinal arteries
9	Semispinalis cervicis	37	Ventral rootlets of spinal nerve
10	Lamina of axis	38	Dural sheath over dorsal root ganglion
11	Greater occipital nerve	39	Vertebral artery
12	Obliquus capitis inferior	40	Lamina of axis
13	Longissimus capitis	41	Lateral atlanto-axial joint
14	Transverse process of atlas	42	Posterior arch of atlas
15	Obliquus capitis superior	43	Atlanto-occipital joint
16	Vertebral artery	44	Zygapophysial joint
17	Dorsal ramus of first cervical nerve	45	Vertebral artery
18	Posterior arch of atlas	46	Dorsal ramus } of fourth cervical nerve
19	Posterior atlanto-occipital membrane	47	Ventral ramus }
20	Splenius capitis	48	Anterior tubercle } of transverse process
21	Basilar part of occipital bone and position of attachment of tectorial membrane	49	Posterior tubercle }
22	Superior longitudinal band of cruciform ligament	50	Body of fourth cervical vertebra
23	Hypoglossal nerve and canal	51	Intervertebral disc
24	Alar ligament	52	Dorsal root ganglion of fifth cervical nerve in intervertebral foramen
25	Transverse ligament of atlas	53	Groove for (ventral ramus of) spinal nerve
26	Superior articular surface of axis	54	Spinous process of fifth cervical vertebra
27	Inferior longitudinal band of cruciform ligament	55	Extradural space
28	Tectorial membrane	56	Subarachnoid space

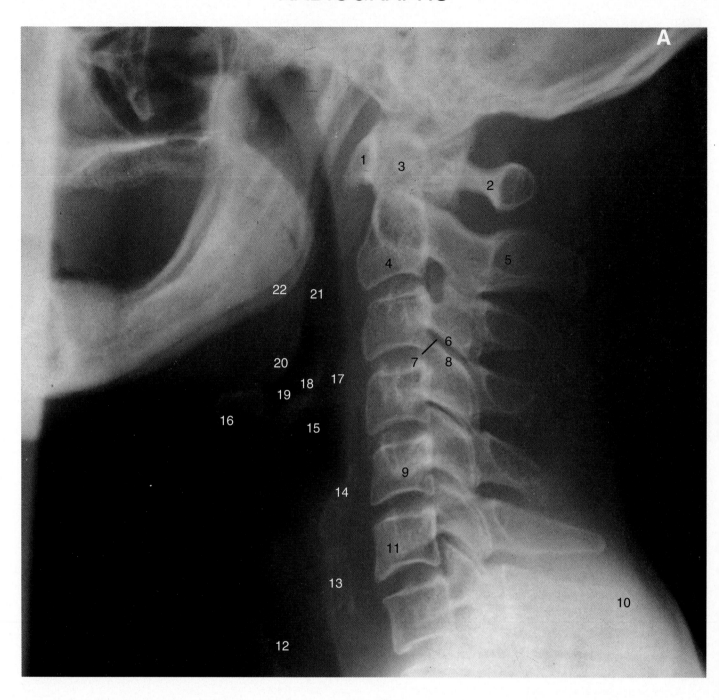

VERTEBRAL COLUMN
Cervical vertebrae
A Lateral view
B Atlas and axis, from the front
C Anterior oblique view

The side view in A shows the vertebral bodies (as at 11) and the obliquely-angled zygapophysial joints (as at 7). The anterior and posterior arches of the atlas (1 and 2) are clearly seen but the dens of the axis (3) is largely obscured in this view (see B). Note the large size of the spine of the axis (5; compare with page 82, C6), and that the spine of C7 vertebra (10) projects farther back than the others. In front of the vertebral column there is translucency due to the air-filled pharynx, larynx and trachea (21, 15 and 12).

In B the picture is taken with the mouth opened wide, the standard radiological method of visualising the dens of the axis (3) and the lateral atlanto-axial joint (24).

The oblique view in C is taken with the neck rotated about 45°, to display the boundaries of an intervertebral foramen (29).

1 Anterior arch ⎱ of atlas **2** Posterior arch ⎰	**17** Tip of greater horn of hyoid bone
3 Dens ⎱ **4** Body ⎬ of axis **5** Spinous process ⎰	**18** Epiglottis **19** Vallecula **20** Base of tongue
6 Inferior articular process of third cervical vertebra	**21** Oral part of pharynx
7 Zygapophysial joint	**22** Angle of mandible
8 Superior articular process of fourth cervical vertebra	**23** Inferior articular surface of lateral mass of atlas
9 Transverse process of fifth cervical vertebra	**24** Lateral atlanto-axial joint
10 Spinous process of seventh cervical vertebra	**25** Superior articular surface of axis
11 Body of sixth cervical vertebra	**26** Bifid spinous process of axis
12 Trachea	**27** Body ⎱ of fourth cervical vertebra **28** Pedicle ⎰
13 Calcification in cricoid cartilage	**29** Intervertebral foramen
14 Calcification in thyroid cartilage	**30** Pedicle ⎱ of fifth cervical vertebra **31** Body ⎰
15 Vestibule of larynx	
16 Body of hyoid bone	

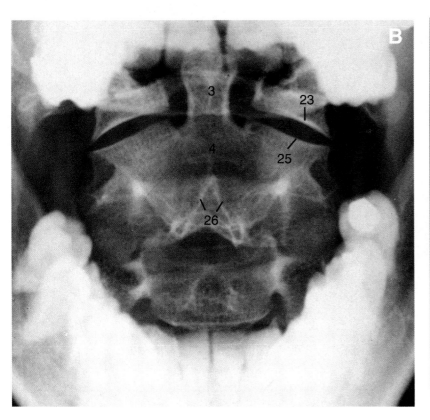

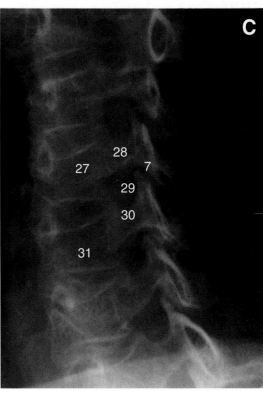

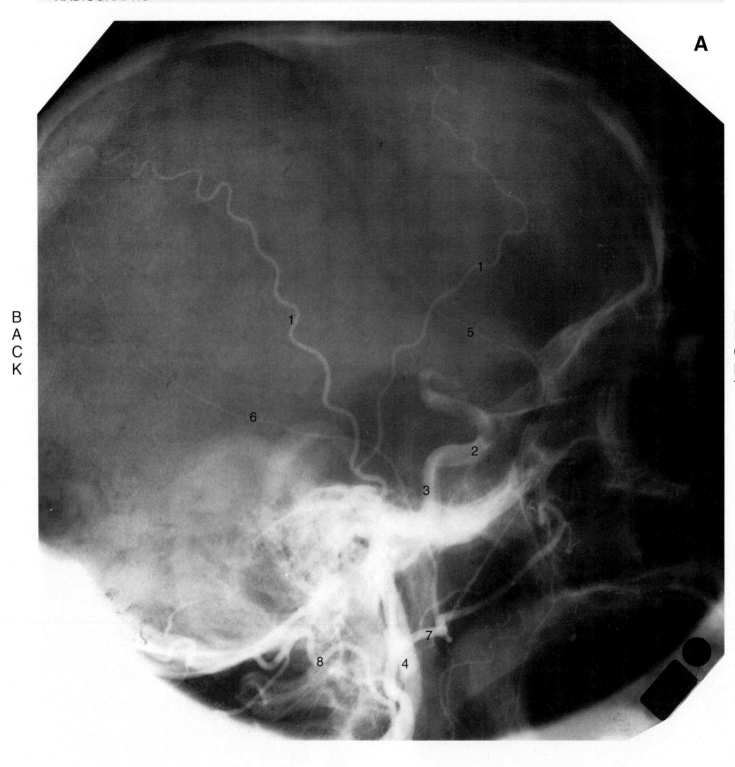

B
A
C
K

A

B

CAROTID ARTERIOGRAM AND VENOGRAM OF THE NECK
A Carotid arteriogram, right side, lateral view
B Venogram, left side, anterior view

In A various branches of the external carotid artery are seen as well as the cervical, petrous and cavernous parts of the internal carotid (4, 3 and 2). Branches of the superficial temporal artery (1) are prominent, as well as the rather smaller anterior and posterior branches of the middle meningeal artery (5 and 6), which arises from the maxillary artery (7).

The central vessels in the venogram in B are the anterior jugular veins (15), mostly outlined against the translucency of the trachea (14). The left internal jugular vein (12, with a catheter passed high up into it and indicated by the asterisks) receives the superior thyroid vein (11), above which the facial and lingual veins can be identified (9 and 10). The middle thyroid vein (13) is prominent at a lower level.

1	Branches of superficial temporal artery
2	Cavernous part ⎫
3	Petrous part ⎬ of internal carotid artery
4	Cervical part ⎭
5	Anterior branch ⎫ of middle meningeal artery
6	Posterior branch ⎭
7	Maxillary artery
8	Occipital artery
9	Facial vein
10	Lingual vein
11	Superior thyroid vein
12	Internal jugular vein
13	Middle thyroid vein
14	Margins of trachea
15	Anterior jugular vein

• In lateral carotid arteriograms the internal corotid artery in and above the cavernous sinus appears like the letter U on its side (as at 2 in A), and is often called the carotid siphon.

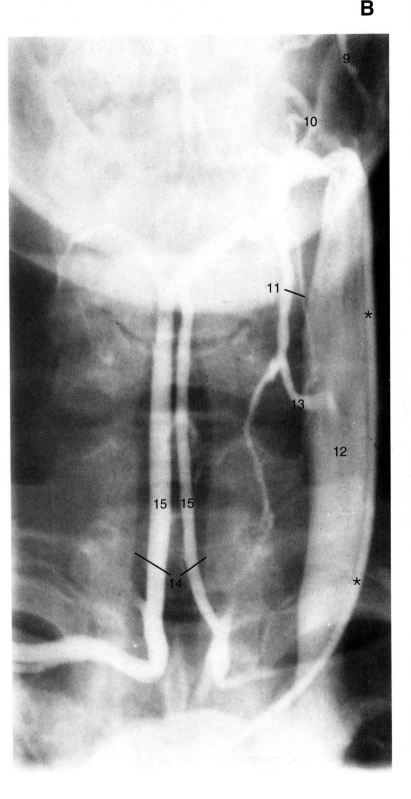

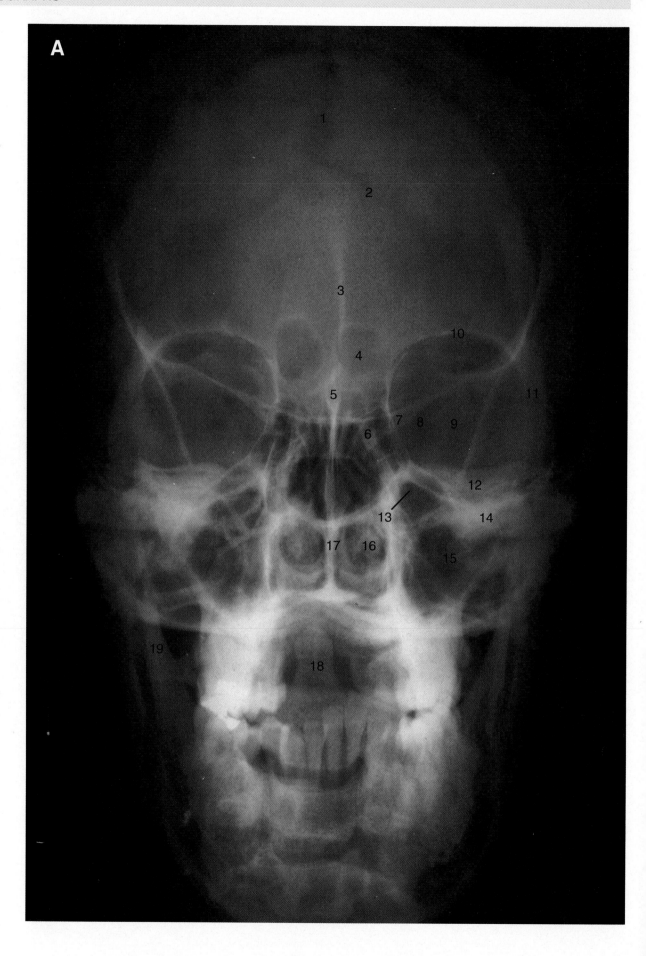

1 Sagittal suture
2 Lambdoid suture
3 Calcification in falx cerebri
4 Frontal sinus
5 Crista galli
6 Ethmoidal air cells
7 Lesser wing of sphenoid bone
8 Superior orbital fissure
9 Greater wing of sphenoid bone
10 Supra-orbital margin
11 Frontozygomatic suture
12 Infra-orbital margin
13 Foramen rotundum
14 Petrous part of temporal bone
15 Maxillary sinus
16 Inferior nasal concha
17 Nasal septum
18 Dens of axis
19 Coronoid process of mandible
20 Zygomatic bone
21 Zygomatic arch

SKULL
The skull and paranasal sinuses
A Postero-anterior view
B Occipitomental view

In a complicated structure such as the skull there is considerable overlapping of bony structures. The more obvious features in a standard anterior view (A) are the orbits (upper and lower margins at 10 and 12) and the nasal septum (17), with the crista galli at a higher level (5). The frontal sinuses are small (4) and there is some calcification in the falx cerebri (3) which would otherwise not be visualised. Ethmoidal air cells (6) lie medial to the orbit, through which are seen the lesser wing of the sphenoid and the superior orbital fissure (7 and 8). At a lower level the foramen rotundum is visible (13), with below it the translucency of the maxillary sinus (15).

The view in B, where the chin is tilted upwards at 45°, is taken to emphasise the frontal sinuses (4) above and medial to the orbits, and the maxillary sinuses (15) below the orbits.

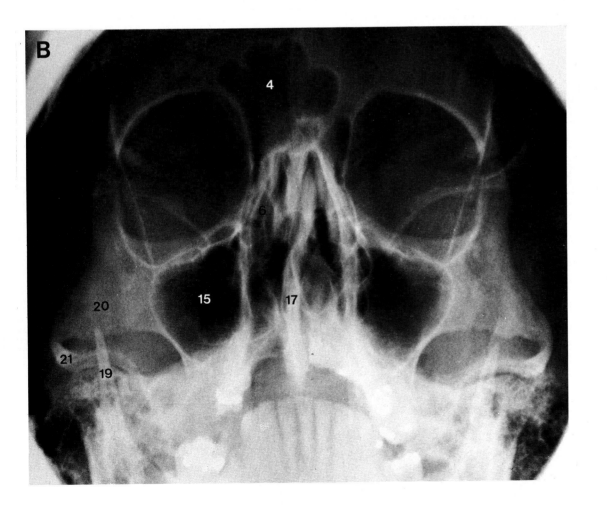

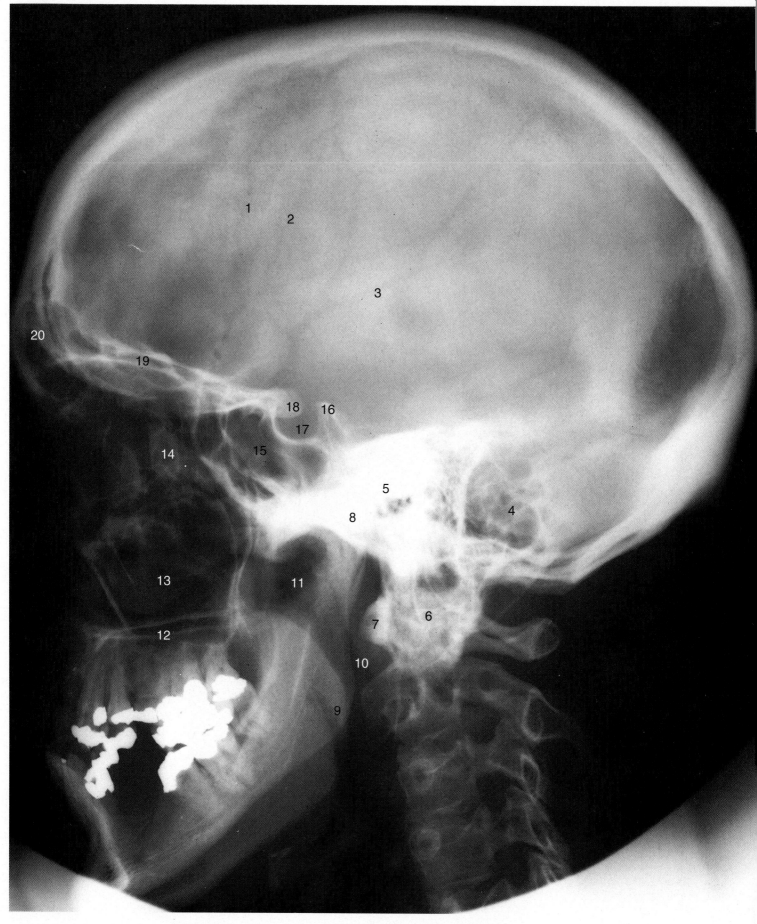

SKULL
Lateral view
The central feature is the pituitary fossa (17), with the anterior and posterior clinoid processes (18 and 16). In the vault of the skull, suture lines (as at 1) must not be confused with vascular markings (as at 2 and 3). The position of the external acoustic meatus is indicated (5), and so is the head of the mandible (8); the density of overlapping bones, especially the petrous temporal, obscures details in this region, but towards the back the honeycomb of mastoid air cells (4) is clear. The opacities in the teeth are dental fillings.

1 Coronal suture
2 Frontal branch ⎫
3 Parietal branch ⎭ of middle meningeal artery
4 Mastoid air cells
5 External acoustic meatus
6 Mastoid process
7 Anterior arch of atlas
8 Head ⎫
9 Angle ⎭ of mandible
10 Oral part ⎫
11 Nasal part ⎭ of pharynx
12 Hard palate
13 Maxillary sinus
14 Ethmoidal air cells
15 Sphenoidal sinus
16 Posterior clinoid process
17 Pituitary fossa
18 Anterior clinoid process
19 Floor of anterior cranial fossa
20 Frontal sinus

ARTERIOGRAMS
Carotid arteriograms (digitally subtracted arterial phase of carotid arteriograms)
A Oblique view, right side
B Anteroposterior view

Digital subtraction arteriography (DSA) is a technique that allows unwanted background material to be reduced, thus emphasising the image of the blood vessels. In the oblique view in A the upper (cervical) part of the internal carotid artery in the neck (1) can be visualised entering the carotid canal in the petrous part of the temporal bone, within which it takes a right-angled turn forwards and medially(2). It then curves upwards along the carotid groove of the sphenoid bone (3) within the cavernous sinus and emerges as the cerebral part (4) which divides into the anterior and middle cerebral arteries (5 and 6). Note the ophthalmic artery (7) passing forwards into the orbit.

In the anteroposterior view in B the characteristic T-shaped division of the internal carotid artery (4) into anterior and middle cerebral branches (5 and 6) is clearly seen.

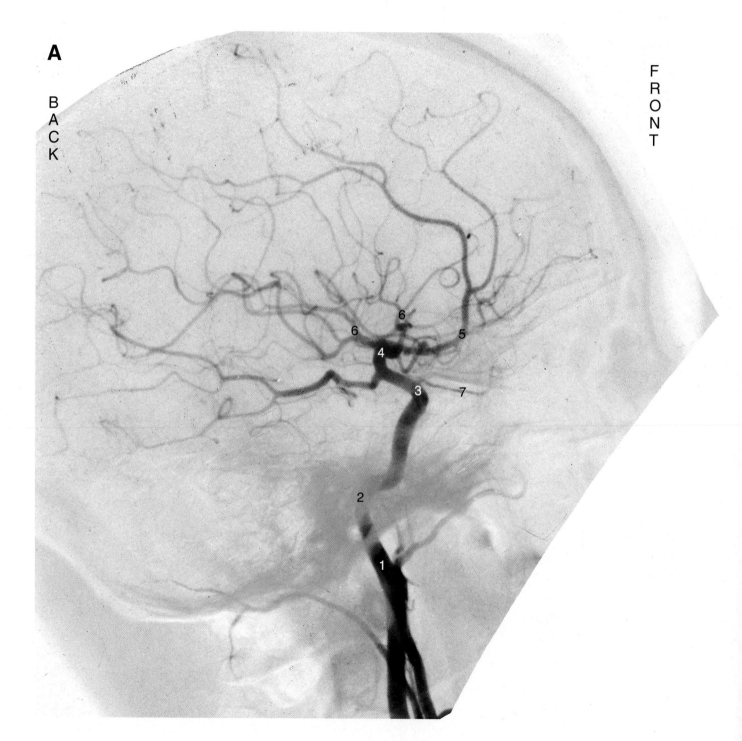

A

BACK

FRONT

1 Cervical ⎫
2 Petrous ⎪ part of internal
3 Cavernous ⎬ carotid artery
4 Cerebral ⎭
5 Anterior cerebral artery
6 Branches of middle cerebral artery
7 Ophthalmic artery
8 Middle cerebral artery

B

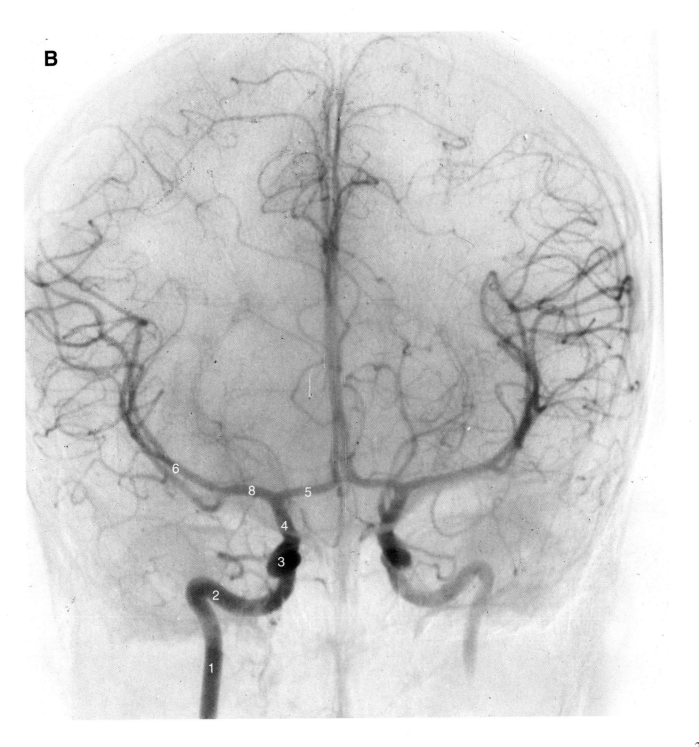

ARTERIOGRAMS
Vertebral arteriograms (digitally subtracted arterial phase of vertebral arteriograms)
A Anterior view of both sides
B Lateral view, left side, from the left

In A each vertebral artery is first labelled (1) after emerging from the foramen in the transverse process of the atlas and taking a right-angled turn medially to lie on the posterior arch of the atlas. After entering the foramen magnum (where both vessels are here unusually tortuous) they unite to form the basilar artery (2) after giving off the posterior inferior cerebellar arteries (3). The basilar artery divides at its upper end into the posterior cerebrals (4) after giving off the superior cerebellar arteries (5).

The lateral view in B emphasises the mass of vessels converging on the cerebellum and the posterior direction of the posterior cerebral artery (4).

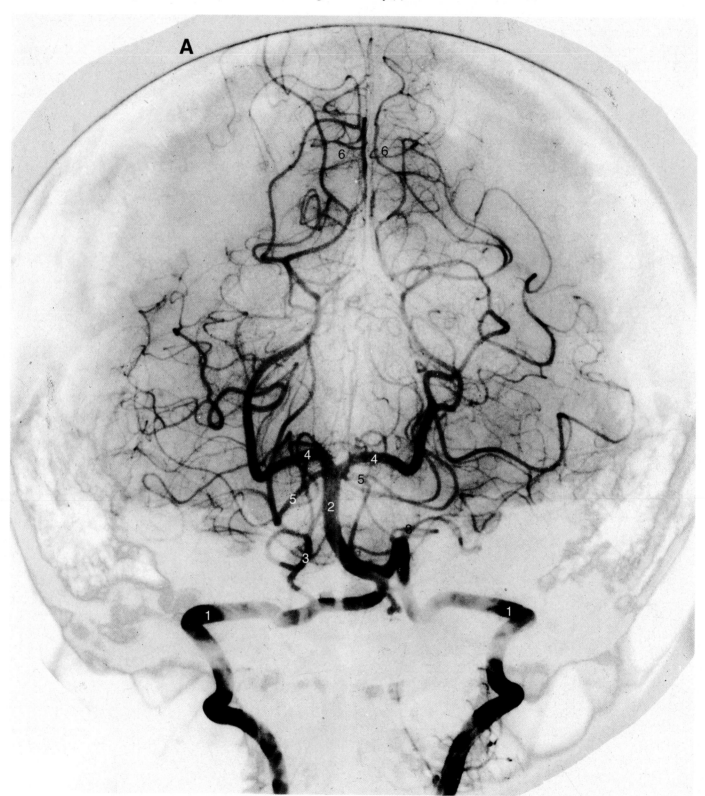

1 Vertebral artery
2 Basilar artery
3 Posterior inferior cerebellar artery
4 Posterior cerebral artery
5 Superior cerebellar artery
6 Occipital and calcarine branches of posterior
   cerebral artery

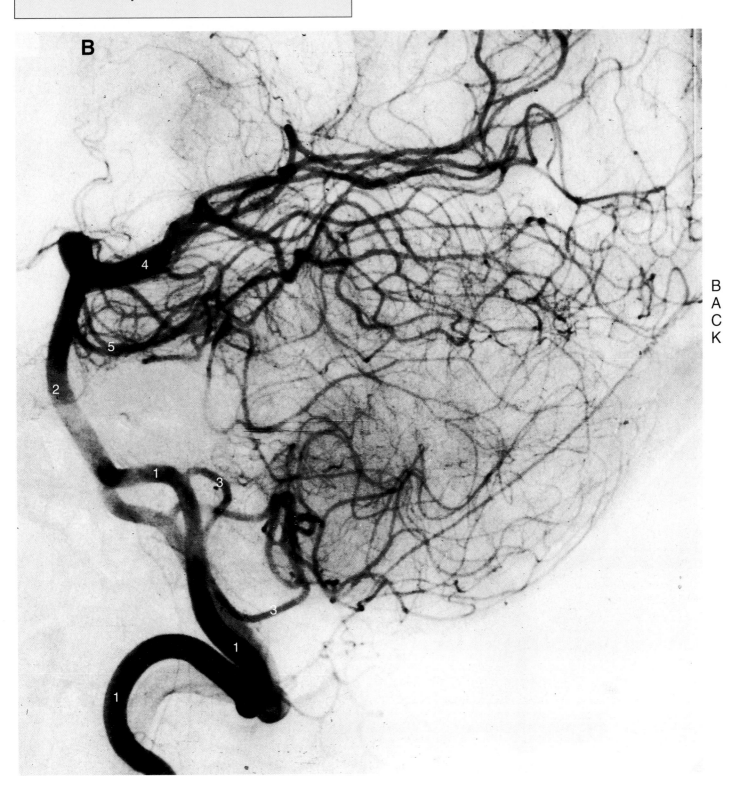

B

BACK

RADIOGRAPHS
Dural venous sinuses (digitally subtracted venous phase of carotid arteriograms)
A Lateral view
B Anteroposterior view

In A the superior sagittal sinus (1) can be traced backwards to the confluence of the sinuses (6) where it runs laterally to become a transverse sinus (usually the right, 7). The other transverse sinus is continuous with the straight sinus (5), into which drain the inferior sagittal sinus (only a small part of which is seen faintly at 11) and the great cerebral vein (4). The transverse sinus turns down to become the sigmoid sinus (8) which leaves the jugular foramen to enter the neck as the internal jugular vein (9).

In B the superior sagittal sinus (1) continues laterally as the right transverse sinus (7). There is a large but fainter confluence of the sinuses (6), above which the inferior sagittal sinus is seen (11).

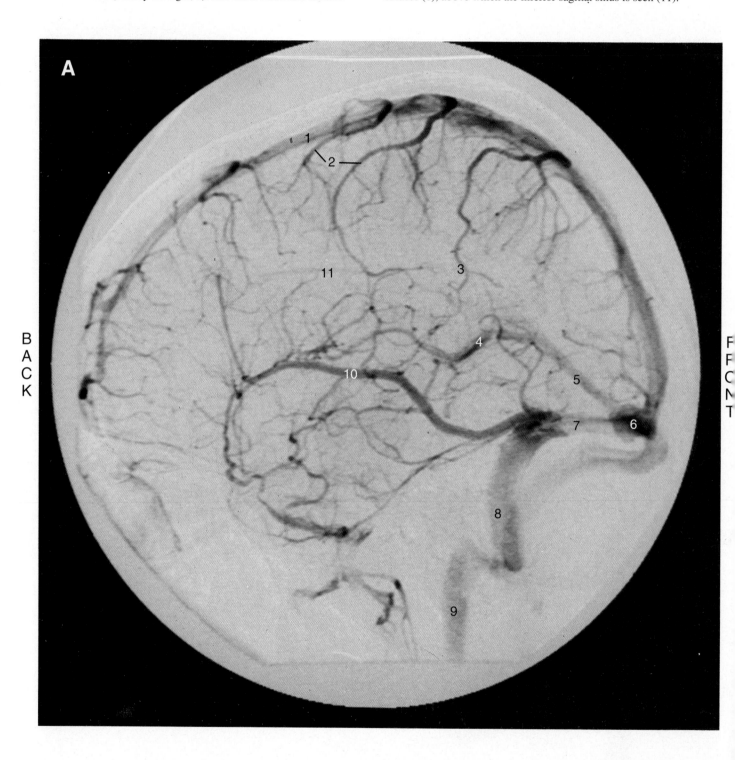

1 Superior sagittal sinus
2 Superior cerebral veins
3 Superior anastomotic vein
4 Great cerebral vein
5 Straight sinus
6 Confluence of sinuses
7 Transverse sinus
8 Sigmoid sinus
9 Internal jugular vein
10 Superficial middle cerebral vein
11 Inferior sagittal sinus

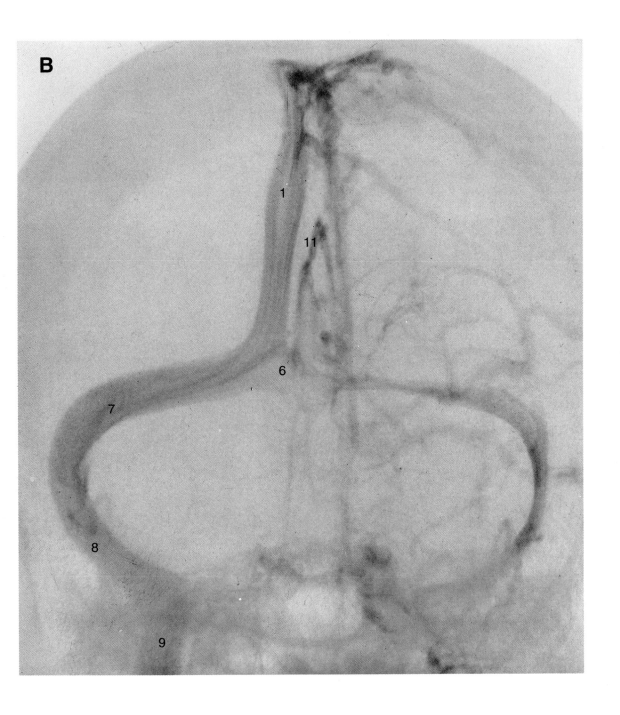

B

Appendix I: Dental Anaesthesia

In dental practice, anaesthesia of teeth and gingivae is achieved either by infiltration or regional nerve block. In *infiltration anaesthesia*, the anaesthetic solution is injected into the area concerned, and the anaesthetic agent diffuses through the tissues to anaesthetise local nerve fibres. In *regional nerve block* the injection is given to affect the nerve(s) supplying the area, which may be at some distance from the operative site.

The bone of the alveolar part of the maxilla, especially that of the buccal (outer) surface, is relatively porous, and anaesthetic solution that can penetrate to the region of the apex of a tooth (where the root canal opens and the nerve enters the pulp) will effectively anaesthetise the tooth and surrounding gingiva. Infiltration anaesthesia of the buccal aspect of the jaw is usually effective for all the upper teeth and will allow painless drilling, but painless extraction will require anaesthesia of the palatal (inner) aspect as well.

For the teeth of the lower jaw, infiltration anaesthesia is usually effective only for the incisors. The other mandibular teeth are embedded in bone that is denser and does not allow sufficient penetration of anaesthetic; for these teeth, a block of the inferior alveolar nerve is required. Again for tooth extraction it is necessary to block the lingual and buccal nerves as well in order to anaesthetise the adjacent soft tissues.

The notes that follow describe the anatomical background to the above two common methods of dental anaesthesia, together with some other nerve blocks that may be required.

It is essential that prior to any injection of local anaesthetic, an attempt is made to aspirate blood into the syringe. A positive aspiration indicates that the needle has inadvertently entered a blood vessel. Direct intravascular injection results not only in failure of the local anaesthetic to work but causes a variety of cardiovascular effects depending on the agent used.

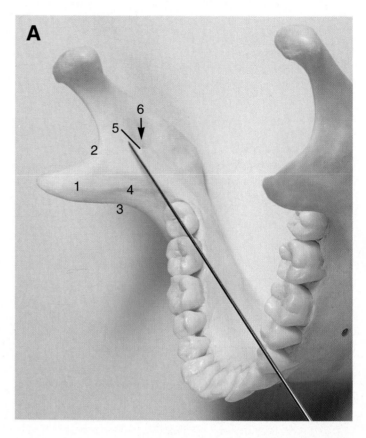

INFERIOR ALVEOLAR AND LINGUAL NERVE BLOCK

After branching off from the mandibular nerve just below the foramen ovale, the inferior alveolar and lingual nerves pass down between the lateral and medial pterygoid muscles (see page 116, A and B). The inferior alveolar nerve enters the mandibular foramen (with the companion artery behind it), lying at this level immediately lateral to the medial pterygoid muscle and to the sphenomandibular ligament which is attached to the lingula and overlaps the opening of the foramen. Within the mandible the nerve supplies the pulps of all the teeth of its own side and part of the periodontal ligament, and through its mental branch it innervates the lower lip and skin of the chin. The lingual nerve emerges from between the two pterygoid muscles about 1 cm in front of and medial to the inferior alveolar nerve. Running downwards across the medial pterygoid, it enters the mouth by passing under the lower border of the inferior constrictor of the pharynx, lying in contact with the periosteum of the mandible below and behind the third molar tooth. It is the sensory nerve to the anterior part of the tongue, the floor of the mouth and the lingual aspect of the mandible, including the gingivae. It also contributes to the innervation of the periodontal ligament.

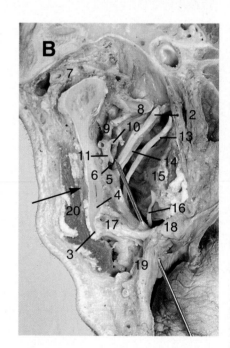

Inferior alveolar nerve block, which invariably includes lingual nerve block, is achieved by introducing the anaesthetic solution through the lateral side of the mouth into the fat of the pterygomandibular space—the region between the ramus of the mandible laterally and the medial pterygoid medially.

Through the open mouth the anterior border of the ramus of the mandible (the external oblique ridge) and the ridge of mucous membrane overlying the pterygomandibular raphe are identified. For right-sided anaesthesia this is done by the operator laying the index finger of the left hand on the occlusal surfaces of the molar teeth and moving it backwards to feel first the external oblique ridge (a rather sharp border) and then, slightly behind and more medially, the internal

1 Coronoid process
2 Mandibular notch (sigmoid notch)
3 Coronoid notch (external oblique ridge)
4 Internal oblique ridge
5 Lingula
6 Mandibular foramen
7 Parotid gland
8 Styloid process
9 Maxillary artery
10 Inferior alveolar vein
11 Inferior alveolar artery
12 Inferior alveolar nerve
13 Lingual nerve
14 Sphenomandibular ligament
15 Medial pterygoid
16 Buccal nerve
17 Temporalis insertion
18 Pterygomandibular raphe
19 Buccinator
20 Masseter
21 Lateral pterygoid
22 Parotid duct

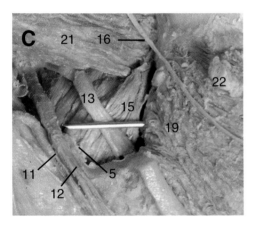

oblique ridge (usually a rather rounded margin). More medially still and with the mouth opened wide, the pterygomandibular raphe is stretched (between its attachments to the pterygoid hamulus of the medial pterygoid plate and the posterior end of the mylohyoid line) to form a ridge in the overlying mucous membrane which can be seen and palpated. With the barrel of the syringe lying over the opposite premolar teeth, the needle is inserted into the mucous membrane 1 cm above the occlusal surface of the third molar tooth and immediately lateral to the ridge over the raphe, i.e. between the ridge medially and the internal oblique line laterally. The needle then pierces the buccinator and about 0.5 cm deeper lies lateral to the lingual nerve, where a small injection is made. After insertion for a further 1 cm the needle tip lies just above the lingula where the main injection is made.

A **Mandible, obliquely from the left, in front and above, with a needle showing the line of approach to the right mandibular foramen**
B **Horizontal section of the right infratemporal fossa, from above, to show the path of the needle**
C **Right infratemporal fossa, from the right, with part of the mandible and fat removed, with the needle tip adjacent to the inferior alveolar nerve**

In A a long needle has been used to indicate that the line of approach to the right mandibular foramen (6) is from the left premolar region. This line takes the needle almost parallel to the slope of the ramus between the internal oblique line (4) and the mandibular foramen; the foramen is 1 cm behind the oblique line. The picture has been placed at this oblique angle, rather like looking into the mouth obliquely, in order to line up the path of the needle with that in B; in both, the needle tip lies just above the opening of the mandibular foramen.

The section in B is about 1 cm above the mandibular foramen. The fat of the pterygomandibular space has been removed to show the needle tip lying above the mandibular foramen (6), with the inferior alveolar nerve (12) entering it.

The arrow shows the direction of view of the dissection in C, with the needle traversing the pterygomandibular space after piercing the buccinator (19).

• If the needle tip is too far lateral it may enter the temporalis muscle insertion (B17) or come into contact with the internal oblique ridge of the mandible (B4).

• If the needle is too far medial it may enter the medial pterygoid muscle (B15) and so lie medial to the sphenomandibular ligament (B14) instead of lateral to it. With the needle tip correctly lateral to the ligament, the ligament and the lingula make a kind of funnel directing the anaesthetic solution into the foramen.

• If the needle passes too far back it may enter the parotid gland (B7) and part or all of the facial nerve may be paralysed. Even correctly placed injections may sometimes percolate through the inferior orbital fissure and cause transient visual disturbances by affecting the nerve supply of the extra-ocular muscles.

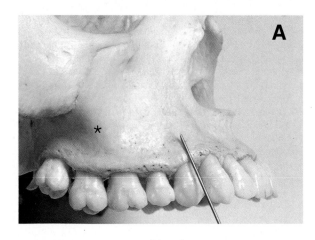

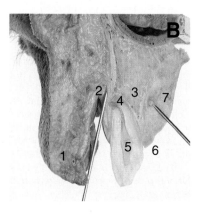

INFILTRATION ANAESTHESIA OF THE UPPER TEETH

For infiltration anaesthesia on the buccal aspect of the jaw, the needle is inserted into or just below the buccal fold (where the mucous membrane is reflected from the jaw to the cheek) opposite the appropriate tooth. The tip of the needle is directed upwards to the level where the apex of the tooth is considered to lie.

For infiltration of the cheek teeth on the palatal aspect, the needle is inserted midway between the gingival margin and the midline of the palate opposite the appropriate tooth. As a submucosa is present in this region, anaesthetic solution can be readily accommodated.

A Right maxilla and position of needle for anaesthesia of the first premolar tooth
B Coronal section of maxilla and cheek through the first premolar tooth

In A the needle is being advanced to the level of the apex of the first premolar, the position for depositing the anaesthetic solution for anaesthesia of this tooth. The asterisk indicates the lower part of the root of the zygomatic process (see note below).

In the coronal section in B the needle on the buccal side is shown penetrating the mucous membrane (2), with the tip lying against the periosteum at the level of the apex of the tooth. Note the presence of a submucosa here. The needle on the palatal side is being inserted midway between the gingival margin (6) and the midline.

• The needle must not penetrate the periosteum and strip it off the bone; this causes pain at the time and residual pain when the anaesthesia has worn off.

• The bone of the zygomatic process of the maxilla is denser than that of the alveolar process bearing the teeth, and if the root of the zygomatic process (indicated by the asterisk in A) extends lower than usual it may not allow effective penetration in the region of the first and second molar roots. Further injections in front and behind may be needed.

1	Lip	**11**	Lateral pterygoid
2	Buccal fold of mucous membrane	**12**	Medial pterygoid
3	Alveolar process of maxilla	**13**	Buccal nerve
4	Apex of tooth	**14**	Maxillary artery
5	Pulp cavity	**15**	Posterior superior alveolar nerve and vessels
6	Gingival margin	**16**	Parotid duct
7	Mucoperiosteum of hard palate	**17**	Buccinator
8	Zygomatic arch	**18**	Lingual nerve
9	Lateral pterygoid plate	**19**	Inferior alveolar nerve
10	Posterior surface of maxilla	**20**	Inferior alveolar artery

POSTERIOR SUPERIOR ALVEOLAR NERVE BLOCK

The nerve arises from the maxillary nerve in the pterygopalatine fossa (see page 116, A and B). It runs down in contact with the infratemporal (posterior) surface of the maxilla which it pierces about halfway down, to lie under the mucous membrane of the maxillary sinus and take part in the formation of the superior dental plexus, usually supplying the three molar teeth (except for the mesiobuccal root of the first molar). It is accompanied by corresponding branches of the maxillary vessels.

Posterior superior alveolar nerve block is rarely necessary because of the ease of infiltration anaesthesia of the molar teeth, but if required it can be achieved through the vestibule of the mouth by advancing the needle upwards along the posterior surface of the maxilla.

The needle is inserted through the buccal fold level with the second upper molar tooth, in a direction upwards and backwards at an angle of 45° to the vertical and occlusal planes. The needle is advanced for 2 cm, keeping as close as possible to the maxillary periosteum (10). At this level the tip should be in the region where the nerve enters the bone.

C Right infratemporal region and maxilla, from behind and below
D Dissection of the right infratemporal fossa, with needle piercing buccinator (17) to lie on the posterior surface of the maxilla

• If the needle is not kept close to the maxilla, the lateral pterygoid muscle or the pterygoid venous plexus may be entered.

• If vessels in the pterygoid venous plexus are damaged by the passage of the needle, a painful haematoma (bruise) will ensue, with limitation of jaw opening due to reflex pterygoid muscle spasm.

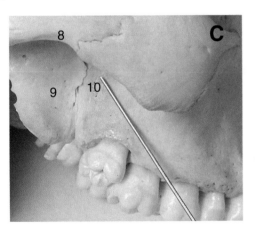

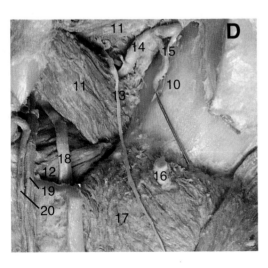

NASOPALATINE NERVE BLOCK

The nasopalatine nerve runs downwards and forwards under the mucous membrane of the nasal septum, and passes through the incisive foramen and incisive fossa to enter the roof of the mouth (see page 135, C). It supplies the hard palate and palatal alveolus in the region of the incisor and canine teeth of its own side and the teeth themselves.

The nerve can be blocked as it emerges from the incisive fossa (A1). The injection is made in an upward and slightly medial direction just lateral to the midline above the gingival margin. The incisor teeth of the nerve's own side and possibly the canine will be affected. For procedures involving the adjacent bone of the maxilla, the needle can be pushed up into the incisive canal (B) for 1 cm in a line parallel with the long axis of the central incisor tooth. However, this procedure results in intense pain until the anaesthetic takes effect.

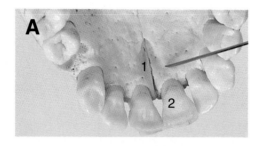

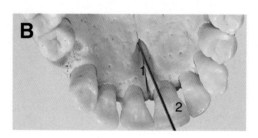

A Upper jaw, from below, with needle tip adjacent to the incisive fossa
B Upper jaw, from below, with needle advanced into the incisive canal
In A the needle is in the normal position for tooth anaesthesia, and in B the needle is being advanced up the incisive canal (1) for more extensive anaesthesia.

• The site of insertion of the needle into the mucoperiosteum is made slightly lateral to the midline (A), because the midline tissue over the incisive fossa is very sensitive, so that the initial injection more laterally is less painful.

• There is no submucosa in this region, the oral mucosa being tightly bound down to the underlying periosteum (mucoperiosteum). Only a small amount of anaesthetic solution is required and only a small amount can be accommodated. If too much is injected too rapidly, the mucosa may be forcibly stripped off the bone, causing considerable postoperative pain.

GREATER PALATINE NERVE BLOCK

The greater palatine nerve (page 129, D29) emerges through the greater palatine foramen, at the level of the second molar tooth about 1 cm above the gingival margin. It runs forwards in a groove on the under surface of the hard palate at the junction of the alveolar and palatine processes of the maxilla, usually reaching as far forward as the canine tooth and forming a plexus with the nasopalatine nerve. (The accompanying artery enters the incisive fossa and foramen to reach the nasal septum, but the nerve does not.)

The nerve can be blocked in front of its foramen (C5). The needle is inserted in an upward and lateral direction—level with the second molar tooth, midway between the gingival margin and the midline of the palate—and directed to just in front of the expected position of the foramen. The block should produce anaesthesia of teeth as far forward as the first premolar; the canine is in the region of cross-innervation between the greater palatine and nasopalatine nerves, and the effects on this tooth are variable.

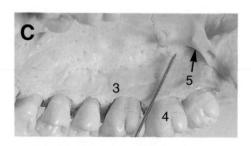

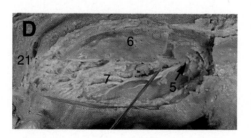

C Hard palate, from the left and below, with needle tip in front of the right greater palatine foramen
D Dissection of palatal mucoperiosteum to show the greater palatine nerve
In C the needle tip lies in the desired position in front of the greater palatine foramen (5) where, as seen in D, it is adjacent to the greater palatine nerve (7).

• Injection too far back may affect the lesser palatine nerves supplying the tonsillar area and soft palate; this is often an unpleasant sensation.

MENTAL AND INCISIVE NERVE BLOCK

The mental nerve supplies the skin of the lower lip and chin and the adjacent mucous membrane and gingiva. The incisive nerve supplies the first premolar, canine and incisor teeth and gingiva. In mental and incisive nerve block, the object is to deposit anaesthetic so that it flows into the mental foramen, thus affecting the mental nerve that emerges from the foramen and runs upwards, and the incisive nerve that continues forwards within the mandible. Since the opening of the mental foramen faces upwards and backwards, the needle must approach it from above and behind so that the tip can enter the opening.

Through the open mouth and with the angle of the mouth retracted, the needle is inserted through the mucous membrane in the depth of the sulcus between the mandible and cheek in the line of the second premolar tooth. After a small mucosal injection, the needle is advanced into the opening of the foramen.

E Right mental foramen
F Dissection

In E the tip of the needle has been advanced vertically from above, in the line of the second premolar tooth, to lie at the opening of the mental foramen (9). In the dissection in F the fibres of depressor anguli oris (10) have been separated to show the needle tip at the opening of the mental foramen (9), from which the mental nerve and vessels (12) emerge and pass upwards.

1	Incisive fossa leading to incisive canal
2	Central incisor tooth
3	Alveolar process of maxilla
4	Second molar tooth
5	Greater palatine foramen
6	Mucoperiosteum
7	Greater palatine nerve
8	Second premolar tooth
9	Mental foramen
10	Depressor anguli oris
11	Depressor labii inferioris
12	Mental nerve and vessels

• The attachment of depressor labii inferioris (E11) lies in front of the mental foramen (E9), and that of depressor anguli oris (E10) below it. Injected solution may enter these muscles if the needle tip is not at the opening of the foramen.

• As this injection results in profound numbness of the lower lip, it is important to warn the patient of the risk of biting the lip until the

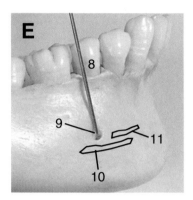

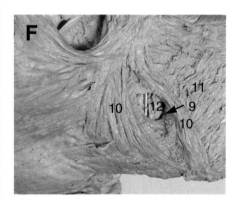

Appendix II Reference Lists

The following lists are included to provide 'at-a-glance' reference to muscle groups, branches of nerves and arteries, tributaries of veins, and to lymph nodes. The nerves and vessels have been grouped to provide quick identification of parent trunks and branches, according to the indentation of the listed names. Thus the superior laryngeal artery is a branch of the superior thyroid, which in turn is a branch of the external carotid.

An arrow indicates a continuity with a change of name, not a branching.

The inclusion of items here does not necessarily imply that they are all illustrated in the atlas. Many of the smaller vessels and nerves in particular are not shown but have been included to provide a record of generally accepted terms as far as the anatomy of the head and neck is concerned.

A list of skull foramina with the structures that pass through them is also included but some students may find that the simplified list of the more important items on page 25 is sufficient for their purpose.

Muscles

MUSCLES OF THE HEAD

Muscles of the scalp
Epicranius
Occipitofrontalis
Occipital belly
Frontal belly
Temporoparietalis

Muscles of the auricle
Extrinsic
Auricularis anterior
Auricularis superior
Auricularis posterior
Intrinsic
Helicis major and minor
Tragicus
Antitragicus
Transversus auriculae
Obliquus auriculae

Muscles of the nose
Procerus
Nasalis
Transverse part (compressor naris)
Alar part (dilator naris)
Depressor septi

Muscles of the eyelids
Orbicularis oculi
Orbital part
Depressor supercilli
Palpebral part
Lacrimal part
Corrugator supercilli
Levator palpebrae superioris (see Muscles of the orbit)

Muscles of mastication
Temporalis
Masseter
Lateral pterygoid
Medial pterygoid

Muscles of the mouth
Levator labii superioris
Levator labii superioris alaeque nasi
Zygomaticus major
Zygomaticus minor
Levator anguli oris
Buccinator
Orbicularis oris
Risorius
Mentalis
Depressor labii inferioris
Depressor anguli oris
Transversus menti

MUSCLES OF THE NECK

Superficial and lateral muscles
Platysma
Trapezius (see Upper limb)
Sternocleidomastoid

Anterior vertebral muscles
Longus colli
Longus capitis
Rectus capitis anterior
Rectus capitis lateralis

Lateral vertebral muscles
Scalenus anterior
Scalenus medius
Scalenus posterior

Suprahyoid muscles
Digastric
Stylohyoid
Mylohyoid
Geniohyoid

Infrahyoid muscles
Sternohyoid
Sternothyroid
Thyrohyoid
Omohyoid

MUSCLE GROUPS IN HEAD AND NECK

Muscles of the pharynx
Superior constrictor
Middle constrictor
Inferior constrictor
Stylopharyngeus
Palatopharyngeus
Salpingopharyngeus

Muscles of the palate
Palatoglossus
Palatopharyngeus
Tensor veli palatini
Levator veli palatini
Musculus uvulae

Muscles of the larynx
Cricothyroid
Posterior crico-arytenoid
Lateral crico-arytenoid
Transverse arytenoid
Oblique arytenoid
Aryepiglottic
Thyro-arytenoid and vocalis
Thyro-epiglottic
(Superior thyro-arytenoid)

Muscles of the tongue
Extrinsic
Genioglossus
Hyoglossus and chondroglossus
Styloglossus
Palatoglossus
Intrinsic
Superior longitudinal
Inferior longitudinal
Transverse
Vertical

Muscles of the orbit
Levator palpebrae superioris
Orbitalis
Muscles of the eyeball
Superior rectus
Inferior rectus
Medial rectus
Lateral rectus
Superior oblique
Inferior oblique

MUSCLES OF THE TRUNK

Suboccipital muscles
Rectus capitis posterior major
Rectus capitis posterior minor
Obliquus capitis inferior
Obliquus capitis superior

Deep muscles of the back
Splenius capitis
Splenius cervicis
Erector spinae
Iliocostalis cervicis
Iliocostalis thoracis
Iliocostalis lumborum
Longissimus capitis
Longissimus cervicis
Longissimus thoracis
Spinalis capitis
Spinalis cervicis
Spinalis thoracis
Transversospinalis
Semispinalis capitis
Semispinalis cervicis
Semispinalis thoracis
Multifidus
Rotatores
Interspinal
Intertransverse

MUSCLES OF THE UPPER LIMB

Connecting limb and vertebral column
Trapezius
Latissimus dorsi
Levator scapulae
Rhomboid major
Rhomboid minor

Connecting limb and thoracic wall
Pectoralis major
Pectoralis minor
Subclavius
Serratus anterior

Scapular muscles
Deltoid
Subscapularis
Supraspinatus
Infraspinatus
Teres minor
Teres major

Nerves

CRANIAL NERVES AND BRANCHES

I Olfactory (from olfactory mucous membrane)

II Optic (from retina)

III Oculomotor
- Superior branch (to superior rectus and levator palpebrae superioris)
- Inferior branch (to medial rectus, inferior rectus and inferior oblique)
    - Oculomotor root to ciliary ganglion

IV Trochlear (to superior oblique)

V Trigeminal
- Sensory root
    - Trigeminal ganglion
- Motor root (joining mandibular nerve)
- Ophthalmic
    - Tentorial
    - Lacrimal
        - Communicating branch with zygomatic
    - Frontal
        - Supra-orbital
        - Supratrochlear
    - Nasociliary → anterior ethmoidal → external nasal
        - Communicating branch with ciliary ganglion
        - Long ciliary
        - Posterior ethmoidal
        - Anterior ethmoidal
            - Lateral and medial internal nasal
            - External nasal
        - Infratrochlear
            - Palpebral
- Maxillary → infra-orbital
    - Meningeal
    - Ganglionic branches to pterygopalatine ganglion
        - Orbital
        - Nasal (lateral and medial posterior superior nasal and nasopalatine)
        - Pharyngeal
        - Greater palatine
            - Posterior inferior nasal
        - Lesser palatine
    - Zygomatic
        - Zygomaticotemporal
        - Zygomaticofaciall
    - Infra-orbital
        - Superior alveolar
            - Posterior, middle and anterior superior alveolar
                - Superior dental plexus
                    - Superior dental
                    - Superior gingival
        - Inferior palpebral
        - External nasal
        - Internal nasal
        - Superior labial
- Mandibular see next column

- Mandibular
    - Meningeal
    - Masseteric
    - Deep temporal
    - Nerve to lateral pterygoid
    - Nerve to medial pterygoid
        - Nerve to tensor veli palatini and tensor tympani via otic ganglion
    - Buccal
    - Auriculotemporal
        - Nerve to external acoustic meatus
        - Tympanic membrane
        - Communicating branches with facial nerve
        - Anterior auricular
        - Superficial temporal
    - Lingual
        - Faucial
        - Communicating branches with hypoglossal nerve
        - Communicating branches with chorda tympani
        - Sublingual
        - Lingual
        - Ganglionic branches to submandibular ganglion
    - Inferior alveolar
        - Mylohyoid
        - Inferior dental plexus
            - Inferior dental
            - Inferior gingival
        - Mental
            - Mental
            - Inferior labial

VI Abducent (to lateral rectus)

VII Facial
- Greater petrosal
- Nerve to stapedius
- Chorda tympani
- Communicating branch with tympanic plexus
- Communicating branch with vagus nerve
- Posterior auricular
    - Occipital (to occipital belly of occipitofrontalis)
    - Auricular (to auricular muscles)
    - To digastric (posterior belly)
    - To stylohyoid
    - Communicating branch with glossopharyngeal nerve
- Parotid plexus

Temporal	⎫ to frontal belly of
Zygomatic	⎪ occipitofrontalis,
Buccal	⎬ muscles of facial
Marginal mandibular	⎪ expression and
Cervical	⎭ platysma

VIII Vestibulocochlear
Cochlear (from coils of cochlea)
Vestibular (from utricle, saccule and ampullae of semicircular canals)

IX Glossopharyngeal
Tympanic
    Tubal
    Caroticotympanic
    Lesser petrosal
Carotid sinus
Pharyngeal
Muscular (to stylopharyngeus)
Tonsillar
Lingual

X Vagus
Meningeal
Auricular
Pharyngeal (to muscles of pharynx and soft palate except stylopharyngeus and tensor veli palatini)
Superior cervical cardiac
Carotid body
Superior laryngeal
    Internal laryngeal
    External laryngeal (to cricothyroid)
Inferior cervical cardiac
Recurrent laryngeal
    Tracheal
    Oesophageal
    Inferior laryngeal (to muscles of larynx except cricothyroid)
Thoracic cardiac
Bronchial
Oesophageal plexus
Anterior vagal trunk
    Gastric
    Hepatic
Posterior vagal trunk
    Coeliac
    Gastric

XI Accessory
Trunk of accessory
    Internal ramus (cranial or vagal part, from cranial roots, to muscles of palate, except tensor veli palatini, and larynx via fibres joining vagus nerve)
    External ramus (spinal part, from cervical roots, to sternocleidomastoid and trapezius)

XII Hypoglossal
Lingual (to muscles of tongue except palatoglossus)
Muscular (derived from cervical nerves and including upper root of ansa cervicalis, to geniohyoid, thyrohyoid, sternohyoid, sternothyroid and superior belly of omohyoid. See cervical plexus, page 226)

SOME HEAD AND NECK NERVE SUPPLIES

All the muscles of	Supplied by	Except	Supplied by
Pharynx	Pharyngeal plexus*	Stylo-pharyngeus	Glosso-pharyngeal nerve
Palate	Pharyngeal plexus	Tensor veli palatini	Nerve to medial pterygoid
Larynx	Recurrent laryngeal nerve	Crico-thyroid	External laryngeal nerve
Tongue	Hypoglossal nerve	Palato-glossus	Pharyngeal plexus
Facial expression (including buccinator)	Facial nerve		
Mastication	Mandibular nerve		

*The cricopharyngeus part of the inferior constrictor may sometimes be supplied by the recurrent or external laryngeal branches of the vagus nerve.

Nerves

CERVICAL PLEXUS AND BRANCHES
Lesser occipital C2
Great auricular C2, 3
Transverse cervical C2, 3
Supraclavicular C3, 4
Phrenic (to diaphragm) C3, 4, 5
Communicating (with vagus and hypoglossal nerves and superior cervical sympathetic ganglion)
Muscular (to rectus capitis lateralis, rectus capitis anterior, longus capitis and longus colli, and by lower root of ansa cervicalis to sternohyoid, sternothyroid and inferior belly of omohyoid) C1, 2, 3

BRACHIAL PLEXUS AND BRANCHES
Supraclavicular branches
From the roots
    To scalenes and longus colli C5, 6, 7, 8
    To join phrenic nerve C5
    Dorsal scapular (to rhomboids) C5
    Long thoracic (to serratus anterior) C5, 6, 7
From the upper trunk
    Nerve to subclavius C5, 6
    Suprascapular (to supraspinatus and infraspinatus) C5, 6

Infraclavicular branches
From the lateral cord
    Lateral pectoral (to pectoralis major and minor) C5, 6, 7
    Musculocutaneous C5, 6, 7
    Lateral root of the median C(5), 6, 7
From the medial cord
    Medial pectoral (to pectoralis major and minor) C8, T1
    Medial root of the median C8, T1
    Medial cutaneous of arm C8, T1
    Medial cutaneous of forearm C8, T1
    Ulnar C(7), 8, T1
From the posterior cord
    Upper subscapular (to subscapularis) C5, 6
    Thoracodorsal (to latissimus dorsi) C6, 7, 8
    Lower subscapular (to subscapularis and teres major) C5, 6
    Axillary C5, 6
    Radial C5, 6, 7, 8, T1

Lymphatic System

THORACIC DUCT AND RIGHT LYMPHATIC DUCT
Thoracic duct
    Left jugular trunk
    Left subclavian trunk
    Left bronchomediastinal trunk

Right lymphatic duct
    Right jugular trunk
    Right subclavian trunk
    Right bronchomediastinal trunk

Cisterna chyli
    Left lumbar trunk
    Right lumbar trunk
    Intestinal trunks

LYMPH NODES OF THE HEAD AND NECK
Deep cervical
    Superior (including jugulodigastric)
    Inferior (including jugulo-omohyoid)

Draining superficial tissues in the head
    Occipital
    Retro-auricular (mastoid)
    Parotid
    Buccal (facial)

Draining superficial tissues in the neck
    Submandibular
    Submental
    Anterior cervical
    Superficial cervical

Draining deep tissues in the neck
    Retropharyngeal
    Paratracheal
    Lingual
    Infrahyoid
    Prelaryngeal
    Pretracheal

Arteries

AORTA AND BRANCHES
Ascending aorta → arch of aorta → thoracic aorta → abdominal aorta

Ascending aorta
Right coronary
    Marginal
    Posterior interventricular
Left coronary
    Circumflex
    Anterior interventricular

Arch of aorta
Brachiocephalic trunk
    Right common carotid
        Right internal carotid
        Right external carotid
    Right subclavian → axillary → brachial
    Thyroidea ima (occasional)
Left common carotid
    Left internal carotid
    Left external carotid
Left subclavian → axillary → brachial

SUBCLAVIAN ARTERY AND BRANCHES
Subclavian → axillary → brachial
Vertebral
    Prevertebral part
    Transversarial (cervical) part
        Spinal (radicular)
        Muscular
    Atlantic part
    Intracranial part
        Anterior and posterior meningeal
        Anterior spinal
        Posterior inferior cerebellar
            Choroidal of fourth ventricle
            To cerebellar tonsil
            Medial and lateral medullary
            Posterior spinal
Basilar (from union of both vertebrals)
    Anterior inferior cerebellar
    Labyrinthine
    Pontine
    Mesencephalic
    Superior cerebellar
    Posterior cerebral
        Precommunicating part
            Posteromedial central
        Postcommunicating part
            Posterolateral central
            Thalamic
            Medial and lateral posterior choroidal
            Peduncular
        Terminal (cortical) part
            Lateral occipital
                Anterior, middle and posterior temporal
            Medial occipital
                Dorsal corpus callosal
                Parietal
                Calcarine
                Occipitotemporal
Thyrocervical trunk
    Inferior thyroid
        Inferior laryngeal
        Glandular
        Pharyngeal
        Oesophageal
        Tracheal
        Ascending cervical
            Spinal
    Superficial (transverse) cervical
    Suprascapular
        Acromial
Internal thoracic
Costocervical trunk
    Deep cervical
    Superior intercostal
        First posterior intercostal
        Second posterior intercostal
            Dorsal
            Spinal
Dorsal scapular

CAROTID ARTERIES AND BRANCHES
Internal carotid
- Cervical part
  - Carotid sinus
- Petrous part
  - Caroticotympanic
  - Pterygoid canal
- Cavernous part
  - Basal and marginal tentorial
  - Meningeal
  - To trigeminal and trochlear
  - Cavernous sinus
  - Inferior hypophysial
- Cerebral part
  - Superior hypophysial
  - Ophthalmic
    - Central of retina
    - Lacrimal
      - Anastomotic branch with middle meningeal
      - Lateral palpebral
    - Short and long posterior ciliary
    - Muscular
      - Anterior ciliary
    - Anterior and posterior conjunctival
    - Episcleral
    - Supra-orbital
    - Posterior ethmoidal
    - Anterior ethmoidal
      - Anterior meningeal
    - Medial palpebral
    - Supratrochlear
    - Dorsal nasal
  - Anterior cerebral
    - Precommunicating part
      - Anteromedial central (thalamostriate)
      - Short central
      - Long central (recurrent)
      - Anterior communicating
    - Postcommunicating part (pericallosal)
      - Medial frontobasal (orbitofrontal)
      - Callosomarginal
        - Anteromedial frontal
        - Intermediomedial frontal
        - Posteromedial frontal
        - Cingular
      - Paracentral
      - Precuneal
      - Parieto-occipital
- Middle cerebral see next column

- Middle cerebral
  - Sphenoidal part
    - Anterolateral central (thalamostriate)
      - Medial and lateral (striate)
  - Insular part
    - Insular
    - Lateral frontobasal (orbitofrontal)
    - Anterior, intermediate and posterior temporal
  - Terminal (cortical) part
    - To central sulcus
    - To precentral sulcus
    - To postcentral sulcus
    - Anterior and posterior parietal
    - To angular gyrus
- Anterior choroidal
  - Choroidal of lateral ventricle
  - Choroidal of third ventricle
  - To anterior perforated substance
  - To optic tract
  - To lateral geniculate body
  - To internal capsule
  - To globus pallidus
  - To tail of caudate nucleus
  - To tuber cinereum
  - To hypothalamic nuclei
  - To substantia nigra
  - To red nucleus
  - To amygdaloid body
- Posterior communicating (joining posterior cerebral)
  - Chiasmatic
  - To oculomotor nerve
  - Thalamic
  - Hypothalamic
  - To tail of caudate nucleus

External carotid
- Superior thyroid
  - Infrahyoid
  - Sternocleidomastoid
  - Superior laryngeal
    - Cricothyroid
- Ascending pharyngeal
  - Posterior meningeal
  - Pharyngeal
  - Inferior tympanic
- Lingual
  - Suprahyoid
  - Sublingual
  - Dorsal lingual
  - Deep lingual
- Facial
  - Ascending palatine
  - Tonsillar
  - Submental
  - Glandular
  - Inferior labial
  - Superior labial
  - Angular
- Occipital
  - Mastoid
  - Auricular
  - Sternocleidomastoid
  - Meningeal
  - Occipital
  - Descending
- Posterior auricular
  - Stylomastoid
  - Posterior tympanic
    - Mastoid
    - Stapedial
  - Auricular
  - Occipital
- Superficial temporal
  - Parotid
  - Transverse facial
  - Anterior auricular
  - Zygomatico-orbital
  - Middle temporal
  - Frontal
  - Parietal
- Maxillary see next column

Maxillary
- Deep auricular
- Anterior tympanic
- Inferior alveolar
  - Dental
  - Mylohyoid
  - Mental
- Middle meningeal
  - Accessory meningeal
  - Petrosal
  - Superior tympanic
  - Frontal
  - Parietal
  - Orbital
  - Anastomotic branch with lacrimal
- Masseteric
- Deep temporal
- Pterygoid
- Buccal
- Posterior superior alveolar
  - Dental
- Infra-orbital
  - Anterior superior alveolar
    - Dental
- Pterygoid canal
- Descending palatine
  - Greater palatine
  - Lesser palatine
- Sphenopalatine
  - Posterior, lateral and septal nasal

Veins

TRIBUTARIES OF MAJOR VEINS
Superior vena cava
Left brachiocephalic
- Left internal jugular
- Left subclavian
- Left vertebral
- Left supreme (first posterior) intercostal
- Left superior intercostal (2-4)
- Inferior thyroid
- Thymic
- Pericardial

Right brachiocephalic
- Right internal jugular
- Right subclavian
- Right vertebral
- Right supreme (first posterior) intercostal

Azygos

Internal jugular
Inferior petrosal sinus
Pharyngeal
Lingual
Facial
Superior thyroid
Middle thyroid

External jugular
Posterior auricular
Posterior branch of retromandibular
Occipital
Posterior external jugular
Suprascapular
Transverse of neck
Anterior jugular

Retromandibular
Superficial temporal
Maxillary
Transverse facial
Pterygoid plexus
- Middle meningeal
- Greater palatine
- Sphenopalatine
- Buccal
- Dental
- Deep facial
- Inferior ophthalmic

Anterior branch to join facial
Posterior branch to external jugular

Facial
Supratrochlear
Supra-orbital
Superior ophthalmic
Palpebral
External nasal
Labial
Deep facial
Submental
Submandibular
Tonsillar
External palatine (paratonsillar)

DURAL VENOUS SINUSES
Posterosuperior group
Superior sagittal
Inferior sagittal
Straight
Transverse
Sigmoid
Petrosquamous
Occipital

Antero-inferior group
Cavernous
Intercavernous
Inferior petrosal
Superior petrosal
Sphenoparietal
Basilar
Middle meningeal veins

EMISSARY VEINS
The most common are found in the
Parietal foramen
Mastoid foramen
Foramen lacerum
Foramen ovale
Venous (emissary sphenoidal) foramen
Carotid canal
Hypoglossal canal
Condylar canal

CEREBRAL VEINS
Superficial cerebral veins
- Superior cerebral
- Superficial middle cerebral
  - Superior anastomotic
  - Inferior anastomotic
- Inferior cerebral

Deep cerebral veins
- Great cerebral
  - Internal cerebral
    - Thalamostriate
    - Choroidal
  - Basal
    - Anterior cerebral
    - Deep middle cerebral
    - Striate

Skull Foramina

INSIDE THE SKULL

MIDDLE CRANIAL FOSSA
Optic canal: in the sphenoid between the body and the two roots of the lesser wing
Optic nerve
Ophthalmic artery

Superior orbital fissure: in the sphenoid between the body and the greater and lesser wings, with a fragment of the frontal bone at the lateral extremity
Oculomotor, trochlear and abducent nerves
Lacrimal, frontal and nasociliary nerves
Filaments from the internal carotid (sympathetic) plexus
Orbital branch of the middle meningeal artery
Recurrent branch of the lacrimal artery
Superior ophthalmic vein

Foramen rotundum: in the greater wing of the sphenoid
Maxillary nerve

Foramen ovale: in the greater wing of the sphenoid
Mandibular nerve
Lesser petrosal nerve (usually)
Accessory meningeal artery
Emissary veins (from cavernous sinus to pterygoid plexus)

Foramen spinosum: in the greater wing of the sphenoid
Middle meningeal vessels
Meningeal branch of the mandibular nerve

Venous (emissary sphenoidal) foramen: in 40% of skulls, in the greater wing of the sphenoid medial to the foramen ovale
Emissary vein (from the cavernous sinus to the pterygoid plexus)

Petrosal (innominate) foramen: occasional, in the greater wing of the sphenoid, medial to the foramen spinosum
Lesser petrosal nerve (if not through foramen ovale)

Foramen lacerum: between the sphenoid, apex of the petrous temporal and the basilar part of the occipital
Internal carotid artery (entering from behind and emerging above)
Greater petrosal nerve (entering from above and behind, and leaving anteriorly as nerve of pterygoid canal)
Nerve of pterygoid canal (leaving through anterior wall)
A meningeal branch of the ascending pharyngeal artery
Emissary veins (from the cavernous sinus to the pterygoid plexus)

Hiatus for the greater petrosal nerve: in the tegmen tympani of the petrous temporal, in front of the arcuate eminence
Greater petrosal nerve
Petrosal branch of the middle meningeal artery

Hiatus for the lesser petrosal nerve: in the tegmen tympani of the petrous temporal, about 3mm in front of the hiatus for the greater petrosal nerve
Lesser petrosal nerve

ANTERIOR CRANIAL FOSSA
Foramina in the cribriform plate of the ethmoid
Olfactory nerve filaments
Anterior ethmoidal nerve and vessels

Foramen caecum: between the frontal crest of the frontal bone and the ethmoid in front of the crista galli
Emissary vein (between nose and superior sagittal sinus)

POSTERIOR CRANIAL FOSSA
Internal acoustic meatus: in the posterior surface of the petrous temporal
Facial nerve
Vestibulocochlear nerve
Labyrinthine artery

Aqueduct of the vestibule: in the petrous temporal about 1cm behind the internal acoustic meatus
Endolymphatic duct and sac
A branch from the meningeal branch of the occipital artery
A vein (from the labyrinth and vestibule to the sigmoid sinus)

Jugular foramen: between the jugular fossa of the petrous temporal and the occipital bone
Glossopharyngeal, vagus and accessory nerves
Meningeal branches of the vagus nerve
Inferior petrosal sinus
Internal jugular vein
A meningeal branch of the occipital artery

Hypoglossal canal: in the occipital bone above the anterior part of the condyle
Hypoglossal nerve and its (recurrent) meningeal branch
A meningeal branch of the ascending pharyngeal artery
Emissary vein (from the basilar plexus to the internal jugular vein)

Condylar canal: occasional, from the lower part of the sigmoid groove in the lateral part of the occipital bone to the condylar fossa on the external surface of the occipital bone behind the condyle
Emissary vein (from the sigmoid sinus to occipital veins)
A meningeal branch of the occipital artery

Mastoid foramen: in the petrous temporal near the posterior margin of the lower part of the sigmoid groove, passing backwards to open behind the mastoid process
Emissary vein (from the sigmoid sinus to occipital veins)
A meningeal branch of the occipital artery

Foramen magnum: in the occipital bone
Apical ligament of the odontoid process of the axis
Tectorial membrane
Medulla oblongata and meninges (including first digitations of denticulate ligament)
Spinal parts of the accessory nerves
Meningeal branches of upper cervical nerves
Vertebral arteries
Anterior spinal artery
Posterior spinal arteries

Skull Foramina

IN THE BASE OF THE SKULL EXTERNALLY

Foramen lacerum
Foramen ovale
Foramen spinosum
Jugular foramen   } see INSIDE THE SKULL
Hypoglossal canal
Condylar canal
Mastoid foramen
Foramen magnum

Inferior orbital fissure – see IN THE ORBIT

Lateral incisive foramen: opens into the incisive fossa, in the midline at the front of the hard palate
Nasopalatine nerve
Greater palatine vessels

Greater palatine foramen: between the maxilla and the palatine bone at the lateral border of the hard palate behind the palatomaxillary fissure
Greater palatine nerve and vessels

Lesser palatine foramina: two or three, in the inferior and medial aspects of the pyramidal process of the palatine bone
Lesser palatine nerves and vessels

Palatovaginal canal: between lower surface of the vaginal process of the root of the medial pterygoid plate and the upper surface of the sphenoidal process of the palatine bone
Pharyngeal branch of the pterygopalatine ganglion
Pharyngeal branch of the maxillary artery

Vomerovaginal canal: occasional, medial to the palatovaginal canal, between the upper surface of the vaginal process of the root of the medial pterygoid plate and the lower surface of the ala of the vomer
Pharyngeal branch of the sphenopalatine artery

Petrosquamous fissure: between the squamous temporal and the tegmen tympani
Petrosquamous vein

Petrotympanic fissure: between the tympanic part of the temporal bone and the tegmen tympani
Chorda tympani
Anterior ligament of the malleus
Anterior tympanic branch of the maxillary artery

Cochlear canaliculus: in the petrous temporal, at the apex of a notch in front of the medial part of the jugular fossa
Perilymphatic duct
Emissary vein (from the cochlea to the internal jugular vein or inferior petrosal sinus)

Carotid canal: in the inferior surface of the petrous temporal
Internal carotid artery
Internal carotid (sympathetic) plexus
Internal carotid venous plexus (from the cavernous sinus to the internal jugular vein)

Tympanic canaliculus: in the inferior surface of the petrous temporal, on the ridge of bone between the carotid canal and the jugular fossa
Tympanic branch of the glossopharyngeal nerve
Inferior tympanic branch of the ascending pharyngeal artery

Mastoid canaliculus: in the inferior surface of the petrous temporal, on the lateral wall of the jugular fossa
Auricular branch of the vagus nerve

Stylomastoid foramen: between the styloid and mastoid processes of the temporal bone
Facial nerve
Stylomastoid branch of the posterior auricular artery

IN THE ORBIT

Superior orbital fissure
Optic canal } see INSIDE THE SKULL

Frontal notch or foramen: in the supra-orbital margin of the frontal bone one fingerbreadth from the midline
Supratrochlear nerve and vessels

Supra-orbital notch or foramen: in the supra-orbital margin of the frontal bone two fingerbreadths from the midline
Supra-orbital nerve and vessels

Anterior ethmoidal foramen: in the medial wall of the orbit between the orbital part of the frontal bone and the ethmoid labyrinth
Anterior ethmoidal nerve and vessels

Posterior ethmoidal foramen: occasional, 1-2cm behind the anterior ethmoidal foramen
Posterior ethmoidal nerve and vessels

Zygomatico-orbital foramen: in the orbital surface of the zygomatic bone
Zygomatic branch of the maxillary nerve

Nasolacrimal canal: at the front, lower, medial corner of the orbit formed by the lacrimal bone and maxilla
Nasolacrimal duct

Inferior orbital fissure: towards the back of the orbit, between the maxilla and the greater wing of the sphenoid
Maxillary nerve
Zygomatic nerve
Orbital branches of the pterygopalatine ganglion
Infra-orbital vessels
Inferior ophthalmic veins

Infra-orbital canal: in the orbital surface of the maxilla
Infra-orbital nerve and vessels

MISCELLANEOUS

Infra-orbital foramen: the anterior opening of the infra-orbital canal, in the maxilla below the infra-orbital margin
Infra-orbital nerve and vessels

Mental foramen: on the outer surface of the body of the mandible below the second premolar tooth or slightly more anteriorly
Mental nerve and vessels

Mandibular foramen: on the inner surface of the ramus of the mandible, overlapped anteriorly and medially by the lingula
Inferior alveolar nerve and vessels

Foramina in the infratemporal (posterior) surface of the maxilla
Posterior superior alveolar nerves and vessels

Pterygomaxillary fissure: between the lateral pterygoid plate and the infratemporal (posterior) surface of the maxilla, and continuous above with the posterior end of the inferior orbital fissure
Maxillary artery (entering pterygopalatine fossa)
Maxillary nerve (entering inferior orbital fissure)
Sphenopalatine veins

Sphenopalatine foramen: at the upper end of the perpendicular plate of the palatine between its orbital and sphenoidal processes and (above) the body of the sphenoid; in the medial wall of the pterygopalatine fossa (viewed laterally through the pterygomaxillary fissure) and lateral wall of the nasal cavity (viewed medially)
Nasopalatine and posterior superior nasal nerves
Sphenopalatine vessels

Foramina in the perpendicular plate of the palatine
Posterior inferior nasal nerves

Pterygoid canal: at the root of the pterygoid process of the sphenoid in line with the medial pterygoid plate, leading from the anterior wall of the foramen lacerum to the posterior wall of the pterygopalatine fossa (and only clearly seen in a disarticulated sphenoid)
Nerve of the pterygoid canal
Artery of the pterygoid canal

Musculotubular canal: at the lateral side of the apex of the petrous temporal, at the junction of the petrous and squamous parts, and divided by a bony septum into upper and lower semicanals
Tensor tympani (upper semicanal)
Auditory tube (lower semicanal)

Parietal foramen: in the parietal bone near the posterosuperior (occipital) angle
Emissary vein (from the superior sagittal sinus to the scalp)

Index

Page numbers refer to items in notes as well as those illustrated